MW00978122

Cluttering

Very few people are aware of the significant negative impact that cluttering—a communication disorder that affects a person's ability to speak in a clear, concise and fluent manner—can have on one's life educationally, socially and vocationally. Although different from stuttering, it is often related to this more well-known disorder. This book treats cluttering as a serious communication disorder in its own right, providing an in-depth examination of the critical factors surrounding its assessment, treatment and research.

Using evidence-based data as well as information regarding the assessment and treatment of cluttering within the field of speech-language pathology, the volume includes the latest research findings and work from leading worldwide cluttering experts. Current viewpoints regarding cluttering along with substantiated evidence are provided. Research findings are presented regarding the nature and neurology of cluttering. A range of successful assessment and treatment methodologies are described in the context of disorders that may co-occur with cluttering, such as autism spectrum disorders, learning disabilities, Down syndrome and stuttering. Future directions with regards to the definition, teaching and researching of cluttering are also addressed.

Students, faculty members, researchers and clinicians in the field of speech pathology will find this book an essential and unique source of information on cluttering.

David Ward is a specialist speech and language therapist in disfluency within the NHS and lectures on disorders of fluency at The University of Reading, UK. He is currently Chair of the International Cluttering Association's academic and research committee, and is involved in research into both theoretical and clinical aspects of stuttering and cluttering. His book, *Stuttering and Cluttering* was published by Psychology Press in 2006.

Kathleen Scaler Scott is a practising speech-language pathologist and researcher who specialises in fluency disorders. She has lectured nationally and internationally on fluency disorders and social communication disorders. She is currently Coordinator of the International Cluttering Association, and Assistant Professor in the Department of Speech-Language Pathology at Misericordia University, USA.

Cluttering

A Handbook of Research, Intervention and Education

David Ward and Kathleen Scaler Scott

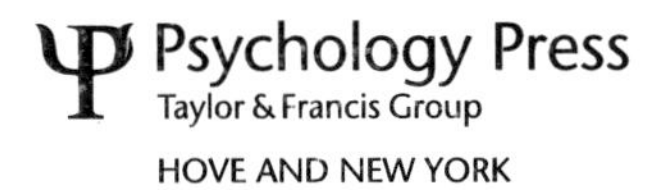

HOVE AND NEW YORK

First published 2011
by Psychology Press
27 Church Road, Hove, East Sussex, BN3 2FA

Simultaneously published in the USA and Canada
by Psychology Press
711 Third Avenue, New York, NY 10017, USA

Psychology Press is an imprint of the Taylor & Francis Group, an informa business

Typeset in Times by RefineCatch Limited, Bungay, Suffolk

Cover design by Andrew Ward

This publication has been produced with paper manufactured to strict environmental standards and with pulp derived from sustainable forests.

British Library Cataloguing in Publication Data
A catalogue record for this book is available from the British Library

Library of Congress Cataloging-in-Publication Data
Cluttering : a handbook of research, intervention, and education / [edited by]
David Ward & Kathleen Scaler Scott.
p. ; cm.
Includes bibliographical references.
ISBN 978–1–84872–029–9 (hbk. : alk. paper) 1. Cluttering (Speech pathology)–Handbooks, manuals, etc. I. Ward, David, 1956 Dec. 9– II. Scott, Kathleen Scaler, 1969–
[DNLM: 1. Speech Disorders. WM 475 C649 2011]
RC424.5.C57 2011
362.196′855–dc22

2010025268

ISBN: 978-1-84872-029-9 (hbk only)

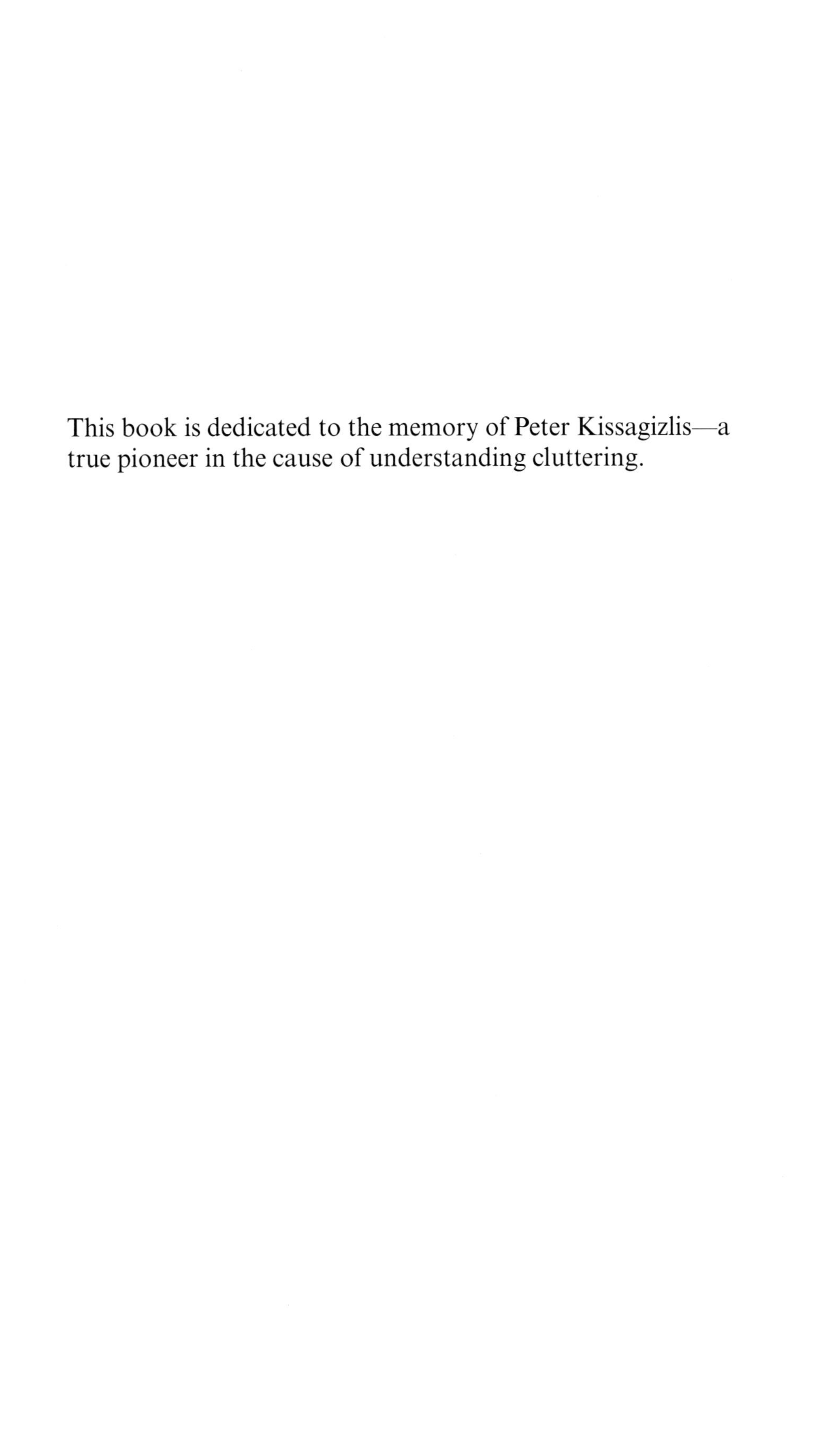

This book is dedicated to the memory of Peter Kissagizlis—a true pioneer in the cause of understanding cluttering.

Contents

Contributors

Per Alm, PhD Uppsala University, Uppsala, Sweden

Klaas Bakker, PhD Department of Communication Sciences and Disorders, Missouri State University, Springfield, Missouri, USA

Ellen Bennett Lanouette, PhD Texas, USA

Stephen Davis, PhD Department of Psychology, University College London, UK

Philipe Dejonckere, PhD University Medical Centre Utrecht, The Netherlands

Jill Douglass, Doctoral Student, Department of Communicative Disorders, University of Louisiana at Lafayette, Lafayette, Louisiana, USA

Juris G. Draguns, PhD Department of Psychology, Pennsylvania State University, University Park, Pennsylvania, USA

Dennis Drayna, PhD National Institute on Deafness and Other Communication Disorders, Bethesda, MD, USA

Peter Howell, PhD Department of Psychology, University College, London, UK

Shoko Miyamoto, PhD Department of Speech, Language and Hearing Therapy, Mejiro University, Saitama, Japan

Florence L. Myers, PhD Department of Communication Sciences and Disorders, Adelphi University, Long Island, New York, USA

Lawrence Raphael, PhD Department of Communication Sciences and Disorders, Adelphi University, Long Island, New York, USA

Isabella Reichel, PhD Graduate Program in Speech and Language Pathology, Touro College, New York, USA

Kathleen Scaler Scott, PhD Department of Speech-Language Pathology, Misericordia University, Dallas, Pennsylvania, USA

Katrin Schulte, PhD Department of Rehabilitation Science/Communication Disorders, Technische Universität Dortmund, Dortmund, Germany

Kenneth O. St. Louis, PhD Department of Speech Pathology and Audiology, West Virginia University, Morgantown, West Virginia, USA

John A. Tetnowski, PhD Department of Communicative Disorders, University of Louisiana at Lafayette, Lafayette, Louisiana, USA

John Van Borsel, PhD Ghent University Hospital, Ghent, Belgium, and Universidade Veiga de Almeida, Rio de Janeiro, Brazil

Yvonne van Zaalen, PhD Fontys University, Eindhoven, The Netherlands

David Ward, PhD Department of Clinical Language Sciences, The University of Reading, Reading, UK

Frank Wijnen, PhD UIL OTS, Utrecht University, The Netherlands

Acknowledgements

We would like to extend our grateful thanks to all our contributors for their wonderful efforts. Thanks are also due to the editorial team at Psychology Press; in particular, Eleanor Jones, Sharla Plant and Kristin Susser, whose thoroughness, patience and guidance we have very much appreciated throughout the book's production. Finally, thanks to our respective families for support and patience throughout this process.

David Ward & Kathleen Scaler Scott

Figures

Tables

Editors' introduction

Background and rationale to the current volume

The bibliography of textbooks on the subject of cluttering is, to put it mildly, short. In marked contrast to the considerable literature on stuttering, only two volumes have ever been produced on cluttering: one by Weiss (1964) and more recently an edited volume by Myers and St. Louis (1992). Both are regarded as seminal works by those studying this complex communication disorder, yet the 28-year gap between them reflects the paucity of data that have been generated on a subject matter that has remained obscure alongside its more visible fluency sibling. The Myers and St. Louis publication was followed in 1996 by a special edition of the *Journal of Fluency Disorders*. This, in turn, led to a further increase in publications on cluttering in the late 1990s and early 2000s.

This burgeoning interest became further distilled when, in May 2007, a group of researchers, clinicians, and consumers came together in Katarino, Bulgaria for the First World Congress on Cluttering. The congress drew people from around the world with a common interest in increasing knowledge and awareness of cluttering. Although interest in cluttering had been steadily increasing in recent years, the congress was an official means of declaring the imminent resurgence of *new* data on this topic. The Congress culminated with the formation of the International Cluttering Association (ICA), an organization whose mission is in part to encourage collaborations among researchers, clinicians, and consumers. It was hoped that projects would emerge out of such collaborations that could provide new evidence and clinical strategies for managing clients with cluttering.

This textbook represents in large part the fruits of those seeds planted in Katarino. Since the Congress and continued development of the ICA, partnerships have been formed within and across countries and continents. The purpose of this book is to bring these projects to light in a way that provides the reader with new data on cluttering *and* practical considerations for applying these data to assessment and treatment.

It was not enough, however, for evidence to be simply 'new'. In the 1996 special cluttering edition of the *Journal of Fluency Disorders*, reviewers called for research projects that represented more than anecdotal evidence, and use of a more narrow and standard definition of cluttering across studies. The chapters in this volume represent the outcome of projects developed with this advice in mind. This textbook aims to acknowledge what is and is not known in cluttering, without overstating applications of evidence. Paired with evidence are new theoretical considerations, ripe for testing by researchers.

The chapters for this text were chosen to fill specific gaps in the literature on cluttering. Recent surveys indicate that clinicians within many countries continue to receive minimal training on this topic at the university level (Di Domenicantonio & Duldulao, 2009; Scaler Scott, Grossman, & Tetnowski, 2010). One of the reasons given for this lack of training is the paucity of evidence-based information to share with students. *Cluttering: a handbook of research, intervention and education* represents a wealth of new, evidence-based information, and has a chapter devoted to guidelines for including this information in a graduate school curriculum.

Perhaps one outcome of the lack of training at the university level has been lack of knowledge of cluttering among speech-language clinicians, resulting in misdiagnoses and lack of services. The practising clinician, whether new to or experienced with cluttering, will find chapters with fresh ideas to bridge this gap in training, including information to help distinguish cluttered speech from other speech and language characteristics of concomitant disorders such as Down syndrome, learning disabilities, and autism spectrum disorders. Given that we are both researchers, educators *and* practising clinicians, it has been our goal to make the information presented in this text a representation of *both* sound evidence for training and research purposes *and* functional ideas for working with clients with cluttering.

Prior cluttering research has not considered the opinions of those who may have the greatest insight into the communication disorder cluttering—namely, those who live with cluttering. This text attempts to capture the lived experiences of adults with cluttering and parents of children with cluttering. It is these experiences that will help the clinician to identify meaningful and functional treatment goals, and the researcher to identify unexplored areas for future investigation.

Finally, many projects related to cluttering are ongoing around the world, yet awareness of such projects has not always been global. We hope through this text that the reader can discover the power of international findings that may be applicable to consumers, clients, researchers, faculty, and students. Additionally, we seek to recognize the worldwide contributions to the field of cluttering that have continued to shape our knowledge of this communication disorder since Deso Weiss' first writings in 1964.

Acknowledgements

These chapters represent the hard and careful work of a talented and passionate group of international researchers, clinicians, and consumers. We thank each and every contributor sincerely for their generosity in sharing their diverse knowledge, for their time and their works; and for their patience and persistence with us as the chapters moved from draft through to final copy. We are grateful for all that they have contributed, and for all that future readers will learn for years to come as a result of their contributions. We go to press with the sincere hope that the recent interest generated in the objective study of cluttering will mean that researchers, clinicians, and consumers alike do not have to wait a further 18 years for the publication of this book's successor.

Some notes on the use of terminology in this book

A recent ICA survey (Scaler Scott, 2007) that sought to identify consumer preferences for terminology of cluttering discovered that, although individual opinions vary, the majority of those surveyed who clutter preferred the term 'people with cluttering' (PWC). We therefore use that term to refer to those who demonstrate the disorder. Recognizing that various terms are used worldwide to describe qualified individuals who treat disorders of fluency, we settled on the term 'clinician' as a cover term for titles such as 'speech language pathologist', 'speech language therapist', 'logopedist', amongst many others. Finally, whenever possible, gender-specific references to male and female clients, research participants, and clinicians have been avoided. Contributors only deviate from this policy when not doing so would result in awkward or cumbersome prose.

David Ward and Kathleen Scaler Scott
June 2010

References

Di Domenicantonio, C., & Duldulao, F. P. (2009, April). *Cluttering education: A survey of Canadian university programs.* A poster presented at the conference of the Canadian Association of Speech-Language Pathologists and Audiologists, London, Ontario.

Myers, F. L., & St. Louis, K. O. (1992). *Cluttering: A clinical perspective.* Leicester: FAR Communications.

Scaler Scott, K. (2007). Results of terminology preference survey. Retrieved June 2, 2010 from http://associations.missouristate.edu/ICA

Scaler Scott, K., Grossman, H. L., & Tetnowski, J. A. (2010, April). A survey of cluttering instruction in fluency courses. *Proceedings of the First World Conference on Cluttering* (pp. 171–179). Katarino, Bulgaria. http://associations.missouristate.edu/ICA

Weiss, D. A. (1964). *Cluttering.* Englewood Cliffs, NJ: Prentice-Hall.

Part I

The nature and neurology of cluttering

1 Cluttering: a neurological perspective

Per A. Alm

Introduction

Background

The term cluttering designates a conglomerate of symptoms and characteristics displayed in varying degrees by affected individuals. No single aspect is sufficient to determine the diagnosis; it is the clustering of certain traits that constitute this syndrome[1] (see St. Louis & Schulte, chapter 14 this volume). Cluttering is a speech-language disorder, but many authors, such as Weiss (1964), have argued that the symptoms also may include non-verbal motor behaviour, temperament, and attention deficits.[2]

Research on cluttering is important in order to provide improved means of treatment, but cluttering may also turn out to be a condition that leads to valuable insights regarding the normal processes underlying speech, language, and attention. Furthermore, understanding of cluttering is essential for the understanding of stuttering, as they are overlapping and yet contrasting disorders. Research on stuttering is complicated by difficulties in determining primary versus secondary aspects. This problem is less apparent in cluttering.

The discussion in this chapter is intended to outline a hypothetical framework of how cluttering may be understood. It should be emphasized that cluttering is a heterogeneous disorder, possibly with different causal mechanisms in different subgroups—partly because of unclear criteria for the diagnosis. Hopefully better understanding of the mechanisms involved will result in a more strict definition of cluttering. It is a conscious decision to make the hypotheses quite detailed, which sometimes means being speculative, in order to allow empirical testing.

A brief overview of this chapter and the conclusions

While the core of cluttering may be seen in the verbal expression of fast and dysrhythmic speech, the understanding of the disorder is likely to involve a very wide range of functions and anatomical structures in the brain related to language, motor control, attention, and intention. There is a lot of information available from current brain research, but there is a need to integrate this, and to relate it to the symptomatology of cluttering. In order to help the reader, the tentative conclusions and suggestions will be summarized here.

It will be proposed that the core of the problems in cluttering is located in the *medial wall* of the left frontal lobe, i.e., the cortex on the wall between the cerebral hemispheres (see Figures 1.1 and 1.2). In brief, the model implies that the medial frontal cortex plays a central role in production of spontaneous speech, in parallel with the more traditional speech and language areas in the lateral part of the left hemisphere, such as the Wernicke's and Broca's areas. The medial cortex is proposed to have a coordinating role in spontaneous speech, related to the motivation to talk; planning of the phrase; retrieval of words, syntactic elements, and phonological code from the lateral cortex regions; execution of the motor sequence, and monitoring of the speech output. The key regions in cluttering appear to be the *anterior cingulate cortex* (ACC), the *preSMA*, and the *SMA proper*, together with the input from the *basal ganglia* circuits. The ACC is proposed to have the functions of a 'central executive', at the core of the initiation of volitional movements and speech, as well as being the centre for wilful attention and high-level error monitoring. The ACC is closely related to the preSMA, which seem to be critical for the 'assembly' of the phrase, from the sequencing to the selection of words and word forms. The model that emerges from current brain imaging data is that the ACC, the preSMA, and the SMA proper constitute a hub or an 'assembly centre' in spontaneous speech, retrieving all the linguistic components from the left lateral cortex regions, such as the Wernicke's and Broca's areas and adjacent zones. The selection of one single word from many competing alternatives is facilitated by the basal ganglia circuits, through a 'winner-take-all' function. The timing of the articulation, and thereby the speech rate, is controlled by the SMA proper with support from the basal ganglia and the cerebellum. The production of speech is monitored on multiple levels, primarily through auditory connections to the ACC and the SMA.

Cluttering may be a heterogeneous disorder, with different (neural) mechanisms in different subgroups. A main mechanism proposed in this chapter is hyperactivation and dysregulation of the medial frontal cortex, which may be secondary to disinhibition of the basal ganglia circuits, for example as a result of a hyperactive dopamine system.

This review and analysis will be divided into main topics that all are intimately interrelated, making the structure somewhat loose. First, the functional anatomy of the medial frontal wall will be briefly presented, in order to provide an anatomical framework. Then the symptoms and characteristics of cluttering will be discussed. Physiological clues from the effect of dopaminergic drugs and abnormalities of EEG lead to a discussion of the possible role of an overactive dopamine system. Thereafter, the review will focus on three main aspects of speech production: (1) *initiation and*

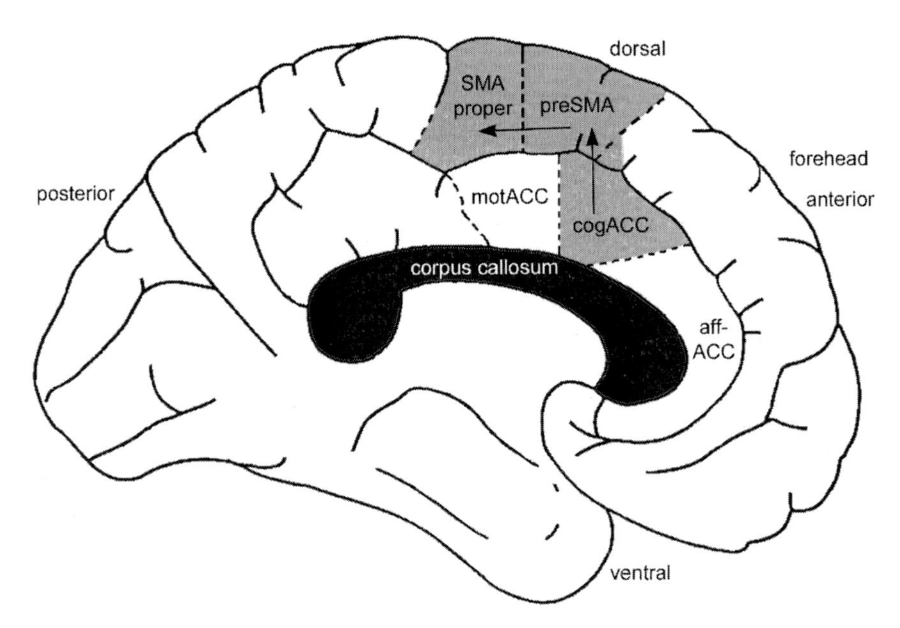

Figure 1.1 The medial wall of the left hemisphere. Regions proposed to constitute an 'executive hub' for speech production are marked in grey: the cogACC, the preSMA, and the SMA proper. (Redrawn from Talairach & Tournoux, 1988, with approximate division of the ACC added, based on Yücel et al., 2003, and review of data from various studies).

sequencing of action; (2) *selection of linguistic items*, such as words and syntactic elements; and (3) *monitoring of speech errors*. The intention is to propose a comprehensive model of speech production, based on current research findings, and relate the symptoms of cluttering to this model.

Functional anatomy of the medial frontal cortex

Functions of the ACC

The connections of the ACC are characterized by convergence—it is a region where drive, cognition, and motor control interface, putting the ACC in a unique position to translate intention to action (Paus, 2001). This key role in volitional behaviour is shown by the fact that bilateral damage to the ACC results in *akinetic mutism*, a state without voluntary motor activity or speech (Paus, 2001).

Attention is a function that may be separated into two different aspects: (1) *spontaneous attention*, elicited by salient stimuli of interest (also known as 'bottom-up', where the stimuli is sufficient to catch the attention) and (2) *effortful attention*, volitionally applied based on motivation to accomplish a certain outcome (or 'top-down', for example when looking for a certain object). The ability to maintain effortful attention seems to be dependent on the ACC, especially in case of divided attention (Loose, Kaufmann, Auer, & Lange, 2003). In fact, it seems likely that the ACC plays a central role in all tasks involving aspects of volitional control and attention, such as suppression of automatic responses, decisions under uncertainty, monitoring of behavioural errors, etc. (see reviews of studies in Botvinick, Cohen, & Carter, 2004; Posner, Rothbart, Sheese, & Tang, 2007; Ridderinkhof, Ullsperger, Crone, & Nieuwenhuis, 2004; Sarter, Gehring, & Kozak, 2006). It has been reported that persons with attention deficit hyperactivity disorder (ADHD) tend to have difficulties activating the ACC in demanding situations (Bush et al., 1999). Furthermore, studies have shown that the ACC also is crucially involved in working memory, in a network with the cortex in, and adjacent to, Broca's area, and maybe other regions (Kaneda & Osaka, 2008; Kondo, Morishita, Osaka, Osaka, Fukuyama, & Shibasaki, 2004; Osaka, Osaka, Kondo, Morishita, Fukuyama, & Shibasaki, 2004).

The ACC receives input related to motivation and drive via multiple pathways, from the limbic system and cortex regions in the lower frontal lobe. Several neuromodulators, like dopamine, influence the ACC, both directly and through projections from the limbic region of the basal ganglia. Strong connections with the prefrontal cortex reflect cognitive functioning. Complex motor behaviours are initiated through the SMA, but the ACC also has more direct motor projections, to the spinal cord and to brain stem nuclei. The more direct motor output from the ACC seems to be responsible for emotional expression, such as laughing and crying (Ackermann, 2008).

Functional divisions of the ACC and the SMA

The ACC may be divided into three functional regions: the *affective, cognitive*, and *motor* ACC (abbreviated *affACC, cogACC, motACC*; Yücel, Wood, Fornito, Riffkin, Velakoulis, & Pantelis, 2003), from the lower frontal end to the upper posterior end (see Figure 1.1). The core region for the ACC functions discussed above is the cogACC.

The SMA is located at the upper border of the cogACC and motACC. Interestingly, also the SMA follows this division, with an anterior cognitive part, the preSMA, connected with the prefrontal cortex, and a posterior motor part, the SMA proper, with motor functions and direct connections both to the primary motor cortex and to the spinal cord (Johansen-Berg et al., 2004; Picard & Strick, 1996). The activation in cogACC has been shown to extend into the preSMA, for example, in studies of response conflict and error monitoring (Botvinick et al., 2004; Ridderinkhof et al., 2004). It has also been shown that this region (SMA and ACC) responds to speech errors and may detect 'spoonerisms' (reversal of sounds) even before they are articulated (Möller, Jansma, Rodriguez-Fornells, & Münte, 2007).

Symptoms and characteristics of cluttering

Trying to understand the symptoms of cluttering from a neurological point of view is not a new endeavour. Miloslav Seeman (1970), phoniatrician of Prague, compared the symptoms of cluttering with other neurological disorders, and proposed that cluttering is the result of a disturbance of the *basal ganglia* system (see Figure 1.2). Similarly, the neurolinguist Yvan Lebrun of Brussels (1996) argued that traits of cluttering after brain damage or disease typically occur after damage to the basal ganglia system, as in Parkinson's disease.

Behavioural symptoms and characteristics

Detailed discussion of the symptoms of cluttering can be found in Weiss (1964) and Luchsinger and Arnold (1965), and more recently in Daly (1993), Myers and St. Louis (1996), Preus (1996), Ward (2006), and St. Louis and Schulte (chapter 14 this volume). Though different authors have a somewhat different focus, the overall picture seems quite consistent. Ward (2006) analyzed the speech errors in cluttering based on Levelt's model of speech and language processing, and found that cluttering affects all levels of this processing: conceptualization, formulation, and articulation. All elements of speech can potentially be affected, from the drive to talk, the sequencing of the message, the selection of words and syntactic elements, the motor output, and the monitoring of speech errors.

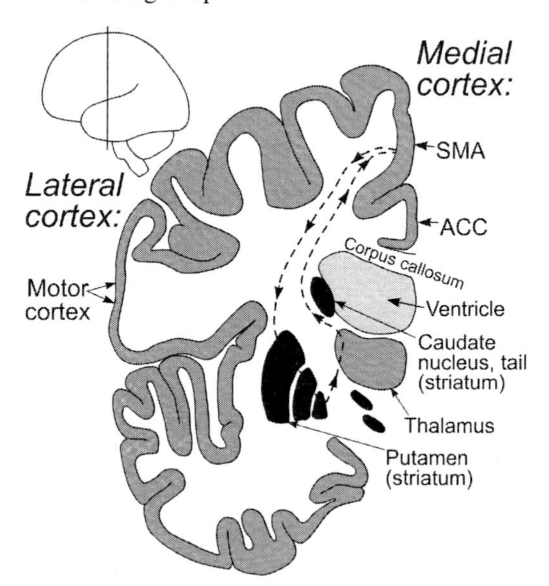

Figure 1.2 Basal ganglia loops, in a cross-section of a single hemisphere. The schematic figure shows a motor loop starting and ending in the supplementary motor area (SMA), passing through the putamen (part of the striatum) and the thalamus. The figure also shows the tail of the caudate nucleus (part of the striatum) in cross-section. ACC: anterior cingulate cortex.

Speech motor aspects

The speech motor symptoms are typically characterized by high speech rate, poor articulation with exaggerated blending of adjacent sounds, phoneme sequencing errors (such as *gleen glass* for *green grass*, or *bo gack* for *go back*; Ward, 2006), and reduced prosody (both timing and pitch range). However, in many cases these symptoms are strongly affected by attention, for example so that speech may sound normal, temporarily, when a tape-recorder is turned on (Daly & St. Louis, 1998). Seeman (1970) mentioned a test he used for diagnosis of cluttering: The patient is asked to repeat the syllable 'tah' as fast and for as long as possible. According to Seeman, many people with cluttering (PWC) are able to do this well at the beginning of the task, but after a while acceleration begins and the articulation loses precision. Some PWC also show motor deficits that are not limited to speech, such as in handwriting and general motor behaviour. For example, Seeman (1970) reported a tendency among PWC for rushed and unexpected movements, and general motor restlessness, also during sleep, of choreiform type (i.e., similar to movements seen in chorea, a type of motor disorder linked to disinhibition of the basal ganglia). Another aspect is that PWC often tend to have difficulties in recognizing and repeating rhythmic patterns (Weiss, 1964). (On motor speech activity in PWC, see Ward, chapter 3 this volume.)

Linguistic aspects

Most descriptions of cluttering include problems with linguistic processing as one aspect (e.g., Myers, 1992; van Zaalen, Ward, Nederveen, Grolman, Wijnen, & DeJonckere, 2009; Ward, 2006; Weiss, 1964), although this does not fall within St. Louis and Shulte's current working definition (St. Louis & Schulte, chapter 14 this volume). From a linguistic point of view cluttering tends to be characterized by difficulties with: (1) word finding; (2) planning of sentences and phrases; and (3) syntactic elements. PWC often speak in short phrases of a few words, or 'bursts'. According to Weiss (1964), this is a reflection of the thought process—that the verbal thoughts of PWC tend to proceed by clusters of two or three words at a time, instead of complete phrases. Repetitions of syllables, words, or phrases are common, as well as fillers like 'eh' and 'um'. These repetitions do not seem to occur because of any motor block, but rather as a result of the difficulties to find words and to create a complete phrase. The word order may be incorrect, and sentences may be left unfinished or continue in a 'maze-like' fashion, leaving the listener behind. Retrieval of words, including names, prepositions, and pronouns, may be inexact, so that an incorrect word is chosen based on similarities in sound or semantic content, such as *plant* for *point*, or *fork* for *knife*. Function words may be omitted and the verb conjugation may be incorrect (Ward, 2006).

Attention, temperament, and social interaction

A typical trait observed amongst PWC seems to be reduced attention to sensory input, displayed as poor monitoring of one's own speech production with limited awareness of cluttered speech, as well as insufficient attention to the listener. The observation that attention to speech often results in temporary normalization indicates that the necessary linguistic and motor functions may be available, but require focused attention.

Regarding personality, Weiss (1964) claimed that PWC are generally of pleasant temperament. Other traits that have been proposed to be frequent among PWC are impulsiveness, impatience, excessive talking, and being short-tempered (Daly, 1993; Weiss, 1964). One way to analyze temperament and motor functions is in terms of *inhibition* versus *disinhibition*. From this viewpoint, the traits mentioned above seem to be associated with disinhibition. However, it is important to avoid generalizing a 'cluttering stereotype', because PWC do differ in these respects (see also Reichel & Draguns, chapter 16 this volume).

Cluttering is defined as a speech-language disorder, but it seems likely that people who primarily have a mood disorder, such as mania, sometimes have been (mis)diagnosed as cluttering because rapid speech is a frequent symptom of the manic state (Geller et al., 2002). It is therefore possible that the descriptions of temperamental traits associated with cluttering have been biased by inclusion of cases with mania, which often is associated with irritability and being short-tempered (Geller et al., 2002). It is important to distinguish between cluttering, as a speech-language disorder, and rapid and pressured speech resulting from a mood disorder. Yet, it may be possible that cluttering and mood disorders co-occur to some extent. Familial co-occurrence of *stuttering* and bipolar disorder has been reported by Hays and Field (1989). There is a need for further research to clarify these issues, also regarding differences and overlap between cluttering and ADHD (Geller et al., 2002).

Physiology of cluttering

The tendency towards disinhibition as a temperamental trait also seems to be reflected in neurophysiological findings based on electroencephalography (EEG) research and response to drugs. Research on the neurophysiology of cluttering emerged in Central Europe in the 1950s and 1960s, and though the results of these studies were quite striking, this line of inquiry has not been continued.

EEG

A high percentage of PWC tend to show abnormalities in their EEG recordings. Langova and Moravek (1970) studied the EEGs of 57 PWC, and classified 50 percent of them as abnormal and 11 percent as atypical. In addition, they noticed relatively low occurrence of alpha waves, suggesting high cortical activation in PWC. The high frequency of abnormalities is in line with other studies, as summarized by Seeman (1970), reporting abnormal EEGs in between 50 and 90 percent of the cases. There is a need for replication with modern techniques, to analyze the anomalies in more detail.

Effect of drugs

Langova and Moravek (1964) also tested the effects of two drugs, one inhibitor and one stimulant. In a group of 13 cases, improvement of speech was reported in 11 cases after treatment with chlorpromazine, a drug that blocks the dopamine receptor type D2 and thereby inhibits the activity of cortex (for a more detailed discussion see Alm, 2004). The stimulant drug (phenmetrazine, which has effects similar to amphetamine, stimulating dopamine) resulted in a worsening effect on speech (details not specified) in all of eight cases. In addition, the subjects complained of internal uneasiness and tension after the stimulant drug. These pharmacological responses are consistent with an elevated level of dopamine in cluttering, as discussed below.

Hyperdopaminergic state in cluttering?

General effects of dopamine

Dopamine is a neurotransmitter with a wide range of complex effects. It is the main factor controlling the flow of signals through the basal ganglia, which in turn modulates the excitatory state of the cortex in the frontal lobe. In short, a high level of dopamine release in the basal ganglia tends to result in a high level of activation of the cortex, with disinhibition of motor behaviour and impulses. Blockade of the dopamine D2 receptors tend to have the opposite effect, with suppression of behavioural impulses and motor activity, as shown in untreated Parkinson's disease.

Below it will be discussed whether elevated effects of dopamine (a *hyperdopaminergic state*) might result in the symptoms shown in some cases of cluttering. The discussion will include effects on timing and speed, motivation and attention, and the physical growth of children. EEG anomalies were discussed above, a symptom that may be compatible with the proposal of a hyperdopaminergic state: Because elevated dopaminergic activity would tend to result in disinhibition of cortical regions, one would expect an increased rate of EEG anomalies.

Dopamine and the control of time and speed

It has been shown that the circuits through the basal ganglia to the frontal cortex have an important role for the perception of time, as well as the timing and speed of motor behaviour (Giros, Jaber, Jones, Wightman, & Caron, 1996; Meck, Penney, & Pouthas, 2008). The effects of these circuits are consistent with the effects of dopaminergic drugs on cluttering, resulting in increased speed with increased dopamine release, and reduced speed with blocking of the D2 receptors (Meck et al., 2008). Two main factors that influence the effect of dopamine in the brain are the amount of dopamine available in the synaptic cleft and the number of receptors for dopamine on the post-synaptic neuron. A high number of receptors can partly compensate for low levels of dopamine. It has been shown, in mice, that overexpression of D2 receptors, or excess release of dopamine (after administration of amphetamine), impairs the ability to estimate time (Drew et al., 2007; Meck et al., 2008). Furthermore, mice in a hyperdopaminergic state show hyperactivity, which is reversed by block of the D2 receptors (Giros et al., 1996).

The hypothesis that the output of the basal ganglia affects the speech rate is supported by earlier work by Guiot, Hertzog, Rondot, and Molina (1961), in which electric stimulation of the ventrolateral (VL) nucleus of the thalamus (see Figure 1.2) resulted in uncontrollable acceleration of speech. The VL nucleus is the link for the output of the basal ganglia motor circuit to the *supplementary motor area* (SMA). This is in agreement with recent brain imaging results, reporting high activity in the VL nucleus of the thalamus in PWC (van Zaalen et al., 2009). High VL activation can be expected to be associated with disinhibition of the SMA.

The articulation rate is the result of the duration of speech sounds. The exact control of the duration of sounds is essential in order to achieve a normal prosody, with longer duration of vowels with stress and emphasis. In order to produce a long sound, the initiation of the next sound has to be delayed. If this delay is insufficient, the result will be excessive speech rate with lack of temporal prosody.

What determines the timing of the next sound, on a neuronal level? Experiments on manual movements in monkeys have shown that delayed movements are initiated when the firing rate in the cortex and the basal ganglia circuits reach a threshold. Before the initiation, the firing gradually increases in a ramp-like fashion, indicating a timing mechanism (Lebedev, O'Doherty, & Nicolelis, 2008; Lee & Assad, 2003). The threshold mechanism is involved also in externally cued movements, but then the firing increases instantaneously after the cue (Lee & Assad, 2003). This mechanism has been shown for delays of about 2 seconds (Lebedev et al., 2008; Lee & Assad, 2003), but it seems possible that the principle applies also to the shorter delays needed when producing long sounds in speech (in the range of tenths of seconds). If the basal ganglia and the cortex are hyperactivated, it seems likely that the firing of the relevant circuits may reach the threshold prematurely, so that the delay is shortened or completely abolished. It has been reported that PWC often show a general hastiness of their movements. It is likely that the hastiness of speech and of general movements have the same neural substrate: impaired ability of the SMA proper to maintain a delay before the initiation of the next motor gesture.

What is the source of normal timing—is there 'a clock'? It has been shown that the basal ganglia circuits play a role in the timing of longer intervals, in the second to minute range, and that the cerebellum is involved in millisecond timing (Ivry & Spencer, 2004). However, Ivry and Spencer concluded that the evidence does not rule out millisecond control also in other parts of the brain, such as the basal ganglia or local cortex regions. Both the basal ganglia and the cerebellum innervate the SMA (Akkal, Dum, & Strick, 2007), but dysfunction of the cerebellum tends to result in symptoms opposite to cluttering, with reduced speech rate and prolongation of short sounds (Ackermann, 2008).

Dopamine and motivation and attention

The exact functions of the dopamine system are still a matter of debate, but there are strong arguments that it has a key role in signalling salient events and rewards (e.g., McClure, Daw, & Montague, 2003; Schultz, 2007). An overactive dopamine system might result in reduced effects of rewards, because of a ceiling effect. For example, hyperdopaminergic mice have been shown to be indifferent to amphetamine and cocaine (Giros et al., 1996), and to have reduced preference for alcohol (Savelieva, Caudle, Findlay, Caron, & Miller, 2002).

It has also been reported that mice with an overactive dopamine system show reduced motivation in operational conditioning tasks (Drew et al., 2007). Weiss (1964) depicted PWC as carefree, careless, lacking in persistence and sense of responsibility, generally with a pleasant temperament, not taking life's problems very seriously (including cluttering treatment), and showing a short attention span. It seems possible that this constellation of traits could be an effect of a hyperactive dopamine system, so that the motivational effect of rewards, or loss of rewards, is reduced. However, it should be emphasized that this is still speculative, and clinical reports indicate that at least in some cases the speech problems in cluttering are unrelated to motivation (D. Ward, personal communication, September 10, 2009).

Children with ADHD are often treated with low doses of stimulants in order to improve attention, though the exact mechanism of action is not known (Solanto, 2002). The results from the pharmacological trials of Langova and Moravek (1964) suggest that PWC show the opposite response to dopaminergic drugs compared with typical cases of ADHD. It is possible that the attention deficits in cluttering and typical ADHD are related to different types of dysregulation, though affecting the same attention system. It may be argued that PWC with attention problems constitute a subgroup of ADHD.

Dopamine in relation to weight and appetite

It has been reported that many children with cluttering tend to be small for their age, and physically immature (Daly, 1993; Weiss, 1964). This may appear to be an odd observation, but could actually make sense within the framework of a hyperdopaminergic state. Reduced growth is a side effect of treatment with dopamine stimulants for childhood ADHD, though final adult stature may not be affected (Faraone, Biederman, Morley, & Spencer, 2008). Dopamine stimulants have been used for weight reduction, by reducing appetite; conversely, weight gain is a frequent side effect of treatment with D2-blockers. It has been shown that peripheral injections of dopamine in human newborns have a strong acute effect in reducing growth hormone secretion (De Zegher, Van Den Berghe, Devlieger, Eggermont, & Velduis, 1993). However, it is not clear whether growth hormone is affected during long-term treatment with stimulants. Another potential mechanism might be elevated metabolism, involving a slight elevation of body temperature, because hyperthermia can be an effect of stimulants (Meredith, Jaffe, Ang-Lee, & Saxon, 2005). In summary, based on observed pharmacological effects, it seems possible that also endogenous hyperdopaminergic states may result in delayed growth.

Summary: hyperdopaminergic state

The hypothesis of a hyperdopaminergic state in PWC may account for a large part of the reported characteristics associated with PWC: (1) the effects of drugs; (2) EEG anomalies; (3) delayed growth; (4) excessive speech rate; (5) short attention span; (6) poor awareness of speech errors; (7) temperamental traits characterized by disinhibition, impulsivity, and a relatively carefree attitude.

A functional hyperdopaminergic state might be caused by several different mechanisms, for example: (1) excessive synaptic release of dopamine; (2) deficient dopamine reuptake from the synaptic cleft; or (3) overexpression of D2 receptors. It is also possible that dysregulation of the dopamine system can be secondary to anomalies in other transmitter systems (Koprich, Johnston, Huot, Fox, & Brotchie, 2009). The indications for hereditary factors in some cases of cluttering calls for genetic investigations, especially focusing genes known to be linked to the dopamine system. A recent finding that may be relevant was published by Lan et al. (2009). They reported that different versions (alleles) of the gene for the D2 receptor increased or reduced the risk for stuttering in a Chinese population. Because of the high reported co-occurrence of stuttering and cluttering (Daly, 1996), it may be possible that this gene is related to traits of cluttering. There seems to be no recent pharmacological trials of treatment of cluttering. However, trials investigating the effects of D2-blockers (including more novel drugs in this family, such as Abilify), as well as low-dose stimulants, would be valuable. Nevertheless, it is important to emphasize that the hypothesis of a hyperdopaminergic state is unlikely to represent a general explanation of cluttering.

Initiation and sequencing of action: The medial frontal cortex

Initiation of action (and speech)

Research consistently indicates a central role of the medial frontal cortex in the initiation of volitional action. As mentioned above, bilateral lesions of the ACC result in akinetic mutism, in which voluntary initiatives to speech or motor activity are absent (Paus, 2001). Also, persons with unilateral lesions often show lack of ideas and initiative (Ferstl & von Cramon, 2002). In fact, based on research data, it has been proposed that non-automatic cognitive processes are initiated and maintained by the medial frontal cortex (Ferstl & von Cramon, 2002).

The dual premotor hypothesis

In the 1980s, Goldberg (1985) and Passingham (1987) proposed that the frontal lobe has two parallel premotor networks, involved in speech and other movements. The medial network, with the ACC/SMA, was suggested to be specialized on volitional execution of well-learnt sequences, without sensory input. The lateral network, with the lateral premotor cortex, was assumed to control actions based on external information. MacNeilage (1998) included this hypothesis in his theory of the evolution of speech, and Snyder (2004), Snyder, Hough, Blanchet, Ivy, and Waddell (2009) and Alm (2005) have discussed this model in relation to stuttering. In 2007, Alm also suggested that the dual premotor model may account for some of the symptoms of cluttering (Alm, 2010).

The proposal by Goldberg and Passingham has been the focus of some empirical studies, with mixed support. The overall pattern emerging from brain imaging studies seems to be that both lateral and medial regions contribute in both externally and internally controlled tasks, with complex interaction (Crosson et al., 2001; Longe, Senior, & Rippon, 2009; Paus, Petrides, Evans, & Meyer, 1993; Tremblay & Gracco, 2006). The recent study by Longe et al. indicated that the cogACC has a direct top-down influence on the lateral prefrontal cortex. Furthermore, it has been shown in monkeys that the medial frontal cortex, including the ACC, have bidirectional connections with temporal auditory areas (Barbas, Ghashghaei, Dombrowski, & Rempel-Clower, 1999), indicating that the medial system actually has direct access to auditory information during speech.

In summary, Goldberg's hypothesis outlined the medial and lateral cortex as two relatively parallel systems, while the current data seem to implicate a more hierarchic relation, with a functionally subordinate lateral system. This will be discussed in more detail later in this chapter.

Sequencing and articulation

In the production of speech the brain has to solve several problems. One main problem is sequencing. An idea can be nonsequential, like an image. In contrast, speech always consists of a linear sequence, on many levels—a sequence of phrases, words, syllables, and sounds. In a very brief and rough summary, based on Levelt's (1999) model, the sequencing of an idea may proceed in the following way: The semantic representation of the idea results in a grammatical frame, providing a sequential overall structure for the utterance. The intended words and the correct grammatical elements are selected and inserted in the grammatical frame. The phonological code, 'the sound', is activated and is structured into syllables (which may pass word boundaries), and the appropriate prosodic pattern is applied. Syllables may be described as 'chunks' of sounds, constituting one opening-and-closing-cycle for the mouth. The role of the syllable in the planning of speech is shown by the observation that when sounds are exchanged between syllables, like *mell wade* for *well made*, the sound almost always move to the same position within the syllable (MacNeilage, 1998).

From this brief outline, it seems clear that the sequencing process must occur simultaneously on many levels, and that the planned sequence has to be temporarily stored in some way, while the segments are articulated in serial order. An example of how the SMA plans movements in advance may be seen in a study by Gerloff, Corwell, Chen, Hallett, and Cohen (1997), in which transcranial magnetic stimulation (TMS) was used to interrupt a well-learnt sequence of complex finger movements in healthy adults. It was found that disturbing the SMA using TMS interrupted the sequence with about 1 second delay.

The preparatory planning of action is also shown by the *readiness potential* (RP, 'Bereitschaftspotential', Shibasaki & Hallet, 2006). The RP is an electric potential preceding volitional movements, and the timing of the potential in various regions shows the order of regional involvement. The early phase of the RP originates bilaterally in the preSMA and the SMA proper, up to 2 seconds before the movement. Shortly thereafter, it spreads to the lateral premotor cortex, also bilaterally. About 0.4 seconds before the movement, the late phase begins, with activation of the contralateral primary motor and premotor cortices (Shibasaki & Hallet, 2006). The same sequence seems to apply for self-initiated speech (Deecke, Kornhuber, Lang, Lang, & Schreiber, 1985).

In a brain imaging study of word production, Alario, Chainay, Lehericy, and Cohen (2006) found that long and unfamiliar utterances activated the posterior part of the preSMA, bilaterally, indicating sequential encoding in this zone, possibly phonological sequence encoding. Articulation activated the SMA proper, but extended into the posterior preSMA (together with bilateral mouth area of the primary cortices).

In summary, the studies with different methods indicate that there is an anterior–posterior gradient within the SMA, bilaterally, with higher level planning and sequencing in the anterior preSMA, sequencing of sounds and syllables in the posterior preSMA, and sequencing of articulation in the SMA proper and the border of preSMA.

Selection of linguistic items: The preSMA

Selection of words

Neurolinguistic theories, for example Levelt (1999), typically describe the linguistic cortex regions as networks of associations, based on semantics, phonology, and so forth. A semantic concept will activate a part of the 'mental lexicon', with many competing words becoming more or less active. When speaking it is essential that one and only one word is selected—this is the problem of word selection. In cluttering, there is an increased risk that a competing but erroneous word is selected.

Brain imaging studies of word selection repeatedly indicate involvement of the left preSMA. This has been shown in word selection based on semantic category as well as initial sounds and rhyming (Crosson et al., 2003; De Carli et al., 2007), and both for nouns and verbs (Warburton et al., 1996). Alario et al. (2006) reported that activation from word selection was limited to the anterior half of the preSMA. Tremblay and Gracco (2010) recently proposed that the preSMA is at the core of a network for volitional selection. Activation extending into the ACC has been reported by Warburton et al. (1996) and by Carreiras, Mechelli, and Price (2006) for low frequency words. It seems possible that accessing such lesser known words would require a higher level of attention, thereby also recruiting the ACC.

Selection of grammatical forms

A role for the preSMA in selection has also been shown for grammatical aspects. In a brain imaging study, Sahin, Pinker, and Halgren (2006) investigated processing related to silent inflection of nouns and verbs, with both regular and irregular forms. In the lateral cortex, the main region was Broca's area, but in the medial cortex, the preSMA and the cogACC also showed involvement. The published images showed higher activation of the cogACC and the preSMA for silent inflection compared with silent reading, and higher activation for irregular verbs compared with regular verbs.

Selection by the basal ganglia?

It is of interest that this type of processing, in which 'the winner takes all', has been described as one of the main functions of the basal ganglia circuits. This principle is presented in Mink (1996), and more recent theoretical accounts and summaries can be found in Gazzaniga, Ivry, and Mangun (2009, pp. 301–302), Leblois et al. (2006), and Houk (2005).

As outlined in Figure 1.2, the basal ganglia can be seen as the main component in a multitude of parallel loops starting and ending in the cerebral cortex. The main cortical input to the loops comes from the same area in which they end, forming closed loops that modify the activity in the target cortical regions. Even though the closed loop seems to be the main principle of these circuits, there also appear to be some integration of inputs from other regions. It is primarily the frontal lobe cortex that is modulated by the basal ganglia, but basal ganglia output has also been found in the temporal lobe (Middleton & Strick, 1996).

It is assumed that the basal ganglia loop highlights the most coherent and consistent activity pattern of the cortex, while rival impulses are inhibited. This is accomplished by the intricate anatomy of the basal ganglia circuits, in which the output activates two competing and intermingled pathways. The *direct pathway* provides focused activation of the strongest pattern in the target cortical region (e.g., the word that is the most strongly activated, and which is in coherence with the activity of other relevant cortex regions). In contrast, the parallel pathways provide a more diffuse and widespread inhibition of the cortex, thereby suppressing the competing impulses.[3] This can be described as a noise filter or a contrast mechanism, allowing the organism to focus on the most important impulse.

Traditionally, the basal ganglia were assumed to only serve motor functions, but it has now become apparent that these structures also are involved in cognitive functions and the processing of language (Booth, Wood, Lu, Houk, & Bitan, 2007; Grahn, Parkinson, & Owen, 2008; Middleton & Strick, 2000; Teichmann et al., 2008). In short, the different regions of the basal ganglia serve the same functions as their cortical targets, with cognitive functions primarily related to the caudate nucleus, sensorimotor functions to the putamen, and affective/motivational functions related to the ventral striatum. In line with this model, Crosson et al. (2003) found that selection of words activated a loop consisting of the left preSMA and the left caudate nucleus of the basal ganglia.

Houk (2005) presented a comprehensive model of how the basal ganglia and the cerebellum may interact with the cerebral cortex, to select and shape cortical activity. According to this view, the same basic principles are involved in the selection and shaping of motor actions as in the selection and shaping of thoughts.

In summary, the basal ganglia circuits are proposed to have the ability to highlight and select cortical activation that is congruent with activation in other parts of the cortex, and to suppress competing activity. This mechanism appears to be ideally suited to support the cortex in making the most appropriate word choice based on a network of semantic associations, or to select the correct preposition or pronoun in a certain context. Dysregulation of the basal ganglia circuits might compromise this function, making the selection less precise. If the cortex in the preSMA is hyperactive, an increased number of words may be passed on to the SMA proper for articulation, including an increased number of selection errors.

An 'executive hub' for speech production

In 1974 Baddeley proposed his classical model of the working memory, with a 'central executive' and 'slave systems' (or subordinate systems) such as the phonological loop and the visuo-spatial sketchpad (Baddeley, 2003). Kaneda and Osaka (2008) argued that the ACC is the main component of the central executive, and that semantic coding in the verbal working memory depends on the ACC.[4]

The studies reviewed above repeatedly point towards a central role of the cogACC, together with the preSMA, for: attention, verbal working memory, initiation of action, control of response conflicts, error monitoring, sequencing of speech, and selection of linguistic items. The model that emerges is that the cogACC and the preSMA constitute an 'executive hub' for cognitive processes and planning of actions. In spontaneous speech, this hub may be viewed as an 'assembly centre', in which all the components of the utterance (retrieved from the lateral cortex regions) are put together in a sequence.

The construction of an utterance requires: (1) the selection of an overall grammatical frame for the utterance, indicating the order of the semantic components; (2) selection of words; (3) selection of grammatical word forms. In all of these processes it is essential that only one alternative is selected, from many competing possibilities. If the cogACC/preSMA region is specialized in selection among competing alternatives, it seems reasonable that this zone actually constitutes a hub for the complete process of spontaneous speech (see schematic outline in Figure 1.3). Within this region there is a gradient from higher to lower level of control—from overall control in the cogACC, to sequential assembly of the utterance in the preSMA, and control of the motor execution in the SMA proper.[5]

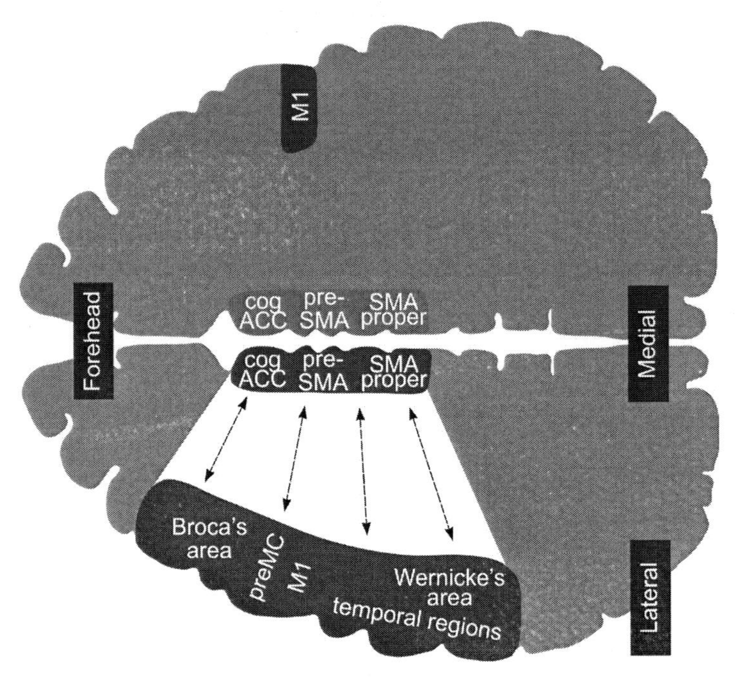

Figure 1.3 Schematic outline of a 'hub-model' of speech production, showing a horizontal cross-section of the brain. The medial hub has the functions of a central executive and an 'assembly centre' for sequencing of the linguistic items selected from the linguistic networks in the left lateral cortex region. M1: Primary motor cortex. PreMC: Premotor cortex.

Lesions resulting in release of subordinate systems

This model of an 'executive hub' in the cogACC/SMA region is supported by symptoms observed after unilateral lesions in the ACC/SMA region (Goldberg, 1992; Jonas, 1981; Suzuki, Itoh, Hayashi, Kouno, & Takeda, 2009). The symptoms are characterized by impaired ability to volitionally initiate an activity, but this function may be involuntarily triggered by external cues. There are reports of this phenomenon in speech (echolalia), reading (hyperlexia), and hand movements ('the alien hand sign'—when one hand is grasping objects and makes purposeful movements that are not volitionally controlled). The common mechanism is that a subordinate system becomes disinhibited after the lesion of the ACC/SMA. It can also be described in terms of rivalry between top-down and bottom-up processes, here resulting in release of the latter (Suzuki et al., 2009).

Suzuki et al. (2009) described a woman who had suffered infarction of the left ACC. Involuntary speech was triggered by written words and by words emanating from unrelated conversations, resulting in repetition. Her right hand showed compulsive manipulation of tools. The woman tried to prevent this by holding the right arm with the left arm.

Monitoring of speech errors

One aspect of cluttering, discussed above, is a tendency to not notice and not correct errors in word selection, speech sounds, or speech rate. Several studies have shown that the cogACC exerts high-level control of errors in the intended outcome of actions (Botvinick et al., 2004; Ridderinkhof et al., 2004). Furthermore, as noted earlier, a study of event-related brain potentials in a task that elicited reversal of sounds ('spoonerisms') showed that the ACC/SMA region responded to these errors even before they were articulated.

Production of speech can be characterized by a series of conversions from higher to lower levels: semantics → words → phonological sequence → motor commands → sound. In principle, higher levels have the information to detect errors in the conversion to a lower level. The level of semantics can detect if an incorrect word has been selected. Likewise, the level that is planning the phonological sequence can detect if a sound is misarticulated. The detection of errors may occur before the sound is produced, called *covert repair* (Postma & Kolk, 1993), based on internal feedback within the brain. Alternatively, errors can be detected from the auditory feedback of the speech sounds.

It is here suggested that the centre of this monitoring is the cogACC/SMA. The functions and connections of this region are ideally suited for this task. If this region constitutes an 'executive hub', all plans for the intended outcome are available here. It has been shown in monkeys that the auditory areas have bidirectional connections with the medial frontal cortex, including the ACC (Barbas et al., 1999). There is little information about these connections in humans, but considering the primary role of spoken language in human evolution, it seems probable that the auditory connections to the frontal lobe have been strengthened rather than weakened. This suggests that auditory feedback is available to the cogACC/SMA.

Weiss (1964, p. 44) wrote that the attention of PWC often is so brief that they may give the impression that hearing is impaired, or that they have a basic disorder in perception. It is important to investigate the underlying mechanisms in more detail, in particular, to determine whether the issue is with attention, or possibly with impaired auditory connections to the medial frontal cortex in some cases. Another hypothetical mechanism is that PWC may have a general problem withholding the next segment (such as sounds, syllables, and words) in a sequence, releasing it prematurely. As discussed above, there are experimental findings indicating that segments in a sequence are initiated when the firing of relevant circuits reach a threshold (Lee & Assad, 2003; Lebedev et al., 2008). If the ACC/SMA region is hyperactivated, the ability to withhold the next segment may be reduced, because the baseline firing rate is close to the threshold for release. In other words, the execution of speech may be 'running away',[6] with impaired volitional control and poor brakes.

It is very important to emphasize that the proposed models are hypotheses, and that their validity must be tested empirically. Hopefully detailed hypotheses will facilitate experimental research.

Summary

A hypothesis of cluttering

When reviewing research on the ACC and the SMA, it is striking how well the functions associated with these regions correspond to the various aspects of 'the cluttering syndrome'. The following is a summary of functions associated with the ACC/SMA:

(1) Drive, motivation, and initiation of action.
(2) Inhibition of impulses.
(3) Attention; monitoring and correction of behaviour.
(4) Planning of sequential behaviour.
(5) Selection of words and word-forms.
(6) Execution and timing of sequential behaviour.

This indicates that dysregulation of the ACC/SMA may account for the full range of symptoms of cluttering. In cases with more limited symptoms, the affected area may be smaller. For example, if the symptoms are limited to speech rate and articulation, without language errors or problems of attention, this would suggest involvement of the SMA proper.

Dysregulation of these cortical regions may be a secondary effect of dysregulation of the basal ganglia circuits, possibly resulting from genetic factors. The indication of genetic heritage in many cases of cluttering implies that cluttering is not typically associated with lesions. The symptoms, the pharmacological effects, and the EEG anomalies may be consistent with hyperactivation of the dopamine system, but this does certainly not exclude other possibilities.

A hypothetical mechanism that may account for the high speech rate is that segments in the speech sequence are initiated when the firing rate of relevant circuits reach a threshold. If the SMA is disinhibited and hyperactive, this threshold may be reached prematurely, resulting in 'runaway speech'.

Implications for treatment?

Medical treatment

Today there is no medical treatment that can be recommended. There is a need for continued research, including trials of dopaminergic drugs, genetic studies, and studies of EEG.[7]

Behavioural and cognitive treatment

This subject is discussed in detail in other chapters of this book. From a neurological point of view, the importance of detailed assessment can be emphasized. Because PWC differ in their profile of impairments and strengths, it may be essential to prepare an individual plan for treatment. Central aspects include awareness, motivation, attention, and the ability to control speech volitionally.

Another possibility for behavioural treatment may be technical aids, similar to hearing aids. The results from studies using delayed auditory feedback (DAF) in cluttering appear to be mixed (Langova & Moravek, 1964; Ward, 2006), with a need for further studies. Another possibility is to amplify the normal auditory feedback, in order to raise attention to the speech outcome.[8] The sound level may be a crucial factor in experiments with auditory feedback in cluttering. With future signal-processing capabilities, it may be possible to design a hearing-aid-type of device that measures the syllable rate and provide reminders to slow down (similar to an analogue device called the Hector Speech Aid in the 1970s; D. Ward, personal communication, September 10, 2009).

Difficulties in achieving a stable improvement may lead to the question of acceptance. Some neurological problems are very resistant to change. Therefore an important clinical task is to individually balance efforts to change versus acceptance.

Acknowledgements

The preparation of this chapter has been supported by grants from The Dominic Barker Trust, Ipswich, UK. I also want to thank Per Östberg and Joseph Donaher for valuable comments.

Notes

1 A syndrome can be defined as a group of symptoms that collectively indicate or characterize a disease, psychological disorder, or other abnormal condition. From Greek, syn-drom, 'running together'.

2 Based on this description of traits linked to cluttering, one might assume that cluttering also affects general intelligence, but this does not seem to be the case. On the contrary, in the literature individuals with cluttering surprisingly often are described as showing very high intelligence, with an aptitude for mathematics and science. For example, Daly (1993) wrote that based on observations, people with cluttering (PWC) are usually average or above average in intelligence, and many PWCs he worked with were exceptionally bright. It is possible these reports are influenced by selection from a university environment, but in any case, it seems that intelligence typically is not an issue in cluttering.

3 The *indirect pathway* in the basal ganglia has been assumed to provide the main inhibition of the frontal cortex. However, it has been suggested that a *hyperdirect*

pathway is more important in this role (Leblois, Boraud, Meissner, Bergman, & Hansel, 2006).

4 The verbal working memory may be viewed as a buffer for planned speech, in which the idea for an utterance is stored in preliminary form. Weiss (1964) claimed that the verbal thoughts of PWC tend to proceed by clusters of two or three words. If this is correct, it seems possible that limitation of the verbal working memory is a main underlying factor.

5 An important source of information has been overlooked in this review, but should be mentioned: the classic book *Speech and brain-mechanisms* by the neurosurgeons Wilder Penfield and Lamar Roberts, from 1959. They summarized systematic observations of the effects of electric stimulation of the brain in awake subjects during brain surgery, and the effects on speech of surgical removal of parts of the brain. They describe the existence of a third cortical speech centre ('the superior speech cortex'), located in the SMA and extending into the adjacent primary sensorimotor cortex. Removal of this region in the dominant hemisphere resulted in transient aphasia which, however, cleared up completely within a few weeks (Penfield & Roberts, 1959). This observation indicates that the medial cortex is necessary for speech production, but also that no essential linguistic information is stored here—the functions of the left SMA is soon compensated by the right SMA. This is consistent with the model proposed in this chapter: The primary linguistic networks are located in the lateral cortex, while the SMA has a main role in the sequencing of information retrieved from the lateral regions.

6 In Swedish, cluttering is called 'skenande tal', which might be translated as 'runaway speech'.

7 Magnetoencephalography (MEG) may be an especially interesting method for the study of the medial wall cortex, because MEG is sensitive to the cortex perpendicular to the skull.

8 If a throat microphone is used, the sounds from surrounding voices and noise are attenuated, which is important if using high amplification. For telephone calls it may be easy to amplify the signal from the telephone microphone to the earpiece.

References

Ackermann, H. (2008). Cerebellar contributions to speech production and speech perception: Psycholinguistic and neurobiological perspectives. *Trends in Neurosciences, 31*, 265–272.

Akkal, D., Dum, R. P., & Strick, P. L. (2007). Supplementary motor area and pre-supplementary motor area: Targets of basal ganglia and cerebellar output. *Journal of Neuroscience, 27*, 10659–10673.

Alario, F. X., Chainay, H., Lehericy, S., & Cohen, L. (2006). The role of the supplementary motor area (SMA) in word production. *Brain Research, 1076*, 129–143.

Alm, P. A. (2004). Stuttering and the basal ganglia circuits: A critical review of possible relations. *Journal of Communication Disorders, 37*, 325–369.

Alm, P. A. (2005). *On the causal mechanisms of stuttering*. Doctoral dissertation, Department of Clinical Neuroscience, Lund University, Sweden. http://theses.lub.lu.se/postgrad/

Alm, P. A. (2010). The dual premotor model of cluttering and stuttering: A neurological framework. In K. Bakker, L. Raphael, & F. Myers (Eds.), *Proceedings of the First World Conference on Cluttering, Katarino, Bulgaria, 2007* (pp. 207–210). http://associations.missouristate.edu/ICA

Baddeley, A. (2003). Working memory and language: An overview. *Journal of Communication Disorders*, *36*, 189–208.

Barbas, H., Ghashghaei, H., Dombrowski, S. M., & Rempel-Clower, N. L. (1999). Medial prefrontal cortices are unified by common connections with superior temporal cortices and distinguished by input from memory-related areas in the rhesus monkey. *Journal of Comparative Neurology*, *410*, 343–367.

Booth, J. R., Wood, L., Lu, D., Houk, J. C., & Bitan, T. (2007). The role of the basal ganglia and cerebellum in language processing. *Brain Research*, *1133*, 136–144.

Botvinick, M. M., Cohen, J. D., & Carter, C. S. (2004). Conflict monitoring and anterior cingulate cortex: An update. *Trends in Cognitive Sciences*, *8*, 539–546.

Bush, G., Frazier, J. A., Rauch, S. L., Seidman, L. J., Whalen, P. J., Jenike, M. A., et al. (1999). Anterior cingulate cortex dysfunction in attention-deficit/hyperactivity disorder revealed by fMRI and the Counting Stroop. *Biological Psychiatry*, *45*, 1542–1552.

Carreiras, M., Mechelli, A., & Price, C. J. (2006). Effect of word and syllable frequency on activation during lexical decision and reading aloud. *Human Brain Mapping*, *27*, 963–972.

Crosson, B., Benefield, H., Cato, M. A., Sadek, J. R., Moore, A. B., Wierenga, C. E., et al. (2003). Left and right basal ganglia and frontal activity during language generation: Contributions to lexical, semantic, and phonological processes. *Journal of the International Neuropsychological Society*, *9*, 1061–1077.

Crosson, B., Sadek, J. R., Maron, L., Gökçay, D., Mohr, C. M., Auerbach, E. J., et al. (2001). Relative shift in activity from medial to lateral frontal cortex during internally versus externally guided word generation. *Journal of Cognitive Neuroscience*, *13*, 272–283.

Daly, D. A. (1993). Cluttering, another fluency syndrome. In R. Curlee (Ed.), *Stuttering and related disorders of fluency* (pp. 179–204). New York: Thieme.

Daly, D. A. (1996). *The source for stuttering and cluttering*. East Moline, IL: LinguiSystems.

Daly, D. A., & St. Louis, K. O. (1998). Videotaping clutterers: How to do it—what to look for. In E. C. Healey & H. F. M. Peters (Eds.), *Proceedings of the 2nd World Congress on Fluency Disorders* (pp. 233–235). Nijmegen: Nijmegen University Press.

De Carli, D., Garreffa, G., Colonnese, C., Giulietti, G., Labruna, L., Briselli, E., et al. (2007). Identification of activated regions during a language task. *Magnetic Resonance Imaging*, *25*, 933–938.

Deecke, L., Kornhuber, H. H., Lang, W., Lang, M., & Schreiber, H. (1985). Timing function of the frontal cortex in sequential motor and learning tasks. *Human Neurobiology*, *4*, 143–154.

De Zegher, F., Van Den Berghe, G., Devlieger, H., Eggermont, E., & Veldhuis, J. D. (1993). Dopamine inhibits growth hormone and prolactin secretion in the human newborn. *Pediatric Research*, *34*, 642–645.

Drew, M. R., Simpson, E. H., Kellendonk, C., Herzberg, W. G., Lipatova, O., Fairhurst, S., et al. (2007). Transient overexpression of striatal D2 receptors impairs operant motivation and interval timing. *Journal of Neuroscience*, *27*, 7731–7739.

Faraone, S. V., Biederman, J., Morley, C. P., & Spencer, T. J. (2008). Effect of stimulants on height and weight: A review of the literature. *Journal of the American Academy of Child and Adolescent Psychiatry*, *47*, 994–1009.

Ferstl, E. C., & von Cramon, D. Y. (2002). What does the frontomedian cortex contribute to language processing: Coherence or theory of mind? *Neuroimage*, *17*, 1599–1612.

Gazzaniga, M. S., Ivry, R. B., & Mangun, G. R. (2009). *Cognitive neuroscience*. New York: WW Norton.

Geller, B., Zimerman, B., Williams, M., Delbello, M. P., Bolhofner, K., Craney, J. L., et al. (2002). DSM-IV mania symptoms in a prepubertal and early adolescent bipolar disorder phenotype compared to attention-deficit hyperactive and normal controls. *Journal of Child and Adolescent Psychopharmacology*, *12*, 11–25.

Gerloff, C., Corwell, B., Chen, R., Hallett, M., & Cohen, L. G. (1997). Stimulation over the human supplementary motor area interferes with the organization of future elements in complex motor sequences. *Brain*, *120*, 1587–1602.

Giros, B., Jaber, M., Jones, S. R., Wightman, R. M., & Caron, M. G. (1996). Hyperlocomotion and indifference to cocaine and amphetamine in mice lacking the dopamine transporter. *Nature*, *379*, 606–612.

Goldberg, G. (1985). Supplementary motor area structure and function. *The Behavioral and Brain Sciences*, *8*, 567–616.

Goldberg, G. (1992). Premotor systems, attention to action and behavioural choice. In J. K. Kien, C. R. McCrohan, & W. Winlow (Eds.), *Neurobiology of motor programme selection* (pp. 225–249). Oxford: Pergamon Press.

Grahn, J. A., Parkinson, J. A., & Owen, A. M. (2008). The cognitive functions of the caudate nucleus. *Progress in Neurobiology*, *86*, 141–155.

Guiot, G., Hertzog, E., Rondot, P., & Molina, P. (1961). Arrest or acceleration of speech evoked by thalamic stimulation in the course of stereotaxic procedures for Parkinsonism. *Brain*, *84*, 363–379.

Hays, P., & Field, L. L. (1989). Postulated genetic linkage between manic-depression and stuttering. *Journal of Affective Disorders*, *16*, 37–40.

Houk, J. C. (2005). Agents of the mind. *Biological Cybernetics*, *92*, 427–437.

Ivry, R. B., & Spencer, R. M. (2004). The neural representation of time. *Current Opinion in Neurobiology*, *14*, 225–232.

Johansen-Berg, H., Behrens, T. E., Robson, M. D., Drobnjak, I., Rushworth, M. F., Brady, J. M., et al. (2004). Changes in connectivity profiles define functionally distinct regions in human medial frontal cortex. *Proceedings of the National Academy of Sciences of the USA*, *101*, 13335–13340.

Jonas, S. (1981). The supplementary motor region and speech emission. *Journal of Communication Disorders*, *14*, 349–373.

Kaneda, M., & Osaka, N. (2008). Role of anterior cingulate cortex during semantic coding in verbal working memory. *Neuroscience Letters*, *436*, 57–61.

Kondo, H., Morishita, M., Osaka, N., Osaka, M., Fukuyama, H., & Shibasaki, H. (2004). Functional roles of the cingulo-frontal network in performance on working memory. *Neuroimage*, *21*, 2–14.

Koprich, J. B., Johnston, T. H., Huot, P., Fox, S. H., & Brotchie, J. M. (2009). New insights into the organization of the basal ganglia. *Current Neurology and Neuroscience Reports*, *9*, 298–304.

Lan, J., Song, M., Pan, C., Zhuang, G., Wang, Y., Ma, W., et al. (2009). Association between dopaminergic genes (SLC6A3 and DRD2) and stuttering among Han Chinese. *Journal of Human Genetics*, *54*, 457–460.

Langova, J., & Moravek, M. (1964). Some results of experimental examinations among stutterers and clutterers. *Folia Phoniatrica, 162,* 290–296.

Langova, J., & Moravek, M. (1970). Some problems of cluttering. *Folia Phoniatrica*, *22*, 325–336.

Lebedev, M. A., O'Doherty, J. E., & Nicolelis, M. A. (2008). Decoding of temporal intervals from cortical ensemble activity. *Journal of Neurophysiology*, *99*, 166–186.

Leblois, A., Boraud, T., Meissner, W., Bergman, H., & Hansel, D. (2006). Competition between feedback loops underlies normal and pathological dynamics in the basal ganglia. *Journal of Neuroscience*, *26*, 3567–3583.

Lebrun, Y. (1996). Cluttering after brain damage. *Journal of Fluency Disorders*, *21*, 289–295.

Lee, I. H., & Assad, J. A. (2003). Putaminal activity for simple reactions or self-timed movements. *Journal of Neurophysiology*, *89*, 2528–2537.

Levelt, W. J. M. (1999). Models of word production. *Trends in Cognitive Sciences*, *3*, 223–232.

Longe, O., Senior, C., & Rippon, G. (2009). The lateral and ventromedial prefrontal cortex work as a dynamic integrated system: Evidence from FMRI connectivity analysis. *Journal of Cognitive Neuroscience*, *21*, 141–154.

Loose, R., Kaufmann, C., Auer, D. P., & Lange, K. W. (2003). Human prefrontal and sensory cortical activity during divided attention tasks. *Human Brain Mapping*, *18*, 249–259.

Luchsinger, R., & Arnold, G. E. (1965). *Voice–speech–language. Clinical communicology: Its physiology and pathology*. Belmont, CA: Wadsworth.

MacNeilage, P. F. (1998). The frame/content theory of evolution of speech production. *Behavioral and Brain Sciences*, *21*, 499–546.

McClure, S. M., Daw, N. D., & Montague, P. R. (2003). A computational substrate for incentive salience. *Trends in Neurosciences*, *26*, 423–428.

Meck, W. H., Penney, T. B., & Pouthas, V. (2008). Cortico-striatal representation of time in animals and humans. *Current Opinion in Neurobiology*, *18*, 145–152.

Meredith, C. W., Jaffe, C., Ang-Lee, K., & Saxon, A. J. (2005). Implications of chronic methamphetamine use: A literature review. *Harvard Review of Psychiatry*, *13*, 141–154.

Middleton, F. A., & Strick, P. L. (1996). The temporal lobe is a target of output from the basal ganglia. *Proceedings of the National Academy of Sciences of the USA*, *93*, 8683–8687.

Middleton, F. A., & Strick, P. L. (2000). Basal ganglia output and cognition: Evidence from anatomical, behavioral, and clinical studies. *Brain and Cognition*, *42*, 183–200.

Mink, J. W. (1996). The basal ganglia: Focused selection and inhibition of competing motor programs. *Progress in Neurobiology*, *50*, 381–425.

Möller, J., Jansma, B. M., Rodriguez-Fornells, A., & Münte, T. F. (2007). What the brain does before the tongue slips. *Cerebral Cortex*, *17*, 1173–1178.

Myers, F. L. (1992). Cluttering: A synergistic framework. In F. L. Myers & K. O. St. Louis (Eds.), *Cluttering: A clinical perspective* (pp. 71–84). Kibworth, UK: Far Communications.

Myers, F. L., & St. Louis, K. O. (1996). Cluttering: issues and controversies. In F. L. Myers & K. O. St. Louis (Eds.), *Cluttering: A clinical perspective* (pp. 11–22). San Diego: Singular Publishing.

Osaka, N., Osaka, M., Kondo, H., Morishita, M., Fukuyama, H., & Shibasaki, H. (2004). The neural basis of executive function in working memory: An fMRI study based on individual differences. *Neuroimage*, *21*, 623–631.

Passingham, R. E. (1987). Two cortical systems for directing movement. *Ciba Foundation Symposium*, *132*, 151–164.

Paus, T. (2001). Primate anterior cingulate cortex: Where motor control, drive and cognition interface. *Nature Reviews*, *2*, 417–424.

Paus, T., Petrides, M., Evans, A. C., & Meyer, E. (1993). Role of the human anterior cingulate cortex in the control of oculomotor, manual, and speech responses: A positron emission tomography study. *Journal of Neurophysiology*, *70*, 453–469.

Penfield, W., & Roberts, L. (1959). *Speech and brain-mechanisms*. Princeton, NJ: Princeton University Press.

Picard, N., & Strick, P. L. (1996). Motor areas of the medial wall: A review of their location and functional activation. *Cerbral Cortex*, *6*, 342–353.

Posner, M. I., Rothbart, M. K., Sheese, B. E., & Tang, Y. (2007). The anterior cingulate gyrus and the mechanism of self-regulation. *Cognitive, Affective & Behavioral Neuroscience*, *7*, 391–395.

Postma, A., & Kolk, H. (1993). The covert repair hypothesis: Prearticulatory repair processes in normal and stuttered disfluencies. *Journal of Speech and Hearing Research*, *36*, 472–487.

Preus, A. (1996). Cluttering and stuttering: Related, different, or antagonistic disorders? In F. L. Myers & K. O. St. Louis (Eds.), *Cluttering: A clinical perspective* (pp. 55–70). San Diego: Singular Publishing.

Ridderinkhof, K. R., Ullsperger, M., Crone, E. A., & Nieuwenhuis, S. (2004). The role of the medial frontal cortex in cognitive control. *Science*, *306*, 443–447.

Sahin, N. T., Pinker, S., & Halgren, E. (2006). Abstract grammatical processing of nouns and verbs in Broca's area: Evidence from fMRI. *Cortex*, *42*, 540–562.

Sarter, M., Gehring, W. J., & Kozak, R. (2006). More attention must be paid: The neurobiology of attentional effort. *Brain Research Reviews*, *51*, 145–160.

Savelieva, K. V., Caudle, W. M., Findlay, G. S., Caron, M. G., & Miller, G. W. (2002). Decreased ethanol preference and consumption in dopamine transporter female knock-out mice. *Alcoholism, Clinical and Experimental Research*, *26*, 758–764.

Schultz, W. (2007). Multiple dopamine functions at different time courses. *Annual Review of Neuroscience*, *30*, 259–288.

Seeman, M. (1970). Relations between motorics of speech and general motor ability in clutterers. *Folia Phoniatrica (Basel)*, *22*, 376–380.

Shibasaki, H., & Hallett, M. (2006). What is the Bereitschaftspotential? *Clinical Neurophysiology*, *117*, 2341–2356.

Snyder, G. (2004). *Exploratory research in the role of cognitive initiation in the enhanced fluency phenomenon*. Unpublished doctoral thesis, East Carolina University, Greenville, NC.

Snyder, G. J., Hough, M. S., Blanchet, P., Ivy, L. J., & Waddell, D. (2009). The effects of self-generated synchronous and asynchronous visual speech feedback on overt stuttering frequency. *Journal of Communication Disorders*, *42*, 235–244.

Solanto, M. V. (2002). Dopamine dysfunction in AD/HD: Integrating clinical and basic neuroscience research. *Behavioural Brain Research*, *130*, 65–71.

Suzuki, T., Itoh, S., Hayashi, M., Kouno, M., & Takeda, K. (2009). Hyperlexia and ambient echolalia in a case of cerebral infarction of the left anterior cingulate cortex and corpus callosum. *Neurocase*, *15*, 384–389.

Talairach, J., & Tournoux, P. (1988). *Co-planar stereotaxic atlas of the human brain*. New York: Thieme.

Teichmann, M., Gaura, V., Démonet, J. F., Supiot, F., Delliaux, M., Verny, C., et al. (2008). Language processing within the striatum: Evidence from a PET correlation study in Huntington's disease. *Brain*, *131*, 1046–1056.

Tremblay, P., & Gracco, V. L. (2006). Contribution of the frontal lobe to externally and internally specified verbal responses: fMRI evidence. *Neuroimage*, *33*, 947–957.

Tremblay, P., & Gracco, V. L. (2010). On the selection of words and oral motor responses: Evidence of a response-independent fronto-parietal network. *Cortex*, *46*, 15–28.

van Zaalen, Y., Ward, D., Nederveen, A. J., Grolman, W., Wijnen, F., & DeJonckere, P. (2009). *Cluttering & stuttering: Different disorders. A neuro-imaging study*. Unpublished manuscript.

Warburton, E., Wise, R. J., Price, C. J., Weiller, C., Hadar, U., Ramsay, S., et al. (1996). Noun and verb retrieval by normal subjects: Studies with PET. *Brain*, *119*, 159–179.

Ward, D. (2006). *Stuttering and cluttering: Frameworks for understanding and treatment*. Hove, UK: Psychology Press.

Weiss, D. A. (1964). *Cluttering*. Englewood Cliffs, NJ: Prentice-Hall.

Yücel, M., Wood, S. J., Fornito, A., Riffkin, J., Velakoulis, D., & Pantelis, C. (2003). Anterior cingulate dysfunction: Implications for psychiatric disorders? *Journal of Psychiatry and Neuroscience*, *28*, 350–354.

2 Possible genetic factors in cluttering

Dennis Drayna

Genetic factors are known to play a role in a number of speech disorders, including dyspraxia and stuttering (Andrews, Morris-Yates, Howie, & Martin, 1991; Felsenfeld et al., 2000; Howie, 1981; Lai, Fisher, Hurst, Vargha-Khadem, & Monaco, 2001; MacDermot et al., 2005). Although no clear data supporting such genetic contributions to cluttering have been published, it is reasonable to hypothesize that genetic factors play a role in this disorder as well. Proof of the existence of such factors will require several types of studies.

First, the basic epidemiology of cluttering is not currently well understood. This has partly been due to differences in the precise clinical criteria used for diagnosis of the disorder. A broadly applicable and widely accepted set of diagnostic criteria will enable estimates of the incidence and prevalence of cluttering (see St. Louis & Schulte, chapter 14 this volume; Ward, chapter 15 this volume). They will also allow estimates of familial recurrence rates, which often provide the first hints of a genetic etiology for a disorder. Another hurdle in our understanding of cluttering epidemiology is the fact that cluttering can co-occur with other speech disorders (see Scaler Scott, chapter 8 this volume; Van Borsel, chapter 6 this volume; Van Zaalen, Wijnen, & Dejonckere, chapter 7 this volume), which injects additional complexity into this task. Clear differentiation of syndromic and non-syndromic presentations of cluttering will be an important starting point for a better understanding of the distribution of this disorder. At this time, what can be said is that cluttering does not appear to be an especially common disorder, and is probably less frequent than stuttering (but see also its heightened occurrence in a small sample of children with Asperger's disorder in Scaler Scott, chapter 8 this volume).

A classical method for distinguishing genetic from non-genetic contributions to a trait is a twin study. There are a number of different twin study designs, but the most common is a comparison of monozygotic (MZ, identical) twin pairs with dizygotic (DZ, fraternal) twin pairs raised together. Such twins share most of their childhood environment, and thus differences between the MZ and DZ groups are likely to arise primarily from differences in genes, or from stochastic factors, including developmental differences. In these studies, the co-occurrence of a trait (such as cluttering) in MZ twin pairs is compared with the rate of co-occurrence in DZ twin pairs. In large sample sizes that tend to average out the contribution of individual stochastic factors, any greater concordance in MZ pairs compared with DZ pairs is evidence for genetic factors in the trait. At this time, no twin studies on cluttering have been published.

While the analysis of twin data is a highly specialized undertaking (Neal & Cardon, 1992; Spector, Sneider, & MacGregor, 2000), a simple example is informative. Let us assume a trait is 100 percent due to a single genetic variant. Because MZ twins share all of their genes, the likelihood that MZ twins will both have the trait (i.e., the MZ concordance rate for this trait) will be 100 percent. In contrast, the concordance rate for this trait in DZ twins, which on average share half their genes, will be 50 percent. Now consider a trait that is 100 percent due to environmental factors during childhood. Such factors could include diet, interactions with siblings and parents, school environment, or even conceivably such things as climate. For such a trait, MZ twins raised together will have a concordance rate of 100 percent, and DZ twins reared together will also have a concordance rate of 100 percent.

While such differences in the MZ versus DZ concordance rates provide a simple estimate of genetic contributions to a trait, a number of sophisticated analytical methods allow partitioning of contributions from shared genes, shared environment, unique environment, and measurement error plus stochastic factors. The final product of such studies is a measure of heritability of the trait, designated h^2, which is the fraction of the variance in a trait (such as speech fluency) that is attributable to shared genes in twin pairs. Heritability values range from 0 to 1, with values <0.3 considered to represent low heritability, values from 0.3 to 0.6 considered moderate heritability, and values above 0.6 representing high heritability. For example, numerous twin studies have produced heritability estimates for stuttering in the range of 0.4–0.7, indicating that this disorder is moderately to highly heritable.

The difficulty with twin studies is that they require a large number of twins pairs in which at least one twin has the trait in question. For a disorder as common as stuttering, finding these is not an especially difficult task. For rare disorders, however, it can be impossible to find sufficient numbers of affected individuals who have a twin. The suspected frequency of cluttering (especially pure cluttering with no concomitant stuttering) suggests that it may be difficult to perform twin studies with high statistical power. However, other study designs have been developed to estimate the heritability of traits.

One such study is an adoption study. These studies typically compare the co-occurrence of traits between parents and their biological versus their adopted children. These studies tend to control for environment, because both biological and adopted children often share the same household during childhood. Higher similarity between parents and their biological children than between parents and their adopted children indicates genetic rather than environmental causes of a trait. Ideally adoption studies also include the biological parents of the adopted children, but because adoption records in the United States have typically been closed, this has not been feasible for large-scale studies. However, several Scandinavian countries have open adoption records, and adoption studies in these countries have a long history of success.

A third method of estimating heritability is by studying the families of individuals who have been identified with a disorder. If a trait is completely genetic, its co-occurrence in family members will be determined by the amount of shared genes between the family members. For example, in the case of a completely genetic trait that is due to a simple single-gene dominant mutation, individuals who share half their genes, such as siblings, will on average share the trait half the time. In contrast, a trait that is completely due to childhood environmental factors will be typically shared by siblings 100 percent of the time. Given the current state of our understanding of cluttering, it appears likely that such family studies may be the most useful for estimating the heritability of this disorder.

It is not possible to predict the heritability of cluttering at this time, because no data that bear on this question have been published. If, however, this disorder is shown to have a high heritability, it does not necessarily mean it will be a simple task to ultimately identify the specific genetic variants involved. In theory, a highly heritable trait could be due to one genetic variant that causes 100 percent of the disorder, or to 100 different genetic variants, each of which constitutes 1 percent of the disorder. In the former case, identification of the causative genetic variant will likely be straightforward with today's technologies. In the latter case, today's technologies may be insufficient to identify any of the 100 causative variants. However, past experience with dyspraxia and stuttering have shown that the situation may be intermediate to the above two extremes. In both these disorders, one genetic variant with a large contribution to the disorder in one or a few families has been observed (Lai et al., 2001), while other causative variants may be rare and cause the disorder in a sporadic fashion (MacDermot et al., 2005; Viswanath, Lee, & Chakraborty, 2004).

In the case of a single genetic variant that plays a major causative role in one or a number of families, the path to identification of genes that cause the disorder is well established. Such efforts traditionally begin with a linkage study performed in families. Linkage studies seek to identify genetic markers, at known chromosomal locations, that are co-inherited (i.e. linked) with the disorder. Such co-inheritance occurs because the markers and the causative genetic variant reside adjacent to each other on the same chromosome. A linkage study typically employs one or more families representing tens to hundreds of individuals, with several hundred to several thousand genetic markers tested in each individual. Because the genetic markers used in linkage studies all reside at known chromosomal locations, once linkage is observed, the approximate location of the causative gene is known. Then, using the Human Genome Sequence (http://www.ncbi.nlm.nih.gov/genome/guide/human/index.shtml) as a reference guide, all of the genes in that region can be determined. These candidate genes can then be sequenced in affected and unaffected individuals, with the goal of identifying a genetic variant that occurs only in affected family members and not in unaffected family members. For this method, it can be seen that the ability to identify genes causing cluttering will depend on the existence of, and participation by, families in which cluttering occurs. At this time, it is not known how frequent such families are, how large they are, and how easily they can be enrolled in genetic research studies.

In the case where many different genetic variants cause a disorder, another type of study has also been used. This study is known as an association study. Association studies are population-based, rather than family-based, and typically enrol large numbers (from hundreds to thousands) of affected cases and a similar number of population-matched normal controls. A very large number of genetic markers, from hundreds of thousands to more than a million, are measured in each of these individuals, with the goal of finding one or more markers that occur more frequently in cases than in controls. Given sufficient numbers of cases and controls, such association studies are capable of identifying genetic variants that account for very small fractions of the disorder, down to a few percent. However, such studies suffer from several weaknesses. First, they require large subject populations. It is not clear that cluttering is sufficiently common or sufficiently easily identified to produce the required number of subjects. Second, association studies are not useful for identifying variants that are due to newly arising mutations in the population. If cluttering is indeed genetic, it is not clear how much is due to *de novo* mutations and how much is due to mutations that have existed in the population for a long period of time.

Overall, genetic methods are generating exciting results in speech and language disorders, and they hold the possibility of providing a new level of understanding of these disorders at the cellular and molecular level. Virtually all human disorders have a non-zero heritability, and it's reasonable to assume that cluttering will indeed have some genetic component. Proving this and estimating the magnitude of the heritability of this disorder are currently the tasks that need to be done. If substantial heritability is found, studies to identify the causative genetic variants can proceed.

References

Andrews, G., Morris-Yates, A., Howie, P., & Martin, N. (1991). Genetic factors in stuttering confirmed. *Archives of General Psychiatry*, *48*, 1034–1035.

Felsenfeld, S., Kirk, K., Zhu, G., Statham, D., Neale, M., & Martin, N. (2000). A study of the genetic environmental etiology of stuttering in a selected twin sample. *Behavioral Genetics*, *30*, 359–366.

Howie, P. (1981). Concordance for stuttering in monozygotic and dizygotic twin pairs. *Journal of Speech and Hearing Research*, *24*, 317–321.

Lai, C. S., Fisher, S. E., Hurst, J. A., Vargha-Khadem, F., & Monaco, A. P. (2001). A forkhead-domain gene is mutated in a severe speech and language disorder. *Nature*, *413*(6855), 519–523.

MacDermot, K. D., Bonora, E., Sykes, N., Coupe, A. M., Lai, C. S., Vernes, S. C., et al. (2005). Identification of FOXP2 truncation as a novel cause of developmental speech and language deficits. *American Journal of Human Genetics*, *76*, 1074–1080.

Neale, M., & Cardon, L. (1992). *Methodology for genetic studies of twins and families*. Dordrecht: Kluwer.

Spector, T., Snieder, H., & MacGregor, A. (2000). *Advances in twin and sib-pair analysis*. London: Greenwich Medical Media.

Viswanath, N., Lee, H., & Chakraborty, R. (2004). Evidence for a major gene influence on persistent developmental stuttering. *Human Biology*, *76*, 401–412.

3 Motor speech control and cluttering

David Ward

Introduction

A recurring theme throughout this book concerns the not inconsiderable difficulty in deciding exactly what cluttering is. Particularly, arriving at a definition that is suitably succinct, but that captures the breadth of the core symptoms and how these might be expressed, remains problematic. Weiss (1964) famously considered cluttering to be just one facet of a bigger syndrome, affecting attention and memory as well speech and language functions. It was, he argued, the verbal manifestation of a 'central language imbalance'. Despite the wide range of speech and non-speech phenomena that Weiss associated with the disorder, one consistently observed feature is that speech output in cluttering appears to be motorically disrupted. Since this, a number of definitions have been proposed, most recently St. Louis and Schulte's lowest common denominator model (St. Louis & Shulte, chapter 14 this volume), yet through the differences of opinion that have persisted in the intervening 45 years, there has been common agreement that cluttering is expressed by an output that sounds motorically disrupted. The key features of inconsistent pacing (and usually fast sounding) speech output, short inappropriately placed pauses, and over co-articulation, all implicate motor speech processing in some shape or form (Daly & Cantrell, 2006; St. Louis & Shulte, chapter 14 this volume; Ward, 2006).

In addition, researchers have commented on the fact that cluttered speech may also show similar problems to other disorders that are acknowledged to be motoric in nature. The limited articulatory range, over co-articulation and increased speech rate seen in Parkinson's speech is often observed in cluttering (Dalton & Hardcastle, 1989, St. Louis & Schulte, chapter 14 this volume; Van Zaalen, Wijnen, & Dejonckere, 2009; Ward, 2006) and the mumbled and indistinct speech output commonly expressed in both disorders may also be subject to festinance (Wohl, 1970). These similarities may seem all the more pertinent when considering that Parkinsonism is related to abnormal levels of dopamine—something that has been considered as possibly related to cluttering (Alm, 2010), as well as stuttering (Alm, 2004; Brady, 1998; Wu et al., 1997). The phoneme and syllable sequencing errors also sometimes seen in cluttering may bear resemblance to those seen in dyspraxic speech. It should not be surprising, then, that cluttering has been likened to both of these disorders (De Hirsch, 1961). Cluttering and stuttering frequently co-occur (Daly, 1993; Myers, 1992; Preus, 1981; St. Louis, Myers, Raphael, & Bakker, 2007; Ward, 2006). The cause(s) of stuttering currently remains obscure, but while the disorder certainly presents as motorically disrupted sound, this is very different from saying that stuttering can be defined as a disorder of motor speech control. Given that the core characteristics of cluttering appear to reflect difficulties with motor control programming and/or execution, it is perhaps surprising that there is remarkably little in the way of controlled studies to demonstrate that those who clutter perform more poorly on tests of motor speech control than those who do not. We will firstly review the little evidence that exists.

Acoustic studies

A number of acoustic parameters have been studied in attempts to identify significant differences between normal and disordered speech. With regard to stuttering, for example, the literature is extensive, and in particular, voice onset time (VOT), voice initiation time (VIT), vowel duration time (VDT), and formant transition time (FTT) have received considerable attention. Fluent and well-coordinated speech is considered to correlate with reduced variability across repetitions of these acoustic phenomena. While some studies found no significant differences between those who stutter and control speakers, generally, findings have demonstrated that those who stutter demonstrate either: (1) longer VOT, VIT, FTT, and extended VDT or (2) greater variability in the windows of change associated with these acoustic events (for a recent review, see Ward, 2006). One possibility is that these findings might simply represent side effects of the fact that those who stutter, on average, speak with a slower than normal speech rate, where, of course, the reverse applies to those who clutter. In stark contrast with findings in stuttering, the literature with regard to the cluttering population is scarce. Recently, Hartinger and Pape (2003) compared VOT and VDT between three adults with cluttering (AWC) and three control speakers. Subjects were asked to repeat consonant (/p/t/k/) + vowel (/a/) syllable strings sequences as fast and as intelligibly as possible over a 10-second time frame. VOTs of two of the three AWCs were found to be longer than those of the controls, a finding that might initially appear counter-intuitive given that increased articulatory speed correlates with reduced VOT. When analysed, however, the consonant vowel (CV) repetition rate of the AWC group was found to be similar to that of the control group, and not quicker, as had been predicted. This finding is consistent with an increasing number of reports that show that, while overall cluttering may be associated with accelerated speech, much of what is considered to be cluttered is actually associated with an output that is perceived by the listener to be fast (or, more accurately, perceived as too fast for that particular speaker) rather than genuinely being fast (again, see St. Louis & Schulte, chapter 14 this volume, for a discussion of this in relation to diagnosis of cluttering). The small subject numbers in this study make interpretation very difficult, but Hartinger and Pape speculate that the AWC were able to focus attention on the task, and reduce their articulatory rate in order to maintain intelligibility. In a similar study, Ward and Bush (2010) compared VOT and VDT between a group of five people who cluttered but did not stutter, a similarly matched group of adults who stuttered (AWS) and control speakers. In contrast to the Hartinger and Pape (2003) study, data were elicited from subjects' reading of a short story, with VOT analyzed from specific /t/ + vowel sequences retrieved from the text. Groups did not differ when analyzed for speech rate, but as a group, the AWC produced significantly shorter VOT times ($p < 0.01$) than either the adults who stuttered, or the control speakers. No significant differences were found between the groups for VDT. Again, numbers are small, but findings may reflect a difference in the task that the groups undertook—suggesting that motor speech control may be more subject to breakdown when vocalizations are more 'meaningful' or, more linguistically based, a finding that has also been observed in the literature on stuttering. Hartinger and Moosehammer (2008) also consider this with reference to the kinematic analysis of cluttered speech (see below).

Kinematic studies of motor speech control

Once again, the literature on cluttering stands in contrast to that of stuttering when considering how coordinated speech movement control (speech kinematics) might be implicated in the disorder. There is currently only one study to date that has examined the physiological components of articulatory control in the speech of PWC. In an adjunct to Hartinger and Pape's (2003) acoustic study described above, Hartinger and Moosehammer (2008) used electromagnetic midsaggital articulography (EMA) to examine the spatial and temporal coordination between the tongue, lip, and jaw in the speech of three people who cluttered. As with the acoustic study, a CV repetition paradigm was used, but in addition, a further task where speakers were required to produce multisyllabic foreign loan words. No significant differences were recorded between the AWC and control groups for the CV repetition task, but the AWC group produced significantly higher coefficients of articulatory variability than the control group, both in temporal and spatial domains in the multisyllabic loan word production task. This difference was interpreted as reflecting specific problems with increasing linguistic complexity, rather than a more generalized inability to control spatial and temporal articulatory movement. As such, this would imply that cluttering may be perceived as a linguistically based disorder, in addition to comprising problems with a compromised motor control system. We should note, however, that although the authors made attempts to match the articulatory complexity of the loan words to the CV structures, further studies are needed to confirm whether those who clutter really do manage speech related tasks involving increased articulatory complexity with equal facility to similarly complex, but non-speech related, tasks.

Speech analysis

Recently, Van Zaalen, Wijnen, et al. (2009) compared the speech of 47 Dutch PWC and PWS with a large control group (N = 327) on a recently developed instrument designed to test word-level motor control (Screening Pittige Articulatie, SPA; for further details of this test, see Van Zaalen, Wijnen, & Dejonckere, chapter 9 this volume). Subjects were required to repeat complex multisyllabic words at a fast rate, and utterances were analyzed for three features: articulatory accuracy, smooth flow (comprising co-articulation and sequencing) and articulatory rate. PWC were found to produce significantly more smooth flow errors than the PWS and the control groups. Controls were also found to produce significantly fewer accuracy errors (p = .0001) than the PWC (Van Zaalen, Wijnen & Dejonckere, 2009).

Non speech motor control in cluttering

Researchers have commented on the apparent association between difficulties with motor control generally, and those specifically controlling motor speech among those who clutter. At a gross motor control level, there has been speculation that PWC may be more clumsy than their normally fluent peers (Daly, 1996), while fine motor skills such as those required when playing a musical instrument, and indeed, even a sense of musicality itself, have also been called into question (Daly, 1996; Daly & Burnett, 1999; Weiss, 1964). Yet again, though, corroborating scientific evidence is currently lacking. With regard to gross motor control, note that cluttering has also been associated with attention deficit hyperactivity disorder (ADHD) and developmental dyspraxia (St. Louis & Myers, 1997; Ward, 2006). It may be that tendencies toward disorders with increased levels of inattentiveness (Daly & Cantrell, 2006) might account for the sometimes observed clumsiness in younger children, rather than any disability related directly to cluttering.

To conclude this section: we speculate, on the basis of empirical observation and the admittedly limited evidence from motor speech studies, that: (1) cluttering appears to be associated with problems of motor speech control; (2) these problems may be more apparent with tasks that place increased demands on language processing; and (3) while problems in motor control outside the speech domain may well co-exist, at present we cannot causally link these to the disorder of cluttering. While identifying a motor control element is a useful start in understanding the disorder of cluttering, this in itself does not help us in determining the nature of that breakdown in the motor speech process. We now turn to this specific question.

The nature of motor speech processing in cluttering

Feedback, speech motor control, and the role of speech processing in cluttering

Traditionally, there have been two schools of thought as to the role of feedback in speech motor control, and feedback in various forms is important to us in any conceptualization of cluttering. Some researchers believe that afferent feedback is unimportant, and that speech is under open loop control. Others argue that, to the contrary, motor movement is continuously controlled by feedback (thus maintaining a closed loop feedback system). There is evidence for this latter view from experiments where speakers have been found to recover articulatory control following the sudden and unexpected introduction of an obstacle to articulatory movement such as a bite block (Gracco & Abbs, 1986). Van der Merwe (2008) points out the current consensus is that both open and closed loop control methods are used, but in a flexible and cooperative manner. Thus feedback is used, but it seems that it can also be switched off when required.

A speech processing model for cluttering

It has been commonly accepted that a speech processing chain is responsible for the conversion of intention and idea into language symbols, and ultimately the acoustic end-product that may be understood by the listener. Within a traditional three-stage model, motor speech planning, programming and execution are seen as representing separate stages in the processing chain. These in turn can be associated with neurological correlates that reflect central and more peripheral processing aspects of speech production. The highest level within this model has also been seen to potentially include some aspects of phonological planning: for example, the notion that problems with phonological sequencing or selection may be responsible for sound substitutions rather than this being a problem of motor speech planning *per se*, and as such, a problem of phonological nature. Under this model, specific speech disorders have been seen to map onto these various levels. The classification of these disorders is significant for us in our study of motor speech control in cluttering for reasons outlined earlier in this chapter, and will again be made apparent, below.

Aquired apraxia of speech (though admittedly still a controversial diagnosis) is generally considered to be associated with problems with speech planning, and implicates cortical structures (Darley, 1980; Duffy, 1995). The issue as to whether the disorder might actually be phonological in nature is consistent with the conceptualization of phonological planning being implicated within the speech planning level. But certain aspects of apraxia, such as the effortful groping for articulatory accuracy commonly reported, may more accurately be explained as a failure of programming, rather than one of planning. Dysarthria, on the other hand, has traditionally been seen to fit under the 'execution' stage of the model, and as a disorder associated with more peripheral processing problems, relating to muscle weakness or incoordination. Yet there are problems with this single-level diagnosis; for example, hypokinetic disarthrias, which implicate subcortical structures of the basal ganglia, might be considered to fall under a programming-level problem as well as execution. A further problem, as Van der Merwe (2008) points out, is that the three-stage model fails to leave room to explain disorders such as cluttering and, for that matter also stuttering, where aetiology is as yet to be confirmed, and where at present a level of motor speech breakdown is currently not identified. Van der Merwe (2008) therefore proposes a four-stage model: (1) to better deal with the potential for multilevel processing explanations of neurological disorders such as apraxia and dysarthria and (2) to allow a more flexible interpretation of speech processing breakdown in disorders such as cluttering and stuttering (where there is less clarity as to the level of breakdown). This four-stage model differs from the three-stage approach mostly in disassociating linguistic and syntactic planning from the final three stages of planning, programming, and execution (see Table 3.1).

All this is of considerable relevance for our study of motor speech aspects of cluttering. As mentioned earlier, cluttering may exhibit a range of characteristics, some of which are core to both dysarthria and apraxia of speech. Under the four-stage model, we can identify potential areas of breakdown at a number of levels.

Linguistic planning level

As mentioned at the start of this chapter, there is very strong agreement among experts that cluttering is characterized by speech that is motorically disrupted, in terms of speech rate, rhythm, and articulation. A number of writers have also commented on the fact that cluttered speech is commonly expressed by disruptions in language output, with errors noted at pragmatic, syntactic, lexical, and phonological levels (Daly, 1996; St. Louis, 1998; Van Zaalen, Wijnen, et al., 2009; Ward, 2004, 2006, 2010). While few would deny a strong association between linguistic and motor determinants in cluttering, there is less of a consensus as to whether language components should be regarded as central to a diagnosis. Some have suggested that speech motor problems might be ultimately responsible for the linguistic errors made in

Table 3.1 Summary of Van der Merwe's (2008) four-level model of speech processing. At first sight this model implies a simple hierarchical structure, but feedback loops allow transmission of processing to be referred to earlier levels

Level of processing	*Primary neurological substrates involved*	*Processing outcome*
1 Linguistic planning	Various	Semantic, syntactic, and phonological specifications for speech production
2 Motor planning	Pre-frontal cortex, Broca's area, Wernicke's area (temporal and parietal lobes)	Identifies overall motor goal, generates overall invariant motor plan
3 Motor programming	Supplementary motor area (SMA), sensori motor cortex (SMC), lateral cerebellum, putamen of basal ganglia	Produces programming algorithms that convert invariant motor plan into motor programmes (including specifications for articulatory goals, such as place and manner of articulation)
4 Motor execution	Motor cortex, thalamus, motor units	Actuation/realization of the speech motor programmes, resulting in the acoustic end-product

cluttered speech; however, the reverse might also be true, with faulty phonological and syntactic aspects of processing existing in their own right, and perhaps even being responsible for, or contributing to, the speech errors seen in cluttering (see Van Zaalen, Wijnen, et al., 2009). It is reasonable to speculate that syntactic and phonological cluttering-related errors may be a result of processing at this level.

Motor planning level

The apraxic-like errors sometimes seen in cluttered speech may reflect breakdown at this level. Unlike apraxia of speech (AOS), however, cluttering is associated with normal or elevated speech rates. Observable, also, is the fact that while inconsistent speech-level errors can be characteristic of cluttering, the effortful articulatory groping characteristic of speech planning difficulties seen in AOS is not observed in cluttering. Sound distortions, on the other hand, are common to both disorders and suggestive of difficulties with the synchronization of articulator sequencing and serial ordering of speech events in cluttering.

Speech planning level

It seems intuitive that cluttering involves a problem in converting a speech motor plan into specific goal-directed behaviour. A breakdown in speech motor programming would be consistent with the evidence that cluttered speech gestures are achieved with less precision than that of control speakers, at least in more linguistically relevant speech sequences (Hartinger & Pape, 2003; Hartinger & Moosehammer, 2008; Van Zaalen, Wijnen, et al., 2009; Ward & Bush, 2010).

Consistent with the outlining of the neurological functioning implicated at this level (see Table 3.1), researchers have speculated that deficiencies in subcortical processing may be at the core of cluttering (Alm, 2010). There is now preliminary evidence to show that the putamen is implicated in the disorder (Van Zaalen, Ward et al., 2009). Disruptions to this subcortical structure are typically associated with difficulties with the inhibition of inappropriate motor activity. It could follow then, that for the person who clutters, loss of inhibitory processes may result in problems with constraining the appropriate specifications for the articulatory programmes. Indeed, this might also be seen as consistent with PWCs' often-reported difficulties in inhibiting racing and sometimes competing thoughts (on this subject also see Alm, chapter 1 this volume).

Motor execution level

As already mentioned, some have commented that cluttered speech may present as dysarthric (Dalton & Hardcastle, 1989; Ward, 2006; Weiss, 1964), with an output characterized by Dalton and Hardcastle as 'over co-articulation'. It is also true that dysarthria can be seen as an execution-level effect. For example, a lower motor neuron (or flaccid) dysarthria implicates the execution of the motor programmes due to a failure of innervation to the motor end plates. In other words, the poor articulation ultimately comes about due to muscle weakness (Duffy, 2005). The situation is, of course, very different in cluttering, where there is no known neurological weakness. Rather, any dysarthic element is likely to more closely resemble that of the hypokinetic dysarthria seen in Parkinsonism, complete with increased speech rate and indistinct articulation. This is not related to damage to the more peripheral lower motor neuron system but to a decrease of dopamine levels as a result of the death of cells that produce this neurotransmitter in the substantia nigra. Again, this would be consistent with the involvement of subcortical structures in cluttering (see Van Zaalen, Ward, et al., 2009).

Summary

Disorders of motor speech where the affected neurological systems have been identified, such as the dysarthrias and apraxia, have generally been thought of as resulting from damage to a single level in the speech processing chain, although van der Merwe's conceptualization challenges this supposition, in the case of some dysarthrias. Cluttering can be described as a disorder of motor speech where multiple levels of processing may be affected, ranging from motor planning all the way to execution. The scope of the processes potentially affected serves to highlight the complexity of the disorder, and reflects the diverse expression of the motor speech disruptions inherent in cluttering.

Conclusion

While the cause(s) of cluttering currently remain obscure, it remains a disorder whose output may be described in terms of a loss of motor speech control. It is proposed that cluttering involves a breakdown in motor speech control that may potentially be seen across a range of processing levels involving planning, programming, and execution. Clearly, further studies are needed to test, more explicitly, the processes that are failing when cluttered speech results, but the limited number of acoustic and kinematic studies support the notion that speech motor control may indeed be compromised. Further, this deficiency in motor speech control needs to be interpreted within the context of language processing systems, as it may have some primacy in the expression of communicative output, and be mediated by language processing variables. At present, the nature of the relationship between motor speech processing and language processing models remains unclear. Further research is needed to verify the nature of any such potential relationships.

References

Alm, P. A. (2004). Stuttering and the basal ganglia circuits: A critical review of possible relations. *Journal of Communication Disorders*, *37*, 325–369.

Alm, P. A. (2010). The dual premotor model of cluttering and stuttering: A neurological framework. In K. Bakker, L. Raphael, & F. Myers (Eds.), *Proceedings of the First World Conference on Cluttering, Katarino, Bulgaria* (pp. 207–210). http://associations.missouristate.edu/ICA

Brady, J. P. (1998). Drug induced stammering: A review of the literature. *Journal of Clinical Psychopharmacology*, *18*, 50–54.

Dalton, P., & Hardcastle, W. (1989). *Disorders of fluency and their effects on communication.* London: Elsevier, North-Holland.

Daly, D. A. (1993). Cluttering: Another fluency syndrome. In R. Curlee (Ed.), *Stuttering and related disorders of fluency* (pp. 6–8). New York: Thieme.

Daly, D. A. (1996). *The source for stuttering and cluttering*, East Moline, IL: LinguiSystems.

Daly, D. A., & Burnett, M. L. (1999). Cluttering: Traditional view and new perspectives.

In R. F. Curlee (Ed.), *Stuttering and related disorders of fluency* (2nd ed.). New York: Thieme.

Daly, D., & Cantrell, R. (2006). *Cluttering: Characteristics identified as diagnostically significant by 60 fluency experts*. Paper presented at the 6th World Congress on Disorders of Fluency, Dublin, Ireland.

Darley, F. L. (1980). *Aphasia*. New York: Saunders.

De Hirsch, K. (1961). Studies in tachyphemia: 4. Diagnosis of developmental language. *Logos, 4*, 3–9.

Duffy, J. (1995). *Motor speech disorders; substrates, differential diagnosis and management*. St. Louis: Moseby.

Duffy, J. (2005). *Motor speech disorders*. St Louis, MO: Mosby Elsevier.

Gracco, V., & Abbs, J. (1986). Variant and invariant characteristics of speech movement. *Experimental Brain Research, 65*, 156–166.

Hartinger, M., & Moosehammer, C. (2008). Articulatory variability and cluttering. *Folia Phoniatrica, 60*, 64–72.

Hartinger, M., & Pape, D. (2003). An articulatory and acoustic study of cluttering. *Proceedings of the 15th International Conference on Phonetic Sciences* (pp. 3245–3248), Barcelona.

Myers, F. L. (1992). Cluttering: A synergistic framework. In F. L. Myers & K. O. St. Louis (Eds.). *Cluttering: A clinical perspective* (pp. 71–84). Kibworth, UK: Far Communications. (Reissued in 1996 by Singular, San Diego, CA.)

Preus, A. (1981). *Identifying subgroups of stutterers*. Oslo: Universitetsforlaget.

St. Louis, K. O. (1998). Linguistic and motor aspects of cluttering symptoms. In E. C. Healey & H. F. M. Peters (Eds.), *Proceedings of the 2nd World Congress on Fluency Disorders* (pp. 40–43). Nijmegen: Nijmegen University Press.

St. Louis, K. O., & Myers, F. L. (1997). Management of cluttering and related fluency disorders. In R. F. Curlee & G. M. Siegal (Eds.), *Nature and treatment of stuttering: New directions* (pp. 312–332). Boston, MA: Allyn & Bacon.

St. Louis, K. O., Myers, F. L., Raphael, L. J., & Bakker, K. (2007). Understanding and treating of cluttering. In R. F. Curlee & E. G. Conture (Eds.), *Stuttering and related disorders of fluency* (3rd ed., pp. 296–326). Stuttgart: Thieme.

Van der Merwe, A. (2008). A theoretical framework for the charaterization of pathological speech sensorimotor control. In M. R. McNeil (Ed.), *Clinical management of sensorimotor speech disorders* (pp. 3–18). Stuttgart: Thieme.

Van Zaalen, Y., Wijnen, F., & Dejonckere, P. (2009). A test of speech motor control on word level productions: The SPA test. *International Journal of Speech-Language Pathology, 11*, 26–33.

Van Zaalen, Y., Ward, D., Nederveen, A. J., Lameris, J. L., Wijnen, F., & Dejonckere, P. (2009). *Cluttering and stuttering: Different disorders and differing functional neurologies*. Presentation at 5th International Fluency Association Congress, Rio de Janeiro.

Ward, D. (2004). *Cluttering and linguistic rhythm: A case report*. Proceedings of the International Fluency Association World Congress, Montreal, Canada, June.

Ward, D. (2006). *Stuttering and cluttering: Frameworks for understanding and treatment*. Hove, UK: Psychology Press.

Ward, D. (2010). Stuttering and normal nonfluency: Cluttering spectrum behaviour as a functional descriptor of abnormal fluency. In K. Bakker, L. Raphael, & F. Myers (Eds.), *Proceedings of the First World Conference on Cluttering, Katarino, Bulgaria* (pp. 261–268). http://associations.missouristate.edu/ICA

Ward, D., & Bush, N. (2010, manuscript in preparation). Voice onset time in cluttering and stuttering.

Weiss, D. (1964). *Cluttering*. Englewood Cliffs, NJ: Prentice-Hall.

Wohl, M. T. (1970). The treatment of non fluent utterances: A behavioural approach. *British Journal of Disorders of Communication*, *5*, 66–76.

Wu, J. C., Maguire, G., Riley, G., Lee, A., Keator, D., Tang, C., et al. (1997). Increased dopamine activity associated with stuttering. *Neuroreport*, *8*, 767–770.

4 A preliminary comparison of speech rate, self-evaluation, and disfluency of people who speak exceptionally fast, clutter, or speak normally

Klaas Bakker, Florence L. Myers, Lawrence J. Raphael, and Kenneth O. St. Louis

Introduction

There is surprisingly little empirical evidence about speech fluency disorders characterized by atypical speech delivery rates. In addition to a recent surge in attention to cluttering, discussed elsewhere in this volume (see also Scaler Scott & St. Louis, 2009) there has been a persistent call for matching levels of empirical clinical research (e.g., Bakker, 1996; Scaler Scott & St. Louis, 2009). The authors of this chapter have initiated a series of empirical research projects centered on the commonly recognized features of cluttering (Daly & Burnett, 1999; Weiss, 1964), notably: (1) speech rate control (Bakker, Raphael, Myers, St. Louis, & MacRoy, 2004; Raphael, Bakker, Myers, & St. Louis, 2007; Raphael et al., 2005; Raphael, Bakker, Myers, St. Louis, & MacRoy, 2001, 2004); (2) self-awareness of rate and clarity (Myers, Bakker, Raphael, & St. Louis, 2005); and (3) speech disfluency (Myers & St. Louis, 1996, 2006; Myers et al., 2004; Myers, St. Louis, Raphael, Bakker, & Lwowski, 2003). As speaking rate is central to our understanding of cluttering-related behaviors, we collected data from clutterers, from individuals who speak perceptually fast but who do not clutter (hereafter referred to as exceptionally rapid speakers, or ERS), as well as from controls (Myers et al., 2004; Raphael et al., 2001).

Of course, the concept of exceptionally rapid speech is not new and has been previously labeled and described as tachylalia (Freund, 1970; Luchsinger & Arnold, 1965; St. Louis & Myers, 1997). The fact that there are individuals who speak at a rapid rate that draws attention to itself but who do not distinguish themselves through other speech- or language-related characteristics is fascinating. One might wonder if cluttering (or tachyphemia) (Arnold, n.d.) and exceptionally rapid speech (or tachylalia) are related, or uniquely different, conditions with accelerated speech delivery rate as a primary and shared clinical sign. If they are related in this sense, one might wonder further if cluttering, exceptionally rapid speech, and normally fluent speech are different points on the same clinical continuum, adding to Ward's (2006) hypothesis that cluttering may be on a continuum with typical speech. However, even if the previous conditions are not related in this sense, comparative descriptive research could still produce important clinical evidence as it points to the need for developing adjusted diagnostic, assessment, and management procedures.

The overall purpose for the present chapter, then, was to compare persons with cluttering (PWC) with exceptionally rapid speakers (ERS) and with those who speak normally, using the same paradigms that have been previously employed for speakers who either do or do not clutter. A specific purpose was for the study to provide an empirical approach to determining if exceptionally rapid speech is a condition potentially related to the fluency disorder of cluttering.

Defining cluttering and exceptionally rapid speech

A unanimously agreed-upon definition of cluttering does not currently exist; therefore, this investigation used our so-called 'working definition' that appears to be widely cited in today's cluttering literature:

> Cluttering is a fluency disorder characterized by a rate that is perceived to be abnormally rapid, irregular, or both for the speaker (although measured syllable rates may not exceed normal limits). These rate abnormalities further are manifest in one or more of the following symptoms: (a) an excessive number of disfluencies, the majority of which are not typical of people who stutter; (b) the frequent placement of pauses and use of prosodic patterns that do not conform to syntactic and semantic constraints; and (c) inappropriate (usually excessive) degrees of coarticulation among sounds, especially in multisyllabic words.
>
> (St. Louis, Myers, Bakker, & Raphael, 2007, pp. 299–300)

Importantly, given the status of empirical research regarding cluttering, this definition continues to be based mostly on the perception of experts. The term 'working definition' designates it as a work in progress, to be adjusted as new evidence is gathered. It should be noted that a slightly revised version of this definition is proposed in St. Louis and Schulte (this volume). The definition presents cluttering primarily as a fluency disorder characterized by a speaking rate that is clinically abnormal in terms of speed and/or regularity; yet, it also ties cluttering to a range of other speech fluency-related differences that frequently co-occur with these problems of speech rate. We submit that the definition points to a breakdown in the organization of communication (primarily manifested in the speech fluency domain) perhaps because of the deleterious effects of a speech rate that exceeds the articulatory capability of the speaker. Other approaches to definition are reviewed by St. Louis and Schulte (chapter 14 this volume).

The authors are not aware of a formal definition of exceptionally rapid speech, which is our choice of terminology to replace tachylalia, an obsolete term previously used in the literature that implies a disorder. For purposes specific to this chapter, exceptionally rapid speech is considered to be speech characterized by a rate that draws attention to itself as being faster than normal and that potentially reduces intelligibility because it occurs faster than some listeners can easily comprehend. We assume that ERS do not present with specific clinically significant characteristics of speech fluency.

As people who speak exceptionally fast, as well as those who clutter, are attempting to 'push the throttle of speech production', it does make sense to compare them in terms of clinical speech fluency characteristics under controlled conditions. For example, PWC and ERS could be on the same clinical continuum and differ only in that PWC are pushing speech rate beyond their ability to maintain the integrity of their speech and language functions (Myers, 1992), whereas ERS may have the speech and language capacities to keep up with their intended rate or are more aware of not exceeding their upper limits for rate.

Another interpretation could be that ERS are most similar to normal speakers, and differ from them only in that they produce speech at the high end of the speech rate dimension. In that perspective, we would not expect them to act differently from normal speakers when tested under conditions that are designed to evaluate unique differences in PWC.

The purpose of this chapter is to provide a first data-based discussion of a range of factors associated with speech fluency and rate-related characteristics of individuals who: (1) clutter, (2) speak exceptionally rapidly but do not clutter, and (3) speak normally. Among the factors considered are: (1) the ability of speakers to produce speech at deliberately varying rates under various controlled conditions; (2) speakers' patterns of typical and atypical forms of speech disfluency; and (3) speakers' ability to evaluate their rate and speech clarity when asked to speak as fast as they can. It should be borne in mind that some of the data presented in this chapter are a portion of those gathered for a larger and ongoing investigation into cluttering.

Method

The study evaluated 24 participants, eight in each of three groups: those who exhibited: (1) exceptionally rapid speech (ERS); (2) cluttering (PWC); and (3) controls. As participant recruitment efforts only produced female participants to represent exceptionally rapid speakers, the decision was made to also select only female participants for the groups of PWC and controls. Classification into one of the three groups was confirmed by the agreement of at least two of the three authors who are certified speech-language pathologists and who specialize in fluency disorders. The classifications were based on recorded samples of connected speech that included conversation and reading of the 'Rainbow Passage', a phonetically balanced reading passage frequently used in speech research in the USA (Fairbanks, 1960), the recitation of nursery rhymes, and the repetition of sentences. For a participant to be classified as ERS, the two authors had to agree that: (1) speech rate was perceived to be high and (2) the speaker did not present with any other features that were of clinical concern, including those cited in the working definition of cluttering discussed above.

Participants classified ERS ranged in age from 19 to 26 years ($M = 22.5$ years; $SD = 2.0$). For each ERS, an age-matched (within 5 years of age) PWC and control were selected of the same sex. Participants classified PWC ($M = 22.4$ years; $SD = 2.3$) also met the criteria specified in the working definition. Based on perceptual judgments, they were considered to have manifested segments of rapid and/or irregular speaking rate and also at least one of the following: (1) excessive disfluencies, a majority of which are unlike those of people who stutter; (2) evidence of pauses in linguistically inappropriate positions; and/or (3) evidence of overly coarticulated speech or omissions of sounds and syllables. The mean age of the eight controls was 22.9 years ($SD = 1.2$).

In addition to conversational spoken material recorded at the beginning of the experiment, the following experimental spoken materials were gathered to analyze participants' ability to control their speech rate: diadochokinetic (DDK) syllable trains and related real words: /pætɪkeɪk/, /tapɪkəl/, /kætəpəlt/, ('pattycake'), ('topical') and ('catapult'); the first paragraph of the 'Rainbow Passage'; a nursery rhyme chosen by the participant; and the repetition of four 10-syllable sentences read by the examiner.

Speech was recorded digitally through use of a digital audio tape recorder (AIWA HD-S1), or solid state digital audio recorder (Marantz PMD660), with comparable specifications (sampling rate at 10 kHz, 16 bits), using Shure PG 81 microphones. The microphone was positioned on a stand 12–15 inches in front of the participant pointed at the mouth but slightly off-center to prevent airflow-related noise artifacts. The resulting recordings were transferred to an acoustic analysis workstation (Computerized Speech Lab (CSL), Model 4500, KayPentax) for analysis of the speech rate-related characteristics. The same recordings were used for analysis of the disfluencies produced by the participants during their conversational speech. Care was taken to reduce unwanted environmental noises during the recordings in a quiet room.

Following approved procedures for acquiring informed consent, each participant entered into conversation with a researcher or a research assistant to obtain a sample of at least 400 syllables from the participant. The recordings were used for the analysis of the frequencies and types of typical and atypical speech disfluencies produced by the participants.

Next, to measure their rate-related capacities, participants were asked to produce the diadochokinetic syllable trains and related real words under four rate conditions: (1) at a self-determined 'comfortable' rate; (2) at a slow rate (modeled at approximately two syllables per second by the examiner); (3) at a maximum rate (Max 1: 'as fast as you can, and don't worry if your syllables get all jumbled up'); and (4) at a rate that was 'even faster' (Max 2) than the rate of the Max 1 condition. If the participants evidenced a breakdown in speech production during Max 1, they were asked to evaluate their speech rate and clarity using a 5-point, Likert-type scale. Otherwise, the evaluation occurred after the Max 2 condition, whether or not there was a breakdown.

Next, the participants engaged in three other tasks. First, they read the first paragraph of the 'Rainbow Passage', initially at a self-selected 'comfortable' rate and then at an unspecified 'faster' rate. Rate analyses were performed on the second and fifth sentences of the paragraph, which are representative for the remainder of the passage. Those sentences, respectively, were 'The rainbow is a division of white light into many beautiful colors' and 'People look, but no one ever finds it'. Second, as in the reading task, subjects were asked to recite a nursery rhyme of their choice from memory at a self-selected 'comfortable' rate, and then at an unspecified 'faster' rate. Most subjects selected either 'Jack and Jill' or 'Humpty-Dumpty', although other nursery rhymes were also selected. Some participants asked to review a written copy of a nursery rhyme to refresh their memory prior to their recitation of the nursery rhyme. In cases where the participants disavowed knowledge of nursery rhymes, they were asked to count from one to ten at 'comfortable' and 'faster' rates. Third, the participants were asked to repeat four sentences modeled at 3.3–5 syllables per second (SPS) by the examiner. This range of rates, modeled by the examiners, is representative for conversational speech in the general population (e.g., Starkweather, 1987). The particular sentences used were from a large USA database (St. Louis, Ruscello, & Lundeen, 1992). Each sentence comprised 10 syllables, e.g., 'Mary ran when she heard the school bell ring.' No directions were given with regard to the rate of the repetition. Syllable rates here were also determined using the aforementioned CSL-based procedure.

The CSL was used to analyze the utterances to be measured in terms of numbers of syllables spoken and articulation time (silences < 500 ms were removed). The raw acoustic wave form and spectrographic displays were used to make the selections. The 'playback' option was used for perceptually verifying identities of the utterances that were analyzed. All acoustic measurements and syllable-rate calculations were made by one examiner and one graduate assistant. In cases where syllable rates differed by more than 0.5 syllables per second, such differences were resolved by re-measurement and consultation between the examiner and graduate assistant. The resulting syllable rate data were analyzed descriptively as well as inferentially. That is, for each condition and subject group, means and standard deviations were determined and individually compared. Possible group differences in speech rate, measured in SPS, among the three subject groups were evaluated using one-way analysis of variance.

From the conversational speech, 400 syllables were transcribed orthographically to determine the frequency and types of disfluencies using the protocol specified by the Systematic Disfluency Analysis (SDA) (Campbell & Hill, 1994). Based on the SDA, unintelligible syllables were not included and disfluencies were categorized as 'more typical' (i.e., disfluencies typical of nonstuttering speakers) or 'less typical' (i.e., stuttering-type disfluencies less typical of normal speakers). The category of 'more typical' disfluencies comprised hesitations, interjections, revisions, unfinished words, phrase repetitions, and word repetitions. The category of 'less typical' disfluencies included syllable repetitions, sound repetitions, prolongations, and blocks. Following training to reach 90 percent inter-judge agreement with the examiner, a graduate research assistant transcribed the speech samples to categorize the disfluencies. The training of the observers was aimed at ensuring a sufficient level of reliability of the observations. In instances where the disfluencies were difficult to categorize, consultation ensued to arrive at consensus. Chi-square tests were applied to determine whether the subject groups differed statistically in distribution of disfluency types.

Results

This study focused on the speech rate characteristics of people who clutter, speak exceptionally rapidly, or normally, in a set of controlled speech rate conditions. In addition, attention was given to speech fluency, and the ability to self-evaluate speech rate and clarity of productions that are very fast.

Speech rate: diadochokinetic tasks (DDKs)

As noted, participants repeated six different syllable trains /pətəkə/, /təpəkə/, /kətəpə/, /pætɪkeɪk/ (or 'pattycake'), /tapɪkəl/ (or 'topical'), /kætəpəlt/ (or 'catapult') at: (1) a self-generated comfortable rate; (2) a slow modeled rate (about 2 syllables per second); and (3) a maximum rate around the point of speech breakdown (with two attempts: Max 1 and Max 2; for Max 2 the subjects were asked to exceed their rate for Max 1). Speech rates in SPS were determined for each syllable sequence separately, and then averaged across utterance type for each participant. Averaging the syllable sequence types was supported by a previous analysis involving participants who do or do not clutter in which it had been demonstrated that speech rate differences across the nonsense and real word syllable sequences were negligible (Raphael et al., 2007). Table 4.1 displays group means and standard deviations of the syllable production rates for each rate condition and for each subject group.

Table 4.1 Descriptive statistics (mean and standard deviation in syllables per second) of speech rates (slow-modeled, at a self-generated comfortable rate, and at fast rates near the point of speech breakdown) for the subject groups (ERS, PWC, and Controls) across six diadochokinetic (DDK) tasks

DDK type	*Comfortable*		*Slow modeled*		*Max 1*		*Max 2*	
	M	*(SD)*	*M*	*(SD)*	*M*	*(SD)*	*M*	*(SD)*
ERS	4.36	(1.23)	2.51	(0.55)	6.76	(0.71)	7.02	(0.39)
PWC	5.00	(0.89)	2.13	(0.60)	7.07	(1.30)	7.12	(1.44)
Controls	4.53	(1.13)	2.25	(0.55)	6.41	(0.81)	7.52	(1.05)

The means did not differ significantly among the subject groups in any of the rate conditions. Specifically, the groups did not differ significantly when producing syllable trains at a comfortable repetition rate ($F = 0.694$, $df = 2$, $p \leq .511$), in their slow modeled productions ($F = 0.884$, $df = 2$, $p \leq .429$), or at either of the maximum rates (MAX1: $F = 0.899$, $df = 2$, $p \leq .423$; MAX2: $F = 0.414$, $df = 2$, $p \leq .668$). Thus, within the constraints of the methodology used in this experiment, DDK repetition rates did not reveal significant differences among ERS, PWC, and controls.

Speech rate: oral reading of the 'Rainbow Passage', recitation of a nursery rhyme, and sentence repetition

As the repetition of meaningless syllables may be somewhat unrepresentative of the rate performance of individual speakers during natural speech, three additional conditions were implemented with linguistically more complete utterances than the simple DDK sequences (on potential differences between meaningless and meaningful stimuli on motor speech control for PWC, see Ward, chapter 3 this volume). Each of the subjects was asked to record the 'Rainbow Passage': (1) at a comfortable self-generated rate and (2) at a faster rate. Syllable production rates were measured only for the two sentences mentioned above (second and fifth). Sentence speech rate data were averaged for each participant.

The same procedure was followed for the syllable rate measurements of the recitation of a nursery rhyme familiar to each participant, but for the nursery rhymes, the entire text of the recitation was used in the analysis of syllable rate.

A descriptive analysis of the means associated with the oral reading conditions, displayed in Table 4.2, shows that ERS and PWC generally produced somewhat faster reading rates than the control subjects. This trend appears to be similar in the comfortable and fast production rate conditions. However, the group differences are statistically significant only for the comfortable rate condition ($F = 8.18$, $df = 2$, $p \leq .003$). The trend is not statistically significant

Table 4.2 Descriptive statistics (means and standard deviations) of oral reading rate in syllables per second (comfortable and fast) of the Rainbow Passage (average SPS of sentences #2 and #5) and recitation rate of a nursery rhyme by participants of the three speaker groups (ERS, PWC, and Controls)

Condition	*Comfortable*		*Fast*	
	M	*(SD)*	*M*	*(SD)*
Oral reading: 'Rainbow Passage'				
ERS	5.91	(0.65)	7.48	(1.63)
PWC	6.51	(0.86)	7.59	(1.48)
Controls	5.21	(0.30)	6.26	(0.34)
Recitation: Nursery rhyme				
ERS	5.19	(0.55)	6.39	(0.90)
PWC	4.99	(1.00)	6.01	(0.86)
Controls	3.98	(0.80)	5.60	(0.90)

in the fast reading condition, most likely due to a higher level of variability in the case of ERS and PWC groups ($F = 2.67$, $df = 2$, $p \leq .09$).

The results of the nursery rhyme recitations parallel those of the oral reading rate conditions. That is, when asked to recite a nursery rhyme at a comfortable speaking rate, ERS and PWC produced the rhymes significantly more quickly than the controls ($F = 4.93$, $df = 2$, $p \leq .02$); in contrast, the fast recitation rate condition did not reveal a statistically significant difference among the subject groups ($F = 1.50$, $df = 2$, $p \leq .25$). Here, the disproportionately higher levels of variability such as those observed during the fast oral reading rates in the case of the ERS and PWC were not evident. This may be related to the difference in the speaking situations between the rote recitation of a nursery rhyme and an oral reading task. A qualitative difference between the tasks is also suggested by the generally slower production rates of the nursery rhymes compared with those of the oral readings. It should be noted that some participants had difficulty in remembering a nursery rhyme and that their uncertainty in reciting them may account, in part, for the slower rate of syllable production for each group.

Finally, each participant was asked to repeat four 10-syllable sentences following a model provided by the examiner. Speech rate data for the examiner, and the repetition rates of the experimental subjects, are displayed in Table 4.3. From the data it appears that while the rates modeled by the examiner for the experimental groups were highly similar across the subject groups and with low levels of rate variability, the sentence repetition rates of the speakers in each of the subject groups were faster than the models. Aside from this general difference, the resulting rates among the individual speaker groups also differed significantly from each other ($F = 5.75$, $df = 2$, $p \leq .01$). The ERS and PWC groups produced the sentences at a faster pace than did the controls. ERS and PWC, in other words, were less accurate in following a

Table 4.3 Descriptive statistics (means and standard deviations) of speech rate in syllables per second of four sentences modeled by the examiner, and repeated by participants of the three speaker groups (ERS, PWC, and Controls). Sentence results were averaged per participant

Subject group	*Examiner models*		*Participant repetition rates*	
	M	*(SD)*	*M*	*(SD)*
ERS	4.05	(0.29)	4.83	(0.40)
PWC	4.12	(0.28)	5.01	(0.42)
Controls	3.91	(0.33)	4.36	(0.36)

modeled rate model than normally fluent speakers, and tended to repeat the modeled speech at faster rates. Perhaps they were less sensitive to a modeled rate, or were less able to reproduce the modeled rate, than individuals who typically speak at normal rates.

Typical and atypical speech disfluencies

According to much of the literature on fluency disorders, PWC may be distinguished from speakers who do not clutter by features other than their speech rate performance, among which is their manifestation of 'excessive numbers of normal disfluencies' (e.g., St. Louis et al., 2007). With respect to ERS, we are unaware of any literature that reports on the types and frequencies of disfluencies. The purpose of our analysis, then, was to conduct a comparison of PWC and ERS with respect to their profiles of speech disfluencies. We also wanted to compare each of these clinical groups to a control group consisting of individuals who presumably are able to control speech rate and who do not clutter.

Conversations between all participants and an examiner at the beginning of the experiment were analyzed for type and frequency of disfluencies using the SDA taxonomy. We doubled the number of analyzed syllables recommended by the SDA manual from 200 to 400. In four cases, the recordings did not contain enough speech to select 400 syllables. In three of these four cases, conversational speech from elsewhere during the protocol was used to complement speech available for the disfluency analysis. Unfortunately, in one case there wasn't enough speech to create a sample of 400 syllables, and the disfluency incidence numbers were prorated to be comparable with data based on 400 syllable samples. This would not likely affect the data much as previous analyses indicated that 200 syllable samples, as recommended in the SDA instructions, were virtually the same as those with 400 syllables (Myers et al., 2004). Table 4.4 displays the means and standard deviations for each disfluency type for the individuals of each participant group.

The data in Table 4.4 reveal that at a descriptive level of analysis there were two disfluency types that occurred much more frequently than others. Interestingly, this was the case for all subject groups. That is, regardless of group, interjections represented 54.4 percent of the total number of disfluencies and revisions 21.9 percent. Two disfluency types, i.e., hesitations and blocks, did not occur in any of the speakers, and prolongations only once for one speaker. The remaining disfluency types, i.e., incomplete utterances, phrase repetitions, word repetitions, syllable repetitions, and sound repetitions, occurred relatively infrequently.

In a descriptive sense, the groups were highly similar in their profiles of speech disfluencies. The similarity was not only in how the disfluencies were distributed within each group (i.e., a high prevalence of interjections and revisions), but also in terms of absolute numbers of disfluencies. The lack of difference in disfluency profiles among the groups was supported by a chi-square test of independence, using only the numbers for disfluencies with incidences higher than zero and therefore excluding hesitations, prolongations and blocks. A chi-square of 9.88, conducted for the remaining disfluencies, failed to meet or exceed the critical value of 21.03 (df = 12; $p \leq .05$). In other words, no group differences among the disfluency profiles were found.

Table 4.4 Means and standard deviations of numbers of more typical and less typical disfluencies as produced by participants of the three speaker groups (ERS, PWC, and Controls). Abbreviations for disfluencies are as follows: hesitations (H), interjections (I), revisions (Rv), unfinished words (U), phrase repetitions (Rp), word repetitions (Rw), syllable repetitions (Rsy), sound repetitions (Rs), prolongations (P), and blocks (B)

Group		*Typical disfluencies*					*Atypical disfluencies*				
		H	*I*	*Rv*	*U*	*Rp*	*Rw*	*Rsy*	*Rs*	*P*	*B*
ERS	M	0.0	9.8	4.9	1.3	0.9	2.0	0.1	0.1	0.0	0.0
	(SD)	(0.0)	(0.6)	(2.4)	(1.4)	(0.8)	(1.6)	(0.4)	(0.4)	(0.0)	(0.0)
PWC	M	0.0	12.1	5.3	1.3	1.0	2.5	0.1	0.5	0.1	0.0
	(SD)	(0.0)	(10.6)	(2.9)	(0.9)	(1.0)	(1.9)	(0.4)	(0.8)	(0.4)	(0.0)
Controls	M	0.0	10.6	3.2	0.8	0.4	2.5	0.3	1.1	0.0	0.0
	(SD)	(0.0)	(4.6)	(2.5)	(0.9)	(0.5)	(1.8)	(0.5)	(1.6)	(0.0)	(0.0)

Self-ratings of speech rate and clarity

An additional aspect of the present analysis was to see how aware the participants were of the relative rate and clarity of their speech at high rates of production. To assess this, all speakers provided self-evaluations of their rate and clarity for one of the two maximum repetition rates of /pətəkə/. This was done, in part, to assess their evaluation of how rapidly and clearly they were able to produce the maximum repetition rate, but also to assess the correspondence of this awareness with the physical production rate. Table 4.5 shows the means and standard deviations of rate and clarity provided by the participants of each group. The endpoints of the rate/clarity scales were: 1 = very slow/unclear and 5 = very fast/clear.

As the data illustrate, the self-evaluations of speech rate were highest for controls and lowest for PWC. The differences among the groups were not statistically significant ($F = 2.22$, $df = 2$, $p = .13$). With respect to reported clarity of the maximum repetition rates, the groups were very close, with the highest clarity rating given by the ERS and the lowest by the controls. Again, the differences among the groups were not statistically significant ($F = 0.03$, $df = 2$, $p = .97$). It cannot be concluded from these findings, then, that ERS or PWC differ from controls in how they judge the clarity of their /pətəkə/ maximum repetition rate productions.

Table 4.5 Means and standard deviations of self-ratings of speech rate in syllables per second and 1–5 scale ratings of clarity regarding the maximum repetition rate of /pətəkə/ for participants of the three speaker groups (ERS, PWC, and Controls)

Subject group	*Rate*		*Clarity*	
	M	*(SD)*	*M*	*(SD)*
ERS	4.44	(0.50)	3.00	(1.55)
PWC	4.25	(0.71)	2.88	(1.13)
Controls	4.79	(0.39)	2.86	(1.07)

Discussion

This study provided preliminary data on people who speak exceptionally rapidly, clutter, and speak normally with respect to: (1) their ability to manage speech rate in a range of controlled conditions; (2) their disfluencies during conversational speech; and (3) their self-reports of speech rate and clarity. This study is unique in that it included a group of speakers who distinguished themselves merely by a tendency to speak very rapidly. There are no specific empirically-based reports on the aforementioned variables for this group, even though its existence has been alluded to in the literature with the term tachylalia (Freund, 1970; St. Louis & Myers, 1997).

Speech rate performance

The most consistent finding of this study was that speech rate differences among the three subject groups were not present when the speakers were challenged to produce speech rapidly, that is, to produce the DDK syllable trains as fast as they could and 'not to worry if the sounds get all jumbled up'. Moreover, ERS and PWC produced similar results across all the rapid speech rate conditions. This finding suggests that there may be a physiological limit to how quickly speech can be produced, and that this limit is the same for ERS, PWC, and typical speakers. If true, this implies that the apparent accelerated speaking rates of ERS and PWC observed in many natural speaking situations are not necessarily indicative of a physiological capacity to speak more rapidly than normally fluent speakers. This would also imply that there may be other than physiological reasons for the rapid rates perceived in cluttered speech, or for much of the speech of people who speak exceptionally rapidly. One possibility is that ERS and PWC more habitually produce speech that is perceived to be fast even when the speaking situation does not require exceptionally fast speech, as when asked to give instructions for using a new cell phone. PWC and ERS could experience a drive, or receive internal triggers, to speak rapidly under all speaking conditions (Alm, 2010).

An examination of the variability of rate within a speaking condition is also of interest. PWC showed the greatest variability across subjects when asked to challenge themselves and produce articulatory rates up to and beyond their maximum limits (i.e., to and beyond the point of articulatory disintegration), but relatively less variability during the self-generated comfortable rate. This may have implications for the maximum capacities of PWC to utter syllabic pulses, but at great expense in terms of a loss of speech intelligibility. Interestingly, though not surprisingly, all three groups showed relatively less variability for the slow modeled rate condition. The latter holds promise for therapy, in that clutterers can slow down when given models of slower speech in highly structured activities, one sentence at a time. The preliminary character of the present study urges replication of these findings employing larger subject groups. Further, rate data need to be analyzed with regard to the types and degrees of articulatory degradations such as vowel neutralizations and syllable deletions that accompany the various rate conditions. Though the two groups of speakers, that is ERS and PWC, share commonalities in rate, speakers in one group, such as PWC, may show more misarticulations leading to reduced speech intelligibility.

Another avenue of research is to design studies that identify individuals' self-perceived thresholds of maximum speaking rate; that is, the self-awareness of one's maximum encoding capacity that would not incur articulatory breakdowns.

One hypothesis, for example, is that PWC exceed this threshold—especially during informal social interactions—because they are not attuned to, nor are they inclined to expend the effort to monitor, their rate threshold and the consequences of exceeding it. Myers (1992, p. 78) postulates that:

> . . . research is needed to test the hypothesis that clutterers might be found to be faster and 'less constrained' in speech patterns. . . . Clutterers

may be found to demonstrate greater variability, but variability which is less modulated, less constrained, and less tempered. The latter is due largely to anomalies in the governance of rate, but possibly also due to a poor servosystem.

A second hypothesis is that within the larger population of PWC, some subgroups may find normalizing—or at least speaking more deliberately—easier than do other subgroups in certain speaking situations (e.g., job interviews) or for utterances of short duration. In this line of reasoning, the normalizing PWC, like typical speakers, would be more aware of their thresholds and find it easier to 'hold back' to rates that are just below their maximum capacities (Starkweather, 1987). They would realize that their communication output would otherwise show telltale signs of breakdowns, such as misarticulations and inappropriate choice of words or wording. Clinicians have also observed that PWC, as a general trend (with exceptions), are not as inclined as typical speakers to repair conversational breakdowns associated with misarticulations and incoherence of narratives and discourse (e.g., St. Louis & Myers, 1997; St. Louis et al., 2007).

The results of this preliminary study also revealed that PWC and ERS produced speech more rapidly than normally fluent speakers in some conditions, but not in others. Their syllable rates were significantly higher than those of the controls in the self-selected comfortable conditions of the nursery rhyme recitations and the reading of the 'Rainbow Passage', as well as in the repetition of the sentences that were modeled by the examiner. In the self-selected comfortable condition of the DDKs, only the PWC syllable rate exceeded that of the controls, whereas in the slow, modeled rate only the ERS syllable rate exceeded that of the controls. Both PWC and ERS had higher rates than the controls in the Max 1 condition, but in the Max 2 condition the controls spoke more quickly than either of the other two groups. The differences in DDK syllable rates among the groups in these conditions were not statistically significant.

It would appear, then, that statistically significant rate differences occurred consistently only in those conditions in which the elicited speech conformed to the semantic and syntactic requirements of English (also see Ward, chapter 3 this volume) and in which speakers either selected a comfortable rate or imitated a modeled rate. It is not possible, however, given the inconsistencies of rate and statistical significance, to say how or to what extent the differences between the DDKs and meaningful language samples or the elicitation of a particular rate affected the production rates of PWC, ERS, and controls.

We should note that, in the sentence repetition condition, all participant groups produced speech that was somewhat more rapid than the examiner model. Perhaps providing an immediate model for the short sentences made the repetition task easier in some way, thereby resulting in faster imitation rates. Given that the participants received no specific instructions to match the examiner's rate, it might also be true that there is a natural tendency to repeat modeled speech at a slightly faster rate than the model.

The results of our rate analysis do suggest the possibility that PWC and ERS speak faster during conditions that are most similar to natural, self-formulated speech. It will require further study with larger populations to test this possibility. The results of further study might provide valuable information relative to identifying the underlying factors contributing to clinically significant, elevated rates.

Self-reports of speech rate and clarity

Participants were asked to report their evaluations of speech rate and clarity in one of the DDK conditions (the production of /pətəkə/) at the maximum production rate and near the point where speech shows signs of breaking down. Interestingly, there were no statistically significant differences between the subject groups in how they judged their rate and speech clarity in this condition. The lack of difference in these judgments is limited to this particular condition.

It is noteworthy that all groups demonstrated similar appreciation of their rate performance and clarity of the /pətəkə/ rapid repetitions. This is not entirely surprising in the case of rate, as actual speech rates of the groups in this condition could not be distinguished either and, in fact, participants were asked to push themselves to their articulatory limits (and beyond). The fact that there was no difference in the self-reported clarity is interesting, but interpretation is limited by the fact that the actual clarity of the repetitions was not determined. Assuming that the DDK repetitions were normal both in rate and clarity, a lack of difference in self-reports would suggest that ERS and PWC have realistic self-observations about speech rate and clarity when required to produce speech rapidly on command, and that they do not differ in this respect from the normally fluent speakers.

A number of methodological issues limit the interpretation of the self-report data on speech rate and clarity. In the case of self-reported rates, all responses were close to the high end of the judgment scale; additionally, responses involved forced selection of integers only, thus limiting variability in responding. Both the fact that the participants were asked to speak as rapidly as possible, even if their syllables 'get all jumbled up' and the fact that the participants were asked to evaluate rate predisposed the speakers to acknowledge that they were speaking extremely fast. There was less of a limitation in the case of self-reports of speech clarity, the majority of which fell in the middle range of the scale. Nonetheless, self-reports were similar across the groups of participants. Finally, it is not possible to generalize the self-report findings to the other rate conditions in this experiment, as self-reports were collected only for the maximum rates of the /pətəkə/ repetitions. It would be interesting, for example, to determine if self-reported rate and clarity deviate from the actual production rate and clarity when conversational speech is accelerated compared to the same speech of normally fluent peers, or when it also contains cluttering. From the present data, it may be concluded that self-reports, made immediately after speech produced rapidly on command, may not differentiate ERS from PWC.

Speech disfluency

The apparent lack of difference in disfluency profiles between the participant groups demands explanation. After all, the fluency characteristics of the speakers were an important factor in their assignment to the subject groups that were investigated. It is important to note that the diagnostic differentiation was made *in a molar perceptual sense* without considering disfluency in the detailed, quantified manner of the present analysis, that is, by counting specific types of speech disfluency. Moreover, excessive disfluency is not even required for a diagnosis of cluttering according to the working definition used (St. Louis et al., 2007).

Even though the frequencies of specific disfluencies were similar across the groups, the individual instances of disfluency may have differed in a qualitative sense. That is, disfluencies could have triggered higher severity judgments if they involved certain grammatical anomalies or co-occurred with a rapid spurt followed by an inappropriate pause for revision of thought. It is reasonable to assume that clinical perception was affected by such factors as syntactic location of the disfluency in the utterance, and the linguistic aspects of the disfluency itself. For example, there may be inherent differences between insertion of a filler such as 'um' in an otherwise linguistically intact sentence and the presence of an incomplete phrase followed by a revision that signals a reformulation of syntax, word choice, or even topic. Other qualitative characteristics may also have been important for the perception of cluttering. For example, disfluent speech fragments could have been produced with atypical forms of prosody, a lack of clarity in production, or have been characterized by unusual aspects of narrative and/or linguistic structure (e.g., narratives that are difficult to follow because they go off on a tangent, are laden with revisions, or lack parts of the story grammar). Finally, some researchers (e.g., Starkweather, 1987) have proposed a distinction between the 'less mature' disfluencies of speakers who produce motoric, stuttering-like breakdowns in the system and the disfluencies of other speakers that can be characterized as attempts to repair communication and thus are 'more mature' (i.e., formulative) in nature (Logan & LaSalle, 1999). This qualitative difference (i.e., types of disfluencies) may contribute more to the perception of cluttering than quantitative differences such as number of disfluencies.

There is additional evidence that cluttered speech in some cases may be judged more by qualitative than quantitative variables. Cluttered speech was judged to be more severe when it occurred in contexts with more disfluency clusters than when it occurred with single disfluencies (Myers, St. Louis, & Faragasso, 2008). Myers and St. Louis (1996) found that, of two youths who cluttered, the more severe clutterer exhibited greater numbers of disfluency clusters (as well as longer strings of clusters) compared to the youth with less severe cluttering. Additionally, speech disruptions characterized by interjections may not be perceived to be as cluttered as speech laden with revisions. The latter significantly disrupt the flow of the information output by aborting a thought and starting anew, hence reducing the predictability of the message and increasing the processing load for the listener (Myers, 1992). Many typical speakers exhibit their share of interjections; while irksome, fillers are not as detrimental to the coherence of the message (Fox Tree, 2001). Clearly, these possibilities indicate that it may be somewhat misleading to study disfluency only by reference to numbers.

We cannot rely exclusively on isolated quantitative measures of individual dimensions of cluttering to determine the nature and severity of cluttering. The multidimensional character of cluttering may, in the end, rely heavily on the *perception* of the degree to which one dimension interacts with another dimension (Myers & St. Louis, 2006; St. Louis, Myers, Faragasso, Townsend, & Gallaher, 2004), influencing the overall coherence and cohesiveness of the message. One possibility for future research, for example, is to examine the loci and type of disfluencies in an utterance. Disfluencies that disrupt the flow of information or meaning of an utterance only to restart with a tangential thought may be perceived as more cluttering-like, contributing to the perception of greater irregularity of flow (or tempo) than two interjections at phrase boundaries. It is interesting, for example, that some of the ERS and controls had their fair share of disfluencies yet were perceived to be typically fluent. Future studies need to examine the role of some of the more qualitative, interactive aspects of cluttering behaviors in determining the diagnosis and severity of cluttering.

Finally, it is possible that the definitions of the various disfluency types imposed by relatively strict adherence to the SDA may have disguised some of the results. For example, whereas the finding of virtually no hesitations in this study are consistent with earlier pilot investigations (Myers et al., 2003, 2004) as well as earlier studies on other PWC (Myers & St. Louis, 1996), it is possible that the requirement of 1 second of silence to score a hesitation may have disguised some potential differences. In fact, hesitations may not be silent and may be perceived at durations of more or less than 1 second. Acoustic verification techniques are needed to supplement perception. Additionally, the SDA was originally developed for use with stuttering clients (Campbell & Hill, 1994). Using a more flexible definition of hesitations, Garnett (2009) found substantially more hesitations amongst PWC than normally speaking controls.

In a different vein, the group similarities in numbers of disfluencies per type could have resulted from a side effect of 'normalizing' in some of the PWC and ERS. The experimental condition of producing conversational speech, while being recorded, could have elicited speech near the normal range of fluency and rate if the participants were more 'on guard' under the laboratory conditions. This, of course, might apply to the control participants as well. To the extent that speech disfluencies may be affected by a speech rate greater than the speaker is able to handle (in the case of PWC), the lack of differences in speech disfluency could be a logical result given the absence of speech rate differences in many conditions during this experiment. In other words, speech produced under less guarded circumstances might have revealed speech accelerations that could subsequently have caused speakers who clutter to produce increased numbers of disfluencies, and of certain types. This conclusion is more tentative in the case of the ERS and perhaps even for typical speakers. While they may have normalized their speech rate, we do not know what the consequences might have been for their speech disfluency profiles. This, then, is in need of further investigation, as it is still possible that PWC and especially the ERS may produce distinct qualitative differences in speech fluency when speaking in less 'guarded situations' and where rate accelerations are also expected to occur. For both clinical and research purposes, it should be noted that PWC who can 'normalize' should be distinguished from those PWC who do not, or cannot, normalize.

The failure to observe significant speech disfluency differences in the present experiment should motivate others who plan to study speech disfluency levels in PWC, or ERS: (1) to take measures that control the tendency to normalize and also (2) to consider qualitative differences among individual instances of disfluency. Likewise, clinicians should consider including qualitative and perceptual strategies (e.g., Bakker & Myers, 2008) to assess the severity of disfluency in cluttered speech, and to differentially diagnose a PWC from an ERS. Unfortunately, the potential tendency to normalize was not systematically controlled in the present study, and in fact is very difficult to control within the constraints of research ethics, which require disclosure of significant details of the experimental procedures.

An intriguing and possibly contaminating issue in terms of subject selection is that of severity level. The subjects in the present study were not subjected to procedures to determine severity of their cluttering, or speech rate deviation. So, the results of the present analysis may (or may not) have been affected by a disproportionate number of participants with relatively low severity levels of either cluttering or of exceptionally rapid speach. Future research could include procedures for determining severity, but this would, for the time being, be limited by a notable absence of quantifiable severity measures for either cluttering or exceptionally rapid speech. It should be noted that development of a severity measure for cluttering (e.g., Bakker & Myers, 2008) is underway and may provide a solution for such research in the near future.

Several issues regarding the subject selection basic to this experiment warrant discussion. PWC and ERS were clinically differentiated as experimental subjects largely through perceptual procedures. That is, the participants were ultimately selected by two of the authors of this work with long-term experience in fluency disorders, and cluttering in particular. When they categorized the participants, their judgments were based on the operational working definition of cluttering (i.e., St. Louis et al., 2007). Unfortunately, there is no systematic literature on how to diagnostically differentiate 'exceptionally rapid speech' other than using largely perceptual procedures. Obviously, there is a strong need for more rigorous and objective methods to differentiate this subject group in order to facilitate future research comparing the characteristics of individuals with clinically compromised speech rate performance. For example, it would be fruitful to compare the speech of these ERS with the speech of news broadcasters, auctioneers, or other highly fluent gifted speakers (Kuiper, 1996).

All participants in this study were female and mostly in their early twenties. The uniform composition of this group according to gender, and age, may have limited the extent to which these findings can be generalized. Future research should attempt to recruit participants of both genders, especially given the report of more males than females who clutter (e.g., Weiss, 1964), and should also consider additional age groups (e.g., young developing speakers and older children). The latter, especially, would have the potential to reveal developments in the interaction between the variables studied.

Another possible threat to the external validity of this experiment could be the noticeable absence of individuals who both clutter and stutter. While, on the one hand, it added to the purity of the group of individuals who clutter, it is also unrepresentative, as many individuals who clutter also stutter (Van Riper, 1971). The recruitment procedure used targeted individuals who demonstrated the features of cluttering, or merely were known for their use of exceptionally rapid speech. This may have caused clinicians who made referrals to not refer individuals who both clutter and stutter, a population that comprises a substantial portion of the entire population of individuals who clutter. In this sense, the present findings and conclusions apply mostly to pure clutterers or individuals who have a pure form of exceptionally rapid speech.

The present investigation was a preliminary attempt to analyze ERS, PWC, and control speakers on multiple dimensions (aspects of speech rate, self-evaluation, and disfluency) and to learn more about: (1) characteristics of people who speak exceptionally rapidly; (2) characteristics of people with cluttering; and (3) how these characteristics interact in ways that are clinically relevant. Interestingly, people who speak exceptionally rapidly in natural unguarded daily situations did not significantly differ from people who clutter in the conditions tested in this experiment. Of course, both groups may have exhibited a tendency to normalize their rates in the speaking situation that was used to determine their respective disfluency profiles; also conversational speech rates were not determined for the situation. Under current US governmental limitations on methodology for studies employing human subjects, it is very difficult to obtain speech in unguarded situations, since doing so requires disclosure of significant aspects of the experimental design. Our findings, however, provide compelling evidence that exceptions to such limitations may be needed in cases where the investigators wish to describe the speech rates and profiles of disfluencies as they exist in typical speaking situations. Participants could be debriefed afterwards and given the option to withdraw their data.

Most of what was learned in the present study is that PWC and ERS differ from typically fluent speakers when they self-select their speech rate; in other words, when these groups have the opportunity to accelerate at will. This difference is reduced when the examiner directs them to accelerate their speech to and beyond their maximum capacity. When maximum production rates are required, they do not have the opportunity to accelerate even further, and the rate performance differences disappear. This suggests a hypothesis that ERS and PWC are somehow driven or triggered to use the accelerated speaking rates rather than that they have a speech mechanism that allows them to speak faster than others. Importantly, considering the specific rate conditions tested in this experiment, ERS and PWC were not different and may stem from a similar clinical population.

With regard to the failure to observe differences among the disfluency profiles of the ERS, PWC, and control speakers, there are at least three emerging explanations. One explanation holds that the group differences in disfluency are not in terms of the numbers or perhaps even types of disfluencies, but rather in other qualities of these individual disfluencies. A second explanation suggests that the participants in this experiment demonstrated a possible tendency to normalize speech during the experiment and did not reveal the disfluency profile that originally caused them to be recruited as participants. A third possibility is that disfluency, *per se*, may be less frequent in cluttering as defined herein than was previously assumed. Our methodology does not permit differentiation of these possibilities. Future research should thus consider using methodologies aimed at further examining these possibilities. Significantly, the disfluency types found in our PWC group were nearly all disfluencies *not* associated with stuttering but with typical speakers. Such data serve as evidence for the differential diagnosis of stuttering from cluttering and has been found repeatedly in other participants either among our larger pool of subjects of the current research project or in participants from other studies on cluttering (Myers & St. Louis, 1996, 2006; Myers et al., 2003, 2004, 2008).

In conclusion, the results of this preliminary reporting of data (from a larger ongoing research project) has revealed some interesting patterns regarding rate, fluency, and (to a lesser extent) self-awareness attributes associated with ERS, PWC, and typical speakers. As with all research, the findings prompted additional questions that have implications for future research, for the assessment and treatment of cluttering, as well as for the theoretical constructs that can serve to contextualize this multidimensional disorder.

References

Alm, P. A. (2010). The dual premotor model of cluttering and stuttering: A neurological framework. In K. Bakker, L. Raphael, & F. Myers (Eds.), *Proceedings of the First World Conference on Cluttering, Katarino, Bulgaria* (pp. 207–210). http://associations.missouristate.edu/ICA

Arnold, G. E. (n.d.). Present concepts of etiologic factors. In *Studies in tachyphemia: An investigation of cluttering and general language disability* (pp. 3–23). New York: Speech Rehabilitation Institute.

Bakker, K. (1996). Cluttering: Current scientific status and emerging research and clinical needs. *Journal of Fluency Disorders*, *21*, 359–365.

Bakker, K., & Myers, F. L. (2008). *A comprehensive measure of cluttering severity*. Paper presented at the annual convention of the American Speech-Language-Hearing Association, Chicago, IL.

Bakker, K., Raphael, L. J., Myers, F. L., St. Louis, K. O., & MacRoy, M. (2004). *DDK production variability in cluttered speech*. Poster presented at the national annual convention of the American Speech Language and Hearing Association, Philadelphia, PA.

Campbell, J. G., & Hill, D. G. (1994). *Systematic disfluency analysis*. Evanston, IL: Northwestern University.

Daly, D. A., & Burnett, M. (1999). Cluttering: Traditional views and new perspectives. In R. F. Curlee (Ed.), *Stuttering and related disorders of fluency* (2nd ed., pp. 222–254). New York: Thieme.

Fairbanks, G. (1960). *Voice and articulation drillbook* (2nd ed.). New York: Harper & Row.

Fox Tree, J. E. (2001). Listeners' uses of um and uh in speech comprehension. *Memory and Cognition*, *29*, 320–326.

Freund, H. (1970). Observations on tachylalia. *Folia Phoniatrica*, *22*, 280–288.

Garnett, E. O. (2009). *Verbal time estimation in clutterers and non-clutterers*. Unpublished master's thesis. Morgantown, WV: West Virginia University.

Kuiper, K. (1996). *Smooth talkers: The linguistic performance of auctioneers and sportscasters*. Mahwah, NJ: Lawrence Erlbaum Associates Inc.

Logan, K. J., & LaSalle, L. R. (1999). Grammatical characteristics of children's conversational utterances that contain disfluency clusters. *Journal of Speech, Language, and Hearing Research*, *42*, 80–91.

Luchsinger, R., & Arnold, G. E. (1965). *Voice–speech–language*. Belmont, CA: Wadsworth.

Myers, F. L. (1992). Cluttering: A synergistic framework. In F. L. Myers & K. O. St. Louis (Eds.), *Cluttering: A clinical perspective* (pp. 71–84). Leicester, UK: FAR Communications. (Reissued in 1996 by Singular, San Diego, CA.)

Myers, F. L., Bakker, K., Raphael, L. J., & St. Louis, K. O. (2005). *Self-ratings of speaking rate and clarity by clutterers following DDK*. Poster presented at the Annual Convention of the American Speech-Language-Hearing Association, San Diego, CA.

Myers, F. L., & St. Louis, K. O. (1996). Two youths who clutter, but is that the only similarity? *Journal of Fluency Disorders*, *21*, 297–304.

Myers, F. L., & St. Louis, K. O. (2006). Disfluency and speaking rate in cluttering: Perceptual judgments versus counts. *Bulgarian Journal of Communication Disorders*, 1, 28–35.

Myers, F. L., St. Louis, K. O., & Faragasso, K. A. (2008). Disfluency clusters associated with cluttering. *Bulgarian Journal of Communication Disorders*, *2*, 10–19.

Myers, F. L., St. Louis, K. O., Lwowski, A., Bakker, K., Raphael, L. J., & Frangis, G. (2004). *Disfluencies of cluttered and excessively rapid speech*. Poster presented at the annual convention of the American Speech-Language-Hearing Association.

Myers, F. L., St. Louis, K. O., Raphael, L. J., Bakker, K., & Lwowski, A. (2003). *Patterns of disfluencies in cluttered speech*. Poster presented at the annual convention of the American Speech-Language-Hearing Association, Chicago, Illinois.

Raphael, L. J., Bakker, K., Myers, F. L., & St. Louis, K. O. (2007). *Syllable rates in the speech of clutterers and controls*. Poster presented at the annual convention of the American Speech-Language-Hearing Association, Boston, MA.

Raphael, L. J., Bakker, K., Myers, F. L., St. Louis, K. O., Fichtner, V., & Kostel, M. (2005). *An update on diadochokinetic rates of cluttered and normal speech*. Poster presented at the annual convention of the American Speech-Language-Hearing Association, San Diego, CA.

Raphael, L. J., Bakker, K., Myers, F. L., St. Louis, K. O., & MacRoy, M. (2001). *Articulatory/acoustic features of DDKs in cluttered, tachylalic, and normal speech*. Paper presented at the annual convention of the American Speech-Language-Hearing Association, New Orleans, LA.

Raphael, L. J., Bakker, K., Myers, F. L., St. Louis, K. O., & MacRoy, M. (2004). *Diadochokinetic rates of cluttered and normal speech*. Poster presented at the annual convention of the American Speech-Language-Hearing Association, Philadelphia, PA.

Scaler Scott, K., & St. Louis, K. O. (2009, July). A perspective on improving evidence and practice in cluttering. *Perspectives on Fluency and Fluency Disorders*, *19*, 46–51.

Starkweather, C. W. (1987). *Fluency and stuttering*. Englewood Cliffs, NJ: Prentice-Hall.

St. Louis, K. O., & Myers, F. L. (1997). Management of cluttering and related fluency disorders. In R. F. Curlee & G. M. Siegel (Eds.), *Nature and treatment of stuttering: New directions* (pp. 313–332). New York: Allyn & Bacon.

St. Louis, K. O., Myers, F. L., Bakker, K., & Raphael, L. J. (2007). Understanding and treating cluttering. In E. G. Conture & R. F. Curlee (Eds.), *Stuttering and related disorders of fluency* (3rd ed., pp. 297–325). New York: Thieme.

St. Louis, K. O., Myers, F. L., Faragasso, K., Townsend, P. S., & Gallaher, A. J. (2004). Perceptual aspects of cluttered speech. *Journal of Fluency Disorders*, *29*, 213–235.

St. Louis, K. O., Ruscello, D. M., & Lundeen, C. (1992). Coexistence of communication disorders in schoolchildren. *ASHA Monograph*, *27*.

Van Riper, C. (1971). *The nature of stuttering*. Englewood Cliffs, NJ: Prentice-Hall.

Ward, D. (2006). *Stuttering and cluttering: Frameworks for understanding and treatment*. Hove, UK: Psychology Press.

Weiss, D. (1964). *Cluttering*. Englewood Cliffs, NJ: Prentice-Hall.

Part II

Cluttering and co-occurring disorders

5 The epidemiology of cluttering with stuttering

Peter Howell and Stephen Davis

Introduction

There are two schools of thought on the relationship between cluttering and stuttering. The first is that cluttering and stuttering are related disorders (Freund, 1934; Hunt, 1870; Preus, 1973; Weiss, 1964). One such theory is that cluttering may lead to stuttering, or as Weiss put it 'stuttering may have its roots in cluttering' (1964, p. 5). In support of this, he cited early work by Freund (1934) and himself (Weiss, 1936). Elsewhere in his monograph, Weiss (1964) referred to the work of Hunt (1870), who maintained that cluttering precedes stuttering. This is also consistent with the view that cluttering can change into stuttering.

One respected clinical reference source also supports a relationship between cluttering and stuttering. Thus, there is no separate index entry for cluttering in DSM-IV-TR (American Psychiatric Association, 2000), which suggests cluttering is not a defined disorder. In an earlier version, DSM-IV (American Psychiatric Association, 1994), cluttering was discussed under the entry for stuttering, which again suggests this authority does not regard cluttering as distinct from stuttering.

Also supporting a relationship is the fact that research into cluttering typically locates cases from speakers previously diagnosed as stuttering. This is shown in the work of Preus (1973, 1992), who looked at a group of speakers with Down syndrome (DS). In his initial report, the speakers with DS were classified as stuttering or not stuttering. Subsequently, Preus (1992) re-examined the data of those considered to be stuttering and sub-divided them into those who were stuttering and those who were cluttering. This research strategy embodies the assumption that cluttering is subordinate to stuttering (not a distinct disorder).

In contrast to this position, researchers who have taken a particular interest in cluttering tend to consider cluttering to be different from stuttering. Ward (2006) commented that the view that cluttering is distinct from stuttering is predominant, and cited in support Daly and Burnett-Stolnack (1994), Myers and St. Louis (1992), St. Louis, Hinzman, and Hull (1985), and van Riper (1992). Further support for this conception can be obtained from the

World Health Organization's International classification of diseases, ICD-9-CM (World Health Organization, 1982). In ICD-9-CM, stuttering was defined under F98.5 and cluttering was defined separately under F98.6.

This chapter approaches the question of whether cluttering and stuttering are related or not by identifying cases of cluttering in a longitudinal sample of children who stutter. All the children were divided into those whose stuttering persisted and those whose stuttering recovered. Each of the children was treated after the initial assessment, so any recovery may be treatment assisted. The three groups of children (children with cluttering and persistent or recovered forms of stuttering, children who persisted in stuttering, and children who recovered from stuttering) were compared on a range of epidemiological, symptomatological, and aetiological factors. The aims were as follows:

(1) To see whether cluttering follows a time course like persistent or recovered forms of stuttering or differs from stuttering.
(2) To see whether cluttering has symptoms like persistent or recovered forms of stuttering or differs from stuttering.
(3) To examine whether cluttering has a different aetiological profile from stuttering (three etiological factors that have been proposed to be behind cluttering are examined).

These three topics are areas where the literature suggests that children who clutter are different from children who stutter (as amplified below). The question addressed for each topic is whether or not there are differences between children who clutter and one or both groups of children who stutter. If there are differences, this would support the idea that children who clutter are different from children who stutter. Alternatively, if no differences are found, there would be no grounds for arguing that the disorders are distinct.

A complicating factor is that there is no agreed definition of cluttering. This affects all investigations into cluttering, not just the present study. In the present study, an extra limitation was that the assessments were based on speech. Some authors discuss essential characteristics such as lack of complete awareness of the problem (Daly & Burnett-Stolnack, 1994). This characteristic was not included as: (1) it is difficult to judge from samples of spontaneous speech that do not discuss awareness of the problem and (2) there is no agreement about this as a criterion of cluttering. In the initial assessments of whether a sample of speech was from a child who clutters or one who stutters, two of Daly and Burnett-Stolnack's (1994) other essential characteristics were used. These were: (1) poorly organized thinking (speaks before clarifying thoughts) and (2) short attention span and poor concentration. Daly and Burnett-Stolnack (1994) also listed an excessive number of whole-word or phrase repetitions as occurring in cluttered speech. This was not used as a criterion for assessing cluttering, as this aspect is considered separately under symptomatology. Speech rate was added to the characteristics even though Daly and Burnett-Stolnack did not include it in their list of characteristics, because it is widely regarded as a feature of cluttering by other authorities (St. Louis, Myers, Bakker, & Raphael, 2007; Weiss, 1964). Daly and Burnett-Stolnack considered a rapid rate of speech to occur frequently, but not invariably, in cluttering.

Using this set of characteristics distilled from a mixture of definitions to identify cluttering is not entirely satisfactory. As an additional assessment, the cases of cluttering were confirmed by international experts on cluttering. One expert specified the characteristics he had used (see method). These were employed next by two experienced listeners to identify samples of cluttering in all the materials.

The judged samples allowed incidence and prevalence of cluttering in a sample of children who stuttered to be established and reported. Cases of pure cluttering were not included. However, this may not be significant, as such cases are reported to be rare (Dalton & Hardcastle, 1989).

The first area examined was onset characteristics and course of the disorder. Age of onset has been reported to be later for cluttering than for stuttering. For example, Diedrich (1984) gives a figure of 7 years for cluttering, whereas stuttering onset is reported to occur between 3 and 4 years (Howell, Davis, & Williams, 2008; Yairi & Ambrose, 2005). The course subsequent to onset was examined in terms of whether the concomitant stuttering persisted or recovered. The distribution of cluttered samples over ages was also examined. This allowed assessment of whether or not cluttering changes into stuttering.

Gender and handedness were also documented. There are more males who stutter than females and there are more left-handers in a sample of stutterers than in the population at large (Howell et al., 2008). Gender and handedness were compared across the three groups to see if there was any evidence that these factors differed for clutterers compared with stutterers, as would be expected if they are different disorders.

The second area examined was symptomatology. The symptoms of cluttering have been considered to be different from those of stuttering. According to St. Louis et al. (2007), part-word repetitions, prolongations, and blocks characterize people who stutter, whereas clutterers have more normal disfluencies. They mention interjections, word repetitions, phrase repetitions, and unfinished words as instances of the latter class. They also state that clutterers typically do not have accessory behaviours. No analysis of separate symptoms has been made on our data to date. However, Stuttering Severity Instrument, Third Edition (SSI-3; Riley, 1994) measures have been made. These include measures of groups of speech symptoms and accessory (or secondary) behaviours. We examined whether the SSI-3 speech symptoms and accessory behaviours differed between the three groups to establish whether cluttering differs from either form of stuttering.

Finally, three selected aetiological factors were examined. St. Louis et al. (2007) reviewed four proposals on the aetiology of cluttering. Their last category (cluttering-stuttering models) was not addressed here. The first proposal of these authors we did examine was based on Dalton and Hardcastle's (1989) view that cluttering may be a reflection of basal ganglia disorder. Their evidence was the similarity between some of the symptoms seen in dysarthrias and cluttering. Stuttering has also been associated with the basal ganglia system (Alm, 2004). However, there is behavioural (Howell et al., 2008) and scanning evidence (Fox et al., 1996) that suggests cerebellar involvement. For the current study, a battery of tests that assess cerebellar functioning were performed with some members of each group, and statistical comparisons performed to see whether there were differences in performance on tests from this battery for the three groups. Any differences would offer some incidental support for different locations underpinning each disorder (the cerebellum for stuttering and possibly basal ganglia for cluttering).

St. Louis et al. (2007) include central auditory problems as a specific cognitive process that may be related to cluttering (a cognitive explanation). Preus (1992) appears to be the first person to speculate that cluttering may be linked to a central auditory processing disorder. Empirical evidence in support of this position was reported by Molt (1996) in a study on three children. An earlier case study by Wolk (1986) reported that a child who had normal auditory ability had difficulty in identifying dichotically presented syllables, which would also be consistent with this view. The most popular current technique for examining central auditory processing disorders is backward masking (Wright et al., 1997). Backward masking thresholds have been reported to differ between persistent and recovered speakers who stutter (Howell, Davis, & Williams, 2006). In the present study, backward masking thresholds were compared between the three groups to see if there was a particular problem for children who clutter.

The last causal explanation offered by St. Louis et al. (2007) that was examined concerns genetic factors. It has been argued that cluttering reflects a genetic predisposition for disfluent speech. There is some evidence that cluttering runs in families (Luchsinger & Arnold, 1965; Weiss, 1964). Genetic factors predispose a child to start stuttering as well (Yairi & Ambrose, 2005). We reviewed family history data for some of the members of each of the three groups to see whether there are any differences in the family profile of stuttering.

Method

Participants

Ninety-six participants who stuttered were used in the study (79 male and 17 female). There were two sets of speech samples for each participant. The first recordings were taken at younger than 12 years and the second at older than 12 years, with a minimum of 12 months between each recording. Spontaneous monologue speech samples, conversation, and reading of a text (see below for details) were obtained using a Sony DAT recorder and Sennheiser K6 condenser microphone. All other information except performance data and information for determining persistence/recovered outcome were obtained on occasion one.

The tests at teenage were made as soon as possible after the child reached 13. The start of teenage was chosen as the upper test age as recovery can happen at any age up to then, but rarely after it (Andrews & Harris, 1964). The mean age at first recording was 10 years, 4 months (*SD* 1 year, 1 month; range 7 years, 8 months–11 years, 11 months). The mean age at second recording was 13 years, 8 months (*SD* 1 year, 11 months; range 12 years 1 month–19 years 8 months). The mean time elapsed between each recording was 3 years, 5 months (*SD* 2 years, 3 months; range 1 year 0 months–11 years, 3 months).

Inclusion criteria for stuttering

Cases were included who were secondary referrals to clinics that specialized in the treatment of stuttering. Stuttering had to be confirmed by a trained and qualified therapist who specialized in childhood stuttering. The child had to be admitted to treatment. All information used for predicting persistence and recovery was obtained before any treatment was received. After the assessments, each participant received a 1- or 2-week intensive course of treatment for stuttering. Locating children showing cluttering through stuttering clinics is the best way of reaching them, as there does not appear to be any clinic that deals specifically with cluttering (St. Louis, personal communication). As indicated earlier, when Preus' work was considered, there is a precedent for doing this.

Classification of participants as persistent or recovered

Case classification at teenage was based on three assessment instruments: (1) a report from one of the parents of the child who stuttered (Parent Report Form); (2) a report from the child who stuttered (Child Report Form); and (3) a set of ratings given by a trained researcher who interviewed the child and a parent for at least 40 minutes (Researcher Report Form). A full description and validation of these instruments, and cut-off points for each instrument, have been published (Howell, Davis, & Williams, 2009).

To be designated as persistent, the participant, parent, and researcher had to assess the participant as still stuttering. To be designated as recovered, the participant, parent, and researcher had to consider the participant as not stuttering. Similar criteria have been used previously by Davis, Shisca, and Howell (2007), Howell (2007), Howell et al. (2006), and Howell et al. (2008).

Procedures for assessing cluttering and reliability of judgements

Cluttering was assessed after the recordings at the two ages had been made. There is no agreed definition of cluttering, which makes its identification problematic. This is doubly difficult when attempting to identify cluttering from speech samples alone. The approach taken was to make these judgements in a variety of ways and see whether they were consistent with each other. The first way was to use a panel that employed the features given below that could be assessed on speech samples. Four listeners with experience of judging disfluent speech, of whom three were female and one was male, reviewed and discussed examples of cluttering not used for the experiment. They then judged the test samples on: (1) poor thinking (e.g. information or stories given out of sequence); (2) short attention span and comprehension (e.g. change of topic in mid utterance); and (3) fast speech. They assessed 45 participants (90 samples). They listened to the 90 samples of spontaneous speech, and nine samples were selected at random. Each judge assessed the speech independently. The responses permitted were 1 = only stuttering, 2 = only cluttering, 3 = both stuttering and cluttering present but more stuttering than cluttering, and 4 = both stuttering and cluttering present but more cluttering than stuttering. The criterion for classifying a participant as exhibiting cluttering was three out of four judges assessing the speech sample as 2, 3, or 4 on the scale. The criterion for classifying a participant as exhibiting stuttering was three out of four judges assessing the speech sample as 1 on the scale. Nine samples of cluttering were identified using these criteria.

The next way was to present these nine samples to two independent experts on cluttering who define cluttering in different ways (St. Louis et al., 2007; Ward, 2006). Thus some disagreement might be expected. The two experts were asked to confirm whether they would judge each sample as cluttered or not. They were not asked to judge all 90 samples because of the time commitment. All samples were confirmed as cluttering by one expert and eight of the nine by the other.

One of the expert judges declared what criteria he would use before making the judgements. He stated that he would look for evidence of a rate that was intermittently or continually too fast or too irregular (jerky), unnatural pauses, over-coarticulation (overly telescoped words, especially multisyllabic words), deletion of weak syllables entirely in rapid speech spurts, and/or excessive 'normal' disfluencies. He also indicated that verbal-mazes (Loban, 1976), along with the preceding characteristics, would make the diagnosis easier, but that he would not diagnose a clutterer based only on language that was incoherent (like the poorly organized thinking of Daly & Burnett-Stolnack, 1994). However, he believed that any stuttering that was present as well might make a cluttering diagnosis difficult because he considered that stuttering often masks cluttering. This did not appear to be the case in eight of the nine samples he judged.

The experts gave consistent classification of the cases that had been identified by the panel of four judges used initially. The judgement criteria that were provided by one of the experts were used on all samples for the final and definitive set of judgements (results reported below) made on all 96 participants (192 samples). The two authors used the criteria given by the expert independently to classify each sample on the 4-point scale used earlier. The classifications of the two expert judges were combined and the criterion for classifying a participant as exhibiting cluttering was that both judges assessed the speech sample as 2, 3, or 4 on the scale. The criterion for classifying a participant as exhibiting stuttering was that both judges assessed the speech sample as 1 on the scale. Twenty-three samples from seventeen participants were judged cluttered and the rest as stuttered.

Reliability of the latter procedure on the initial 45 participants was checked against those judgements made by the original panel. All cases judged cluttered by the initial panel (including the one that one of the experts considered not cluttering) were judged cluttered. No new cases of cluttering were judged to occur.

Epidemiological assessment

The parent of each participant designated as cluttering indicated the age at which fluency problems started. This was based on their assessment of when stuttering symptoms first emerged. This is appropriate as clutterers show the same types of disfluency as speakers who stutter, although events such as interjections, word repetitions, phrase repetitions, and unfinished words may be more frequent in cluttered speech (St. Louis et al., 2007). Parents were asked to date onset based on significant events in their child's personal history, such as at a particular birthday.

Distribution of cluttered samples over persistent and recovered cases and over ages were based on the information collected at the first assessment and teenage. Gender was reported by a parent. Handedness was assessed by establishing which hand the child used for the majority of everyday tasks (McManus, 2002). The children's responses were verified by the parent.

Severity assessment using SSI-3 as a measure of symptoms (occasions one and two)

SSI-3 scores (Riley, 1994) were obtained on both test occasions using the monologue, a dialogue, and an SSI-3 text, each of which had a minimum of 200 syllables. At the time these were recorded, a note was made of distracting sounds, facial grimaces, head movements, and any other body movements. These records were scored using Riley's (1994) guidelines. No attempt was made to distinguish cluttering from stuttering. Physical concomitants (or accessory behaviours) were noted for the SSI-3 assessments. These were examined separately (as well as part of SSI-3), as St. Louis et al. (2007) claim they are less frequent in cluttered speech.

Information collected for models of stuttering etiology

Central nervous system models—balance, posture, and complex movement for assessing cerebellar performance (Fawcett, Nicolson, & Dean, 1996)

Balance, posture, and complex movement were assessed at the time of the second recording, if time permitted. These tests were made for 7 participants who cluttered, for between 10 and 15 of the participants who recovered from their stuttering, and for between 13 and 24 participants who persisted in stuttering, depending on the test. Balance was defined as variation in weight-distribution over time and was measured using a SwayWeigh electronic force platform. Participants took off their shoes and stood upright on the active plate of the SwayWeigh while it was calibrated for their weight. Each participant was blindfolded and stood with the right foot on the active plate and the left foot on the fixed plate. After they were accustomed to the blindfold and weight was equally distributed between both legs, they stood as still as possible for 30 seconds while facing straight ahead. During this period, variation in weight distribution across the plates was recorded on a Picolog data-recording program running on a Dell PC. Variation was used as the dependent variable in the analyses. Balance measurements were obtained with the arms: (1) by the side and (2) outstretched with the palms of the hands facing down.

Procedures were the same in the postural stability conditions, except that participants were pushed lightly on the back and on the arms while they were blindfold, having previously been informed of what to expect. During each 30-second period, the participant was pushed on the back and on the upper arm from the right and left side by the experimenter, using the palm of the hand. Pressure was applied to each point for 1 second and then released. The experimenter exerted a pressure of approximately 2 kg (previously calibrated by practising pushing at 2 kg on kitchen scales). Analysis for reliability of the researcher's pushing pressure showed that this was accurate to ±3 percent. The dependent variable was the variation in weight distribution (from the equilibrium position, described above) over the 30-second period.

The complex movement tasks were past-pointing, finger-to-finger pointing, and finger-to-thumb opposition. In the past-pointing task, a bullseye target with ten concentric rings with radii increasing in 10 mm steps was fastened onto a wall at eye level and at arm's length from the child. A marker pen was held in the dominant hand. The participant had five practice attempts to hit the bullseye with the marker pen. He or she was then blindfolded and made ten test attempts (the pen marks providing a permanent record of performance). Each attempt was scored 10 for the bullseye and the score decreased by 1 for each subsequent ring. The 10 attempts for each participant were summed and gave a score of between 0 and 100.

For the finger-to-finger task, the participant placed the index finger of the non-dominant hand through a 10-mm-radius hole at the centre of a bullseye target. The target had four concentric rings that increased in radius by 10 mm each. Participants brought their index fingers together as quickly as possible. Each participant had two practice attempts and was then blindfolded and made five experimental attempts. Attempts scored five when fingers touched, and scores decreased by one for each ring. Attempts falling outside the target received no points. This gave a score of between 0 and 25 for each participant.

For the finger-to-thumb task, the index finger and thumb of one hand had to be placed on the thumb and finger, respectively, of the other hand. One contacting thumb–finger pair was kept together and the thumb turned clockwise and the finger and thumb of the other pair were released and turned counterclockwise until the finger and thumb touched again. At that point the other thumb and finger were moved in the reverse direction. Participants practised the sequence until they completed five movements fluently. They then performed the successive opposing movements 10 times, as fast as possible. The overall time taken to do this was recorded by stopwatch.

Central auditory processing—peripheral and central auditory assessments

Standard air-conducted pure tone audiograms were obtained at the time of the second recording. These indicated that hearing was within normal limits for all the participants whose data are reported below.

Reports of middle ear infection (otitis media with effusion, OME) were obtained by parental report from all 17 of the children classified as cluttering, and for 28 participants who stuttered who recovered and 29 participants who stuttered who persisted. OME is usually considered a peripheral, not a central, hearing problem. It is considered here that OME can affect communication and may be contributory to central auditory problems (Stephenson & Haggard, 1992).

Three further auditory assessments were made (pure tone threshold, simultaneous masking, and backward masking). The first two are estimates commonly used in assessments of the auditory abilities of participants, while the latter is regarded as an indication of central auditory processing. Pure tone thresholds were estimated for 8 participants who cluttered, 13 participants who recovered, and 15 participants who persisted. Simultaneous masking thresholds were estimated for 7 participants who cluttered, 8 participants who recovered, and 12 participants who persisted. Backward masking thresholds were estimated for 8 participants who cluttered, 13 participants who recovered, and 15 participants who persisted.

For all three conditions, the stimulus tone was a 1-kHz sine wave, 20 ms in duration, including 10 ms raised cosine onset and offset gradients. No masker was presented in the pure tone threshold condition. The masker for the simultaneous masking and backward masking conditions was a 300-ms band-limited white noise (Hartmann, 1979) with a spectrum level of 40 dB *re* 10^{-12} watts per Hz. The masker frequency range was 600–1400 Hz; representing a 1.16 octave-wide band centred at 916 Hz. In the simultaneous masking condition, the stimulus started 200 ms after the masking noise. In the backward masking condition, the 20-ms probe tone was presented immediately before the 300 ms burst of the masker.

The threshold estimation procedure was the same in all three conditions. A set of three test intervals was indicated to the participant on each trial. Two of the three intervals contained no sound and the other one contained the stimulus for the pure tone threshold condition. Two of the three intervals contained just the masking noise and the other one contained the masking noise and stimulus in the simultaneous and backward masking conditions. The position of the sound that contained the stimulus was varied at random for all conditions. An interval was indicated when the expression on one of three faces displayed on a computer screen changed from a neutral to an open-mouthed expression (these appeared in left-to-right sequence). The participant indicated which of the three intervals had contained the stimulus by clicking on the corresponding face graphic. Feedback was given by an appropriate change in the selected graphic (to a smile or a frown). Thresholds were determined using a Levitt (1971) tracking procedure and estimated to within 2 dB. Further details of the procedures are given in Howell et al. (2006).

Genetic models—family history of stuttering

Family history data were obtained from parents of 8 of the 17 children who cluttered, 29 children who recovered from stuttering, and 30 children who persisted in their stuttering. Assessments were made using questionnaires adapted from Janssen, Kloth, Kraaimaat, and Brutten (1996).

Results and discussion

Epidemiology

Judgements about cluttering and stuttering in the sample

Of the 192 samples, 23 (12.0 percent) were judged as cluttered. Out of the 96 participants, there were 17 participants who had at least one sample judged to be cluttered. Samples at the two ages were judged to be cluttered for six participants. Although Preus (1981) reported that about one-third of stutterers also manifested cluttering, the rate of cluttering in the current sample of participants was much lower.

Distribution of cluttered samples over ages, prevalence, and incidence rates in the sample of children who stuttered

Of the 23 samples judged to have been cluttered, 17 were from the first assessment. The null hypothesis is that half the samples should be from the first assessment and half from the second. A Sign test indicated that the observed distribution of instances over assessments was significantly different from 50/50 (p = .017). This supports the view that cluttering is more like forms of stuttering observed at the early, rather than the late, age. This offers incidental support for clutterers being more likely to recover fluency. Point prevalence at age 8 was 17.7 percent (17/96), prevalence at teenage was 6.25 percent (6/96) and incidence from age 8 to teenage was also 17.7 percent (and there were no new cases of cluttering at teenage).

Onset and course of disorder

AGE OF ONSET OF STUTTERING

The mean age of onset of stuttering for the participants who cluttered was 52.59 months (*SD* 20.26) compared with 49.07 months (*SD* 15.06) for the participants who recovered from stuttering and 50.34 months (*SD* 21.10) for the participants who persisted in stuttering. No significant differences were found between the groups by t test. Diedrich (1984) reported that onset of cluttering was later than for stuttering by about 7 years. The direction of age of onset of cluttering was consistent with this (although not significant).

Distribution of cluttered samples over persistent and recovered cases

The samples were next examined to see how the participants who cluttered were classified at the second assessment (i.e. whether they were designated as participants who persisted in, or recovered from, stuttering). Five of the six participants with two samples that were judged cluttered were from participants classified as persistent according to the criteria given in the method. These five participants showed that cluttering can develop into persistent stuttering. Alternatively, it may be that the addition of cluttering to the diagnosis increased the likelihood of stuttering becoming persistent. All 11 of the remaining participants were classified as recovered participants. Although more than twice the number of participants recovered (12) than persisted (5), this was not significantly higher than expected by chance (p = .072 by Sign test).

Recovery rate was examined for the 79 participants classified as stuttering with no signs of cluttering: 39 were classed as recovered and 40 as persistent. Overall recovery rate was 49.4 percent, which is lower than the rate for those judged to clutter (with 12/17 who recovered, or 70.6 percent). However, there was no association by χ^2 between recovery status and whether the participant cluttered or stuttered, $\chi^2(1) = 2.530$, $p = .112$). Although there was no definitive evidence that cluttering is more likely to be associated with recovery than persistence, the two reported effects were approaching significance (rate of recovery in the sample of clutterers and comparison over cluttered and stuttered for recovery/persistence). It seemed, therefore, advisable to compare cluttering participants separately from recovered and persistent stutterers in all remaining analyses where comparison with children who stutter was made.

Gender

Out of the 17 participants who cluttered, 15 (88.2 percent) were male compared with 32 of the 39 (82.1 percent) participants who recovered from stuttering. There was no significant association by χ^2 between gender and whether the participant cluttered or went on to recover from stuttering. Thirty-two out of the forty (80 percent) participants who persisted were male. In this case too, there was no association between gender and whether the participant cluttered or went on to persist in stuttering.

Handedness

Out of the 17 participants who cluttered, 14 (82.3 percent) were right-handed compared with 25 out of the 34 (73.5 percent) of the recovered, and 25 out of the 31 (80.7 percent) of the persistent participants who stuttered for whom we have information. A χ^2 test for association between cluttering and handedness was not significant. It is noteworthy that right-handedness was lower than in the population as a whole (usually considered to be 90 percent; McManus, 2002).

Symptomatology

Similar symptoms would be expected by those authors who see some continuity between cluttering and stuttering. In contrast, St. Louis et al. (2007) emphasize that the symptoms are not the same. The nearest we have to symptomatology are the SSI-3 estimates. As its name suggests, SSI-3 was developed for assessing stuttering severity and, if St. Louis et al. are correct, this instrument may not be ideal for assessing cluttering. To obtain an SSI-3 score, symptom counts are obtained and secondary behaviours are assessed separately. St. Louis et al. (2007) say that clutterers typically do not have accessory behaviours. We tested for differences between SSI-3 scores and for differences between accessory behaviours across test occasions one and two for all three groups.

Symptomatology at first assessment

SSI-3 total scores are presented as box and whisker diagrams for recovered, persistent, and cluttering participants at first and second recordings in Figure 5.1. The top and bottom edges of the boxes indicate interquartile ranges (25–75 percent of scores fall within these points), and the whiskers are the low and high scores (there was one outlier in the cluttering group).

The data from the second test occasion are discussed further below. Examination of SSI-3 total scores on the initial test occasion showed that the participants who persisted in their stuttering had higher scores (SSI-3 = 31.37) than those who recovered (24.25) and those who cluttered (23.88). Using Tukey's honestly significant differences test (HSD) on these SSI-3 total scores showed that participants who persisted had significantly higher scores than those who recovered and those who cluttered, but that the scores of the participants who recovered did not differ significantly from those who cluttered.

The data from the physical concomitants (secondary symptoms) section of the SSI-3 were examined separately. The box and whisker diagrams showing the SSI-3 physical concomitants scores for the persistent, recovered and cluttering participants at first and second assessment are shown in Figure 5.2.

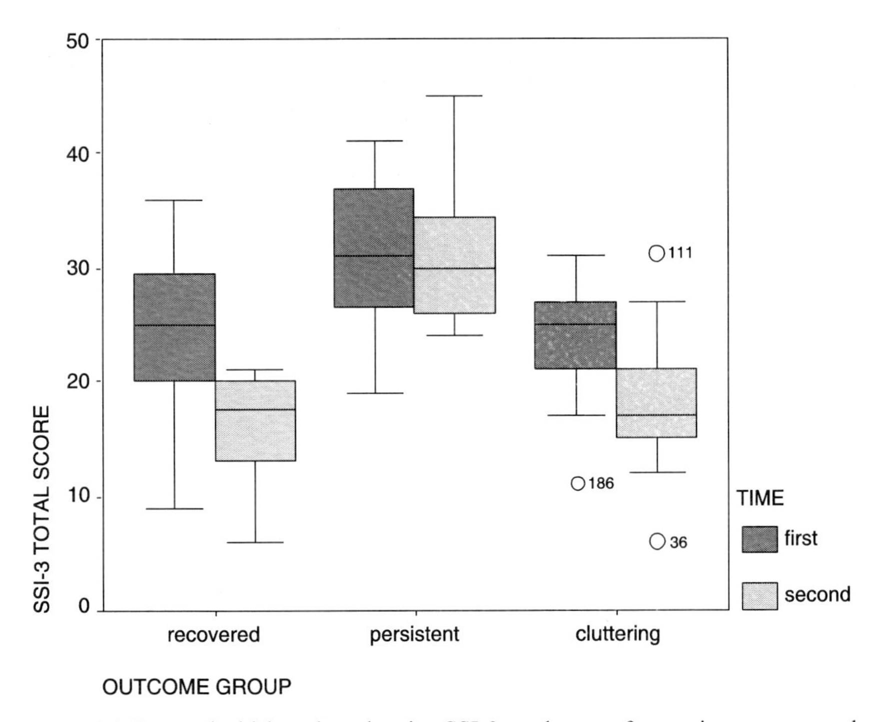

Figure 5.1 Box and whisker plots showing SSI-3 total scores for persistent, recovered, and cluttering groups at first and second assessment.

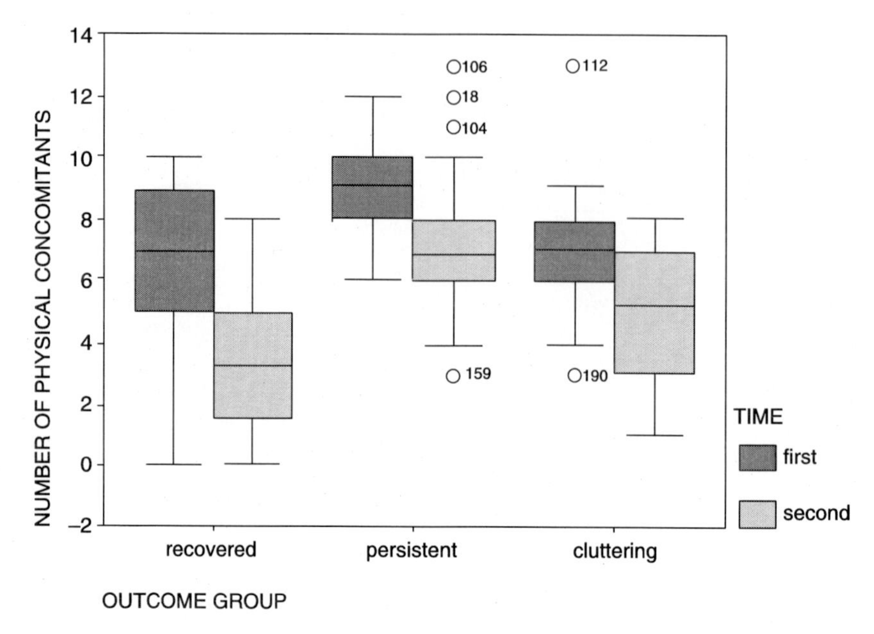

Figure 5.2 Box and whisker plots showing SSI-3 physical concomitants (accessory behaviour) scores for persistent, recovered, and cluttering groups at first and second assessment.

There were two outliers in the cluttering group on the first test occasion and four outliers in the persistent group on the second test occasion.

Examination of SSI-3 physical concomitants scores on the initial test occasion showed that the participants who persisted in their stuttering had higher scores (SSI-3 physical concomitants mean score = 9.05) than those who recovered (6.78) and those who cluttered (7.29). Tukey's HSD confirmed that this pattern was statistically significant (the participants who persisted had significantly higher physical concomitants scores than those who recovered and those who cluttered, but that the scores of the participants who recovered did not differ significantly from those who cluttered).

Symptomatology at teenage

On the second test occasion, SSI-3 total scores showed that the participants who persisted in their stuttering had higher mean scores (SSI-3 = 30.53) than those who recovered (15.92) and those who cluttered (17.82). Tukey's HSD on the SSI-3 total scores showed that participants who persisted had significantly higher scores than those who recovered and those who cluttered, but that the scores of the participants who recovered did not differ significantly from those who cluttered.

Examination of the box and whisker plots in Figure 5.1 showed that little change in SSI-3 total scores occurred across test sessions for the persistent participants (SSI-3 scores remained at the high level, as would be expected if stuttering continued). The profiles of the participants who recovered and those who cluttered were similar, with both groups showing no overlap in the interquartile ranges across test sessions.

Examination of SSI-3 physical concomitants scores on the second test occasion showed that the participants who persisted in their stuttering had higher scores (SSI-3 physical concomitants = 7.42) than those who recovered (3.39) and those who cluttered (4.47). Tukey's HSD showed that participants who persisted had significantly higher physical concomitants scores than those who recovered and those who cluttered, but that the scores of the participants who recovered did not differ significantly from those who cluttered.

Models of cluttering aetiology

It is cautioned that there are limited amounts of data that address the aetiological factors. St. Louis et al. discuss four categories where models of cluttering have been offered: (1) central nervous system function models; (2) cognitive processing capabilities models; (3) genetic models; and (4) models that propose a link between cluttering and stuttering. The first three are commented on here (the fourth was addressed in the symptomatology section).

Central nervous systems models

Dalton and Hardcastle (1989) argued for cluttering being associated with basal ganglia problems on the grounds that clutterers show similarity to people with hypokinetic dysarthria. We have argued (based on some evidence of our own and scanning) for cerebellar problems being involved in stuttering. If cluttering is rooted in basal ganglia problems and stuttering in cerebellar problems, participants who stutter (recovered and persistent) should show differences in performance on tasks that assess cerebellar ability. (Also see Alm, chapter 1 this volume.)

Performance on each of the seven cerebellar performance measures was compared using independent *t* tests. As indicated in the Method section, data were available from 7 participants who cluttered and between 10 and 15 of the participants, depending on the test, who recovered from their stuttering. No significant differences between the two groups were found.

Cerebellar performance was available for the 7 participants who cluttered and for between 13 and 24 participants who persisted in stuttering. Again there were no significant differences between the participant groups.

Cognitive processing capabilities models—central auditory processing

PERIPHERAL HEARING PROBLEMS (OME) THAT MAY IMPACT ON CENTRAL AUDITORY PROBLEMS

Otitis media with effusion (OME) is a problem of the middle ear system that is relatively common in children, and it can affect speech. Out of the 17 participants with cluttering, 5 (29.4 percent) were reported to have experienced repeated middle ear infections compared with 9 out of the 28 (32.1 percent) participants who stuttered who recovered for whom we have information. The χ^2 test for association between cluttering and OME was not significant. Four out of the five (80.0 percent) affected participants who cluttered were fitted with ventilation tubes compared with five out of the nine (55.5 percent) participants who stuttered who recovered.

For the participants who persisted, 7 out of the 29 (24.1 percent) participants had repeated middle ear infections. The χ^2 test that examined the association between cluttering and OME was not significant. Four out of the seven (57.1 percent) participants who persisted had ventilation tubes fitted.

ASSESSMENT OF CENTRAL AUDITORY FUNCTIONING

Threshold estimates for three masking procedures were available for some participants. Data were available from 7 or 8 participants who cluttered and 8–13 participants who recovered from stuttering (depending on the threshold test). Independent *t* tests showed no significant difference between the groups for any of the three procedures.

Masking thresholds were also available on three masking procedures for 12–15 participants who went on to persist in their stuttering. Independent *t*-tests again showed no significant differences between the groups for any of the three procedures.

Genetic models

Family history was reported to be associated more often with cluttering than with stuttering. For example, Freund (1952) reported respective rates of 93 percent and 51 percent.

Family history of stuttering data were available using the modified Janssen et al. (1996) questionnaire. Parents of 8 out of the 17 (47.1 percent) participants who cluttered reported that there were people who stuttered in their immediate family (first, second, or third degree relatives), compared with 16 out of the 29 (55.2 percent) parents of the participants who recovered for whom the information was available. This is in the opposite direction to what Freund reported. Analysis by χ^2 showed that there was no significant association between family history of stuttering and whether the participant cluttered or went on to recover from stuttering.

Out of the 30 participants who persisted in their stutter for whom we have information, 18 (60.0 percent) had a positive family history. Again there was no significant association by χ^2 between family history of stuttering and whether the participant cluttered or persisted in their stuttering.

General discussion

The three different methods for classifying cluttering identified the same cases as clutterers even though the criteria varied. This is not surprising for the judgements made by the two international experts on selected samples and the authors' judgements on all samples, as the latter used the criteria declared by one of the experts. It is more surprising that the characteristic list used in the first assessments, which was drawn from a number of reports, led to similar classification of cases. However, the list did include one criterion that was also used in the other two methods (speech rate). Rate may, in turn, impact on coarticulatory effects that were included as criteria in the last two methods. Also, poorly organized thinking on the list may be related to mazes, which were also included in the last two methods. The similarity in the judgements across methods may, then, be due to similar characteristics being termed differently although they still have the same underlying basis.

Twelve per cent of all samples were judged to be cluttered. Significantly more of these occurred at the younger than the older test ages (17.7 percent versus 6.25 percent). This indicated that cluttering is less common at older ages.

Cluttering had a later onset than stuttering, as Diedrich (1984) reported, although this was not significant. All children were designated with respect to whether they stuttered at teenage or not. Five children were classed as persistent and twelve as recovered. The five cases showed that cluttering can change into stuttering (as argued by: Freund, 1934; Hunt, 1870; Preus, 1973; Weiss, 1964). However, although cluttering can lead to stuttering, this happened in a minority of cases. So proponents of the view that stuttering is distinct from cluttering may draw support from this (Daly & Burnett-Stolnack, 1994; Myers & St Louis, 1992; St. Louis et al., 1985; van Riper, 1992; Ward, 2006). Gender and handedness rates did not differ over the three groups, so there are no grounds for concluding that stuttering differs from cluttering for these factors.

Post-hoc examination of SSI-3 scores obtained at the first test occasion showed that those of the recovered and cluttering participants were lower than those of the persistent ones. The persistent participants showed little change in SSI-3 scores across test occasions. The recovered participants showed a reduction over test occasions, and there was no overlap between SSI-3 scores of this group on test occasion two and the corresponding scores of the persistent group. Davis et al. (2007) reported SSI-3 scores for eight fluent speakers whose ages corresponded with those at the second test occasion here. The scores ranged from 8 (very mild) to 17 (mild). Comparison of these values with those for the recovered speakers on the second test occasion show there is a large degree of overlap. Thus, the recovered participants appear to have SSI-3 scores similar to fluent speakers. The participants who cluttered showed a similar pattern to the recovered participants, though there was some overlap on occasion two, due in part to one of the participants being classed as persistent. On this basis, cluttering again seems more similar to recovered forms of stuttering than it does to persistent forms. This contradicts the observations of Langova and Moravek, who assert that 'Cluttering arises in childhood, worsens in puberty and persists as a rule throughout life' (1970, p. 325). Van Riper and other experienced experts also agree that cluttering gets worse with age. It is possible that the lower SSI-3 scores at intake impacted on the way fluency subsequently developed. The secondary symptoms or accessory behaviours also showed a similar pattern between the cluttering and recovered participants and differences with the persistent participants.

None of the three aetiological factors (central nervous system, central processing problems, and family history) showed any difference across the three groups. Either all three groups are affected equally by these aetiological factors or there is no difference in the aetiologies of cluttering, and persistent and recovered forms of stuttering. The latter interpretation could suggest that cluttering is not distinct from stuttering.

Conclusion

To summarize overall, there were few differences between the clutterers and either group who stuttered. The main differences to emphasize are that more samples were judged cluttered at the earlier age than teenage, and there were marginal suggestions that cluttering tended to be associated with recovered forms of stuttering.

Caveats

Researchers who take different points of view about cluttering could look at different features of these data and draw some support. Thus, instead of comparing cluttering with recovered or persistent stuttering, which supported the idea of a relationship between cluttering and recovered forms of stuttering, other authors could point to the fact that in the majority of cases cluttering progresses into fluent speech and does not turn into stuttering, suggesting that these two forms are not related.

All the cases of cluttering here were obtained through stuttering clinics. As the expert who declared his criteria commented, the presence of concurrent stuttering with cluttering may mask the symptoms of cluttering. If this is so, the only way of studying cluttering would be by using pure cases and these are rare.

This study has focused on participants who stutter and the conclusions are specific to the ages from 8 to teenage. As we have said, there are rare reports of cases of cluttering in adulthood. However, there are no reports about their speech or performance on tasks such as those described here. Pure cluttering needs to be investigated further.

Future research

More extensive tests on participants who clutter are required in order to examine the relationship between cluttering and stuttering, to distinguish between the two views outlined earlier. Ideally, participants who only clutter need to be located. Tests need to be conducted at earlier ages (i.e. younger than 8), as has been done with children who stutter (Yairi & Ambrose, 2005).

Clinical implications

The study has clinical implications. Clinicians need to know if they should attempt a differential diagnosis between cluttering and early forms of stuttering (at around age 8). The present results show that this would be possible using the features employed by the judges.

Acknowledgements

This work was supported by grant 072639 from the Wellcome Trust to Peter Howell. Address correspondence to: Peter Howell, Division of Psychology and Language Sciences, University College London, Gower Street, London WC1E 6BT, England. E-mail: p.howell@ucl.ac.uk Thanks to Drs St. Louis and Ward for giving their time to serve as expert judges on cluttering. Thanks also to Susanne Rosenberger, Charlene Simons, and Eleanor Bailey who helped by making the preliminary assessments.

References

Alm, P. A. (2004). Stuttering and the basal ganglia circuits: A critical review of possible relations. *Journal of Communication Disorders*, *37*, 325–369.

American Psychiatric Association. (1994). *Diagnostic and statistical manual of mental disorders* (4th ed.). Washington, DC: American Psychiatric Association.

American Psychiatric Association (2000). *Diagnostic and statistical manual of mental disorders* (4th ed., text rev.).Washington, DC: American Psychiatric Association.

Andrews, G., & Harris, M. (1964). *The syndrome of stuttering*. Clinics in Developmental Medicine (No. 17). London: Heinemann.

Dalton, P., & Hardcastle, W. (1989). *Disorders of fluency and their effect on communication* (2nd ed.). London: Elsevier North Holland.

Daly, D. A., & Burnett-Stolnack, M. L. (1994). *Differential diagnosis of cluttering and stuttering for individualized treatment planning*. Presented at the annual convention of the American Speech-Language-Hearing Association, New Orleans.

Davis, S., Shisca, D., & Howell, P. (2007). Anxiety in speakers who persist and recover from stuttering. *Journal of Communication Disorders*, *40*, 398–417.

Diedrich, W. M. (1984). Cluttering: Its diagnosis. In H. Winitz (Ed.), *Treating articulation disorders: For clinicians by clinicians* (pp. 307–323). Baltimore, MD: University Park Press.

Fawcett, A. J., Nicolson, R. I., & Dean, P. (1996). Impaired performance of children with dyslexia on a range of cerebellar tasks. *Annals of Dyslexia*, *46*, 259–283.

Fox, P. T., Ingham, R. J., Ingham, J. C., Hirsch, T., Downs, H., Martin, C., et al. (1996). A PET study of the neural systems of stuttering. *Nature*, *382*, 158–162.

Freund, H. (1934). Relationship between stuttering and cluttering. *Monatsschrift für Ohrenheilkunde, LXVIII*.

Freund, H. (1952). Studies in the interrelationship between stuttering and cluttering. *Folia Phoniatrica*, *4*, 146–168.

Hartmann, W. M. (1979). *Signals, sound, and sensation*. New York: AIP Press.

Howell, P. (2007). Signs of developmental stuttering up to age eight and at 12 plus. *Clinical Psychology Review*, *27*, 287–306.

Howell, P., Davis, S., & Williams, R. (2008). Late childhood stuttering. *Journal of Speech, Language and Hearing Research*, *51*, 669–687.

Howell, P., Davis, S., & Williams, R. (2009). The effects of bilingualism on speakers who stutter during late childhood. *Archives of Disease in Childhood*, *94*, 42–46.

Howell, P., Davis, S., & Williams, S. M. (2006). Auditory abilities of teenage speakers who persisted, or recovered, from stuttering. *Journal of Fluency Disorders*, *31*, 257–270.

Hunt, J. (1870). *Stammering and stuttering: Their nature and treatment* (7th ed.). London: Longmans, Green and Co.

Janssen, P., Kloth, S., Kraaimaat, F., & Brutten, G. (1996). Genetic factors in stuttering: A replication of Ambrose, Yairi and Cox's (1993) study with adult probands. *Journal of Fluency Disorders*, *21*, 105–108.

Langova, J., & Moravek, M. (1970). Some problems of cluttering. *Folia Phoniatrica et Logopaedica*, *22*, 325–336.

Levitt, H. (1971). Transformed up-down methods in psychoacoustics. *Journal of the Acoustical Society of America*, *49*, 467–477.

Loban, W. (1976). *The language of elementary school children*. Champaign, IL: National Council of Teachers of English.

Luchsinger, R., & Arnold, G. E. (1965). *Voice–speech–language. Clinical communicology: Its physiology and pathology*. Belmont, CA: Wadsworth.

McManus, I. C. (2002). *Right hand, left hand*. London: Weidenfeld & Nicolson.

Molt, L. F. (1996). An examination of various aspects of auditory processing in clutterers. *Journal of Fluency Disorders*, *21*, 215–223.

Myers, F. K., & St. Louis, K. O. (1992). *Cluttering: A clinical perspective*. Leicester, UK: Far Communications.

Preus, A. (1973). Stuttering in Down's syndrome. In Y. Lebrun & R. Hoops (Eds.), *Neurolinguistic approaches to stuttering* (pp. 90–100). The Hague: Mouton.

Preus, A. (1981). *Identifying subgroups of stutterers*. Oslo: Uniersiteitsforlaget.

Preus, A. (1992). Cluttering and stuttering. Related, different or antagonistic disorders? In F. K. Myers & K. O. St. Louis (Eds.), *Cluttering: A clinical perspective* (pp. 55–70). Leicester, UK: Far Communications.

Riley, G. D. (1994). *Stuttering severity instrument for children and adults* (3rd ed.). Austin, TX: Pro-Ed.

Stephenson, H., & Haggard, M. (1992). Rationale and design of surgical trials for otitis media with effusion. *Clinical Otolaryngology*, *17*, 67–78.

St. Louis, K. O., Hinzman, A. R., & Hull, E. M. (1985). Studies of cluttering: Disfluency and language measures in young possible clutterers and stutterers. *Journal of Fluency Disorders*, *10*, 151–172.

St. Louis, K. O., Myers, F. M., Bakker, K., & Raphael, L. J. (2007). Understanding and treating cluttering. In R. F. Curlee & E. G. Conture (Eds.), *Stuttering and related disorders of fluency* (3rd ed., pp. 297–325). New York: Thieme.

van Riper, C. (1992). Foreword. In F. L. Myers & K. O. St. Louis (Eds.), *Cluttering: A clinical perspective* (p. vii). Leicester, UK: Far Communications.

Ward, D. (2006). *Stuttering and cluttering: frameworks for understanding and treatment*. Hove, UK: Psychology Press.

Weiss, D. A. (1936). Cluttering and its treatment. *Monatsschrift für Ohrenheilkunde, LXX*.

Weiss, D. A. (1964). *Cluttering*. Englewood Cliffs, NJ: Prentice-Hall.

Wolk, L. (1986). Cluttering: A diagnostic case report. *British Journal of Disorders of Communication*, *21*, 199–207.

World Health Organization. (1982). *International statistical classification of diseases and related health problems, ninth revision clinical manual* (ICD-9-CM). Geneva: World Health Organization.

Wright, B. A., Lombardino, L. J., King, W. M., Puranik, C. S., Leonard, C. M., & Merzenich, M. M. (1997). Deficits in auditory-temporal and spectral resolution in language-impaired children. *Nature*, *387*, 176–178.

Yairi, E., & Ambrose, N. G. (2005). *Early childhood stuttering*. Austin, TX: Pro-Ed.

6 Cluttering and Down syndrome

John Van Borsel

Introduction

There is probably no other condition that has been more frequently referred to when discussing the occurrence of cluttering than Down syndrome. Down syndrome (DS), resulting from trisomy 21, is a well-known condition. With an incidence of 1 in 600–700 births, it is the most frequently occurring chromosomal abnormality (Lambert & Rondal, 1979). The condition is characterized by some typical physical characteristics such as a short stature, a flat occiput, small and slanting palpebral fissures, epicanthic folds (skin folds of the upper eyelid covering the inner corner of the eye), a depressed nasal bridge, a small nose, and an overlarge tongue relative to the size of the mouth (Pueschel, 1988). The syndrome is also associated with behavioural characteristics, including the presence of speech and language problems (Rondal & Buckley, 2003).

Already in 1866 John Langdon Down made reference to the speech of individuals with the syndrome called after him in terms that would seem to fit in with a diagnosis of cluttering. Langdon Down characterized the speech of those with DS as 'thick and indistinct' (Down, 1866, p. 261). It was not until the 1950s, however, that more systematic investigation into the speech of individuals with Down syndrome was undertaken, and that the possibility of cluttering as a speech diagnosis was considered. A review of the relevant literature highlights one major recurrent theme, namely the question whether the disfluent speech in Down syndrome represents stuttering or indeed cluttering. At the same time, this literature illustrates the definitional problems of cluttering in general and the problem of diagnosing cluttering in individuals with more complex conditions.

Cluttering or stuttering?

Disfluent speech appears to be very common in individuals with DS, and several authors have reported an unusually high prevalence of stuttering in this population. Figures range between 15 and 48 percent (Bloodstein,

1995). The only exception to this trend is in data reported by Martyn, Sheehan, and Slutz (1969). In their sample of 42 participants, stuttering was found in only one participant (1/42 or 2.3 percent). Several authors have also argued, however, that the disfluent speech in individuals with DS does not represent stuttering but cluttering.

The first study to argue that the disfluent speech in DS represents cluttering appears to be that of Cabanas (1954), who reported speech and voice therapy findings over a 2-year period in 50 individuals with DS (aged 5 to 15 years). Cabanas concluded that the participants in his study demonstrated cluttering rather than stuttering because of the absence of secondary behaviours. Weiss (1964) and Van Riper (1971) expressed the same opinion. According to Van Riper, most of the individuals with DS are not aware that they demonstrate fluency failures. He quotes the example of a child with DS repeating the first syllable of his name 18 times without showing any signs of frustration. Otto and Yairi (1975), in a study that compared the spontaneous speech samples of 19 institutionalized, non-stuttering individuals with DS and 19 normally intelligent individuals, concluded that cluttering more correctly characterized speech in DS. Their conclusion was not based, however, on a lack of awareness of a speech defect but on the high speaking rate observed in many of their participants. Farmer and Brayton (1979) also concluded that the disfluent speech of 6 of their 13 subjects with DS represented cluttering rather than stuttering, but forwarded yet another argument. They refer to their participants' poor ratings of intelligibility.

Apart from the claim that the disfluent speech in DS represents cluttering rather than stuttering, it has also been suggested that both disorders can occur in this population, and that they may even coexist in the same individual. Preus (1973) studied 47 DS participants in two Norwegian institutes for the mentally retarded. He concluded that the disfluencies found in patients with DS may be classified as genuine stuttering. In one-third of his participants, he observed secondary symptoms in the form of body movements, devices of masking (e.g. pretending to cough or changing word order when blocking on a sound), and other postponement and avoidance behaviours, indicating proof of a 'conscious experience of stuttering'. Preus added, however, that the presence of stuttering in the speech of individuals with DS does not rule out the possibility that cluttering may also be found. Only 27.7 percent of the participants were diagnosed as pure stutterers, 12.7 percent were diagnosed as pure clutterers, and 19.2 percent as combined cases. Of the total sample, 40.4 percent displayed neither stuttering nor cluttering.

One logical approach to try to find out if the disfluent speech in individuals with DS represents stuttering or cluttering would be to have a closer look at the disfluencies and other speech patterns to see how these compare to what is typically seen in stuttering and in cluttering respectively. Such an exercise is not as straightforward as it may seem at first, one problem being the scantiness of data.

Comparison with stuttering

As far as the comparison with stuttering is concerned, it appears that the nature of the disfluencies in individuals with DS is not different from that of individuals with developmental stuttering not associated with DS. Cabanas (1954), for instance, found blocks, hesitations, and repetitions in DS participants. Schlanger and Gottsleben (1957) reported the presence of clonic, tonic, and secondary reactions but did not further specify these patterns. Willcox (1988) described repetitions of sounds, syllables, words and phrases, and prolongations. According to Evans (1977), repetitions are most frequent, followed by interjections, prolongations, and blocks. Thus, like in stuttering not associated with DS, patterns signify a combination of both stuttering disfluencies and normal disfluencies.

Looking at the distribution of disfluencies, Cabanas (1954) claimed that in individuals with DS, disfluencies occur not predominantly on consonants, but mostly on vowels. Also disfluencies would not occur systematically on the same sounds, but might occasionally affect any sound. In this respect, Cabanas contends the fluency failures demonstrated by individuals with DS would be different from developmental stuttering. Willcox (1988), however, who examined fluency in five children with DS in relation to those of five developmentally normal subjects matched for language age, found no particular sounds in either group that occurred more frequently in disfluencies. Willcox (1988) also provides details on the frequency of repetitions, duration of prolongations, and the locus of the disfluencies in the five children with DS she studied. All but one participant produced examples of three repetitions of a unit, while two participants demonstrated examples of four or more repetitions of a unit. Three of the five children produced prolongations of more than 1 second. These disfluencies tended to occur on the first stressed element in the head, or on the nucleus of the tone unit, and they almost invariably occurred at the beginning of a word. This would be expected to be the case in most developmental stuttering children as well.

As pointed out above, a number of authors concluded that the disfluencies in individuals with DS differ from those in individuals with developmental stuttering, in that they are not accompanied by secondary behaviours. There is no consensus on this point, however. Others did report the occurrence of secondary behaviours in individuals with DS, such as avoidance and postponement behaviour, and synkinesias such as facial grimaces or blinking the eyes (Devenny and Silverman, 1990; Preus, 1973; Stansfield, 1990). Hence, the presence or absence of secondary behaviours does not clearly differentiate the speech associated with DS from developmental stuttering.

Comparison with cluttering

A comparison of the speech pattern of individuals with DS with what is typically seen in cluttering not only suffers from a lack of data but is moreover hampered by a lack of consensus on what constitutes the distinguishing characteristics of cluttering. In the past, investigators concluding that the speech of individuals with DS represents cluttering have almost always based their conclusion on a limited number of features (for instance, the absence of secondary features, a high speech rate, poor intelligibility), which they assume to be characteristic of the disorder. Currently, the prevailing opinion is that cluttering is a multifaceted disorder that may include a wider range of features (see St. Louis & Schulte, chapter 14 this volume).

In an attempt to investigate the occurrence of cluttering in individuals with DS, taking into account the range of symptoms that may be found in cluttering, Van Borsel and Vandermeulen (2008) recently asked speech-language therapists having clients with DS on their caseload to administer the Predictive Cluttering Inventory (PCI; Daly & Cantrell, 2006). The latter instrument was developed by having 60 recognized fluency specialists educated and trained in different programs around the world rate and rank-order 50 signs and symptoms believed to be characteristic of cluttering. The PCI contains 33 items covering 4 domains (pragmatics, speech-motor, language-cognition, motor coordination-writing problems). Each item is scored on a 5-point rating scale indicating how often the behaviour is observed (1 = almost never, 2 = infrequently, 3 = sometimes, 4 = frequently, 5 = almost always), yielding a total possible score of 165. A score of 80 or more classifies a client as a person with cluttering, while scores from 40 to 79 are believed to indicate a diagnosis of 'clutterer-stutterer'. Twenty-six speech-language therapists completed a total of 76 surveys of individuals with DS, 51 of which were male and 24 of which were female (in one individual gender was not disclosed). Age of these individuals ranged from 3.8 years to 57.3 years (mean 22.8 years). The contributing speech-language therapists were not told that the questionnaire they were invited to complete was an instrument to diagnose possible cluttering, nor that the purpose of the study was to investigate the occurrence of cluttering in individuals with DS.

The results of the investigation were quite impressive. The proportion of participants with a score indicative of cluttering proved extremely high. Of the 76 participants, 60 (i.e. 78.9 percent) obtained a score that classified them as persons with cluttering (PWC) and 13 other participants (i.e. 17.1 percent) qualified as a clutterer-stutterer. These figures are all the more remarkable as the individuals in this study were not selected for the presence of disfluencies in their speech. Moreover, in a considerable number of the questionnaires (> 65 percent), not all items had been scored, thus compromising strict interpretation of the PCI. It is possible that these elevated figures represent a sampling error and that the majority of participants in the study were indeed PWC. A more likely explanation, however, is that these figures reflect the definitional problem that currently still surrounds cluttering. In the PCI, certain deficits in the domain of pragmatics and language-cognition are included as symptoms of cluttering. An analysis of the responses for the individuals who were classified as PWC showed that four of the five items with the highest scores on average belonged to the domains of pragmatics and language-cognition. Furthermore, pragmatics was also the domain with the lowest number of unscored items, followed by the language-cognition domain. It is presently unclear to what extent language and pragmatic problems are really implicated in the diagnosis of cluttering. St. Louis, Raphael, Myers, and Bakker (2003), for instance, did not include language difficulties and pragmatic problems in their working definition of cluttering. Interestingly, Preus (1973) pointed out that his findings did not apply to individuals with DS who have less developed language proficiency than those in his study. The results of the study by Van Borsel and Vandermeulen (2008) thus clearly illustrate the need for a consensus on the symptoms that are essential for a diagnosis of cluttering. They also point to a more general problem, namely that of diagnosing cluttering in individuals with a more complex condition.

Diagnosing cluttering in individuals with a more complex condition

Down syndrome was perhaps the first condition to be associated with a high prevalence of cluttering, but it is certainly not the only condition. Several authors have also suggested that the speech of individuals with Fragile X can be diagnosed as cluttering (Chudley & Hagerman, 1987; Grisby, Kemper, Hagerman, & Myers 1990; Hanson, Jackson, & Hagerman, 1986; Scharfenaker, 1990; Vilkman, Niemi, & Ikonen, 1988). Fragile X syndrome is the second most frequent cause of mental retardation of genetic origin after Down syndrome (Goldson & Hagerman, 1992; Turner, Webb, Wake, & Robinson, 1996) and is caused by a defect on the long arm of the X-chromosome. Disfluent speech is considered such a typical characteristic of Fragile X syndrome that it is among the 13 items of the checklist for screening Fragile X developed by Hagerman (1987). A diversity of labels have been used to characterize the speech of individuals with Fragile X, including a perseverative speech pattern, a repetitive speech pattern, disfluent speech, stuttering, fast speech, disrhythmia, verbal apraxia, developmental apraxia, and also cluttering. Characteristics referred to in respect to a diagnosis of cluttering (see St. Louis & Schulte, chapter 14 this volume) in this population are the fast and fluctuating speech rate, the occurrence of bursts of speech, and slurred articulation. Even less data are available, however, than for DS to substantiate the claim that the disfluencies observed in individuals with Fragile X syndrome represent cluttering. With regard to a fast speech rate, it should at any rate be remarked that this is not a constant feature in this syndrome. In a study investigating the disfluencies in the speech of French-speaking individuals with Fragile X syndrome, Van Borsel, Dor, and Rondal (2008) found a speech rate below the 4 to 6 or 7 syllables per second (which has been recorded as normal for French speakers) in 8 of their 9 participants.

Yet another syndrome with a high prevalence of disfluent speech that to some extent is consistent with a diagnosis of cluttering is Tourette syndrome (TS). Tourette syndrome, named after the French physician, Georges Gilles de la Tourette, is characterized by the presence of multiple motor tics and one or more vocal tics that cause marked distress or significant impairment in social, occupational, or other important areas of functioning (American Psychiatric Association, 1987). Just like in Down syndrome, the fluency failures of those with Tourette syndrome have often been diagnosed as stuttering, and estimates of the incidence of stuttering in this population are remarkably high, ranging from 15.3 percent to 31.3 percent (Comings & Comings, 1993; Pauls, Leckman, & Cohen, 1993). Stuttering is also listed as one of the initial symptoms of the Tourette's complex in t*he Diagnostic and Statistical Manual of Mental Disorders* (*DSM IV*) (American Psychiatric Association, 1987). A number of studies that investigated more closely the nature of the fluency failures in individuals with Tourette syndrome show, however, that the disfluencies displayed do not conform to the classic pattern of stuttering. Rassas Cohn et al. (1983), who studied the disfluencies in a 25-year-old male with Tourette syndrome, reported that in spontaneous speech only one-fifth of their subject's fluency failures were stuttered disfluencies. Similar findings were arrived at by Van Borsel and Vanryckeghem (2000) in an 18-year-old male with Tourette syndrome, in a study involving three Tourette children (aged 9 years 11 months, 12 years 7 months, and 12 years 2 months) (Van Borsel, Goethals, & Vanryckeghem, 2004), and in a larger study of participants with TS (De Nil, Sasisekaran, Van Lieshout, & Sandor, 2005). It is mainly the preponderance of a substantial number of non-stuttering disfluencies such as interjections, phrase repetitions and whole-word repetitions, and also possibly the frequent occurrence of incomplete phrases and revisions (suggestive of disorganized wording), that point to a diagnosis of cluttering in Tourette syndrome.

The observation of a high incidence of fluency failures that somehow resemble cluttering in Down syndrome and in some other syndromes like Fragile X syndrome and Tourette syndrome stands in sharp contrast to the general consensus that cluttering is quite rare (Perkins, 1977; Weiss, 1964). Such observations warrant an explanation.

One possibility is that individuals with a more complex condition such as Down syndrome and others simply display more of the symptoms that have been considered to be part of cluttering. In this respect it is interesting to remember that a meta-analysis of 29 cases reported in a special issue of the *Journal of Fluency Disorders* devoted to cluttering showed reference to over 50 different cluttering symptoms (St. Louis, 1996). The high incidence of cluttering in conditions such as Down syndrome then may be no more than the result of a lack of consensus on which features are essential to a diagnosis of cluttering. As Ward put it, cluttering at the moment constitutes 'a broad church' indeed (2006, p. 151).

Another possibility is that the speech in individuals with DS and other conditions does not represent cluttering. This would imply that there are at least some features that set the speech in such conditions apart from what is normally seen in, or at least is considered typical of, cluttering. As far as DS is concerned, it is perhaps significant that in the study of Van Borsel and Vandermeulen (2008), the proportion of individuals classified as a PWC was slightly higher in the female participants than in the male participants. This is at odds with what has been reported in previous studies and also contradicts the professional opinion about the sex ratio in cluttering. Arnold (1960), for instance, reported a male to female ratio in cluttering of 4 to 1, just like in stuttering. Surveys in the USA by St. Louis and Hinzman (1986) and in the UK by St. Louis and Rustin (1996), involving respectively 156 and 130 speech-language pathologists, have shown that professionals agree that there is a male to female preponderance in cluttering, without agreement, though, about the exact ratio (6.1 to 1 in the former study versus 3.0 to 1 in the latter).

If the speech in individuals with DS and other conditions does not represent cluttering, and as suggested above, is not consistent with patterns of genuine stuttering either, then the question arises how the fluency failures in these conditions should be labelled. Perhaps the fluency disorders associated with certain genetic syndromes constitute a subtype of disfluency of their own. It is not impossible either that the fluency failures in DS (and similarly in other syndromes) are even syndrome specific. Some decades ago, Adler (1976) pointed out the possibility that specific genetic syndromes may cause specific speech and language disorders. It is only recently, however, that research into this area really developed. What seems needed is research that compares the speech of individuals with Down syndrome with that of developmental stutterers, with that of PWC, and with that of individuals with other genetic syndromes, taking into account variables such as age, gender, degree of mental retardation, and the presence of other speech and language disorders. What is equally crucial is, of course, a consensus on what constitutes the essential features of cluttering. Only then can the question be answered as to whether the disfluent speech in Down syndrome really represents cluttering.

Conclusion

More than half a century after Cabanas' (1954) first suggestion that the speech in persons with DS may represent cluttering rather than stuttering, there is still no consensus on which diagnosis applies best to the fluency failures in this population. Studies in the past have often based their diagnosis on a very limited number of symptoms. The more recent recognition, however, that cluttering probably is a multifaceted disorder by no means clarifies the picture. On the contrary, a broader definition of cluttering seems to result in an unusually high incidence of cluttering in DS. Perhaps the fluency failures in persons with DS constitute a pattern that bears some resemblance with both cluttering and stuttering, but is still distinct from either of these. To what extent the speech pattern in DS is syndrome-specific remains to be determined.

References

Adler, S. (1976). The influence of genetic syndromes upon oral communication skills. *Journal of Speech and Hearing Disorders*, *41*, 136–137.

American Psychiatric Association. (1987). *Diagnostic and statistical manual of mental disorders*. Washington, DC: American Psychiatric Association.

Arnold, G. (1960). Studies in tachyphemia. III Signs and symptoms. *Logos*, *3*, 82–95.

Bloodstein, O. (1995). *A handbook on stuttering*. London: Chapman & Hall.

Cabanas, R. (1954). Some findings in speech and voice therapy among mentally deficient children. *Folia Phoniatrica*, *6*, 34–37.

Chudley, A. E., & Hagerman, R. J. (1987). Fragile X syndrome. *The Journal of Pediatrics*, *110*, 821–831.

Comings, D., & Comings, B. (1993). Comorbid behavioral disorders. In R. Kurlan (Ed.), *Handbook of Tourette's syndrome and related tic and behavioral disorders* (pp. 111–147). New York: Dekker.

Daly, D. A., & Cantrell, R. P. (2006). *Cluttering: Characteristics identified as diagnostically significant by 60 fluency experts*. Paper presented at the International Fluency Congress, Dublin, Ireland, July 27.

De Nil, L. F., Sasisekaran, J., Van Lieshout, P. H. H. M., & Sandor, P. (2005). Speech disfluencies in individuals with Tourette syndrome. *Journal of Psychosomatic Research*, *58*, 97–102.

Devenny, D. A., & Silverman, W. P. (1990). Speech dysfluency and manual specialization in Down's syndrome. *Journal of Mental Deficiency Research*, *34*, 253–260.

Down, J. L. H. (1866). Observation on an ethnic classification of idiots. *Clinical lectures and reports by the medical and surgical staff of the London hospital*, *3*, 259–262.

Evans, D. (1977). The development of language abilities in Mongols: A correlational study. *Journal of Mental Deficiency Research*, *21*, 103–117.

Farmer, A., & Brayton, E. R. (1979). Speech characteristics of fluent and dysfluent Down's syndrome adults. *Folia Phoniatrica*, *31*, 284–290.

Goldson, E., & Hagerman, R. J. (1992).The fragile X syndrome. *Developmental Medicine and Child Neurology*, *34*, 822–832.

Grigsby, J. P., Kemper, M. B., Hagerman, R. J., & Myers, C. S. (1990). Neuropsychological dysfunction among affected heterozygous fragile X females. *American Journal of Medical Genetics*, *35*, 28–35.

Hagerman, R. J. (1987). Fragile X syndrome. *Current Problems in Pediatrics*, *17*, 621–674.

Hanson, D., Jackson, A., & Hagerman, R. (1986). Speech disturbances (cluttering) in mildly impaired males with the martin bell/fragile x syndrome. *American Journal of Medical Genetics*, *23*, 195–206.

Lambert, J. L., & Rondal, J. A. (1979). *Le mongolisme*. Bruxelles: Pierre Mardaga.

Martyn, M. M., Sheehan, J., & Slutz, K. (1969). Incidence of stuttering and other speech disorders among the retarded. *American Journal of Mental Deficiency, 74*, 206–211.

Otto, F. M., & Yairi, E. (1975). An analysis of the speech dysfluencies in Down's syndrome and in normally intelligent subjects. *Journal of Fluency Disorders, 1*, 26–32.

Pauls, D., Leckman, J., & Cohen, D. (1993). Familial relationship between Gilles de la Tourette syndrome, attention deficit disorder, learning disability, speech disorders and stuttering. *Journal of the American Academy of Child and Adolescent Psychiatry, 32*, 1044–1050.

Perkins, W. (1977). *Speech pathology: An applied behavioral science*. St. Louis, MO: Mosby.

Preus, A. (1973). Stuttering in Down's syndrome. In Y. Lebrun & R. Hoops (Eds.), *Neurolinguistic approaches to stuttering* (pp. 90–100). The Hague: Mouton.

Pueschel, S. M. (1988). Physical characteristics, chromosome analysis and treatment approaches in Down syndrome. In C. Tingey (Ed.), *Down syndrome: A resource handbook* (pp. 3–21). Boston, MA: College-Hill Press/Little, Brown & Co.

Rassas Cohn, E. R., Shames, G. H., McWilliams, B. J., & Ferketic, M. (1983). *Dysfluency as the predominant speech symptom in a patient with Gilles de la Tourette syndrome*. 19th World Congress of the International Association of Logopedics and Phoniatrics (pp. 591–596).

Rondal, J., & Buckley, S. (2003). *Speech and language intervention in Down syndrome*. London: Whurr.

Scharfenaker, S. K. (1990). The fragile x syndrome. *American Speech and Hearing Association, September*, 45–47.

Schlanger, B. B., & Gottsleben, R. H. (1957). Analysis of speech defects among the institutionalized mentally retarded. *Journal of Speech and Hearing Disorders, 22*, 98–103.

Stansfield, J. (1990). Prevalence of stuttering and cluttering in adults with mental handicaps. *Journal of Mental Deficiency Research, 34*, 287–307.

St. Louis, K. O. (1996). A tabular summary of cluttering subjects in the special edition. *Journal of Fluency Disorders, 21*, 337–343.

St. Louis, K. O., & Hinzman, A. R. (1986). Studies of cluttering: Perceptions of cluttering by speech-language pathologists and educators. *Journal of Fluency Disorders, 11*, 131–149.

St. Louis, K. O., Raphael, L. J., Myers, F. L., & Bakker, K. (2003, November 18). Cluttering updated. *The ASHA Leader*, 4–5, 20–22.

St. Louis, K. O., & Rustin, L. (1996). Professional awareness of cluttering. In F. L. Myers & K. O. St. Louis (Eds.), *Cluttering: A clinical perspective* (pp. 23–35). San Diego/London: Singular Publishing Group.

Turner, G., Webb, T., Wake, S., & Robinson, H. (1996). Prevalence of fragile X syndrome. *American Journal of Medical Genetics, 64*, 196–197.

Van Borsel, J., Dor, O., & Rondal, J. (2008). Speech fluency in fragile X syndrome. *Clinical Linguistics and Phonetics, 22*, 1–11.

Van Borsel, J., Goethals, L., & Vanryckeghem, M. (2004). Disfluency in Tourette syndrome: Observational study in three cases. *Folia Phoniatrica et Logopaedica, 56*, 358–366.

Van Borsel, J., & Vandermeulen, A. (2008). Cluttering in Down syndrome. *Folia Phoniatrica et Logopaedica, 60*, 312–317.

Van Borsel, J., & Vanryckeghem, M. (2000). Dysfluency and phonic tics in Tourette syndrome: A case report. *Journal of Communication Disorders*, *33*, 227–240.
Van Riper, C. (1971). *The nature of stuttering*. Englewood Cliffs, NJ: Prentice-Hall.
Vilkman, E., Niemi, J., & Ikonen, U. (1988). Fragile X speech phonology in Finnish. *Brain and Language*, *34*, 203–221.
Ward, D. (2006). *Stuttering and cluttering. Frameworks for understanding and treatment*. Hove, UK: Psychology Press.
Weiss, D. (1964). *Cluttering*. Englewood Cliffs, NJ: Prentice-Hall.
Willcox, A. (1988). An investigation into non-fluency in Down's syndrome. *British Journal of Disorders of Communication*, *23*, 153–170.

7 Cluttering and learning disabilities

Yvonne van Zaalen, Frank Wijnen, and Philipe H. Dejonckere

Introduction

The co-occurrence of cluttering and learning disabilities has interested researchers for many decades. According to Gregory (1995), the disorder of cluttering provides us with one obvious example of how much speech, language, and learning disabilities have in common. Preus (1996) stated that cluttering has more in common with learning disabilities than with stuttering. The coherence of problems in cluttering and learning disabilities exists, for many researchers, mainly with regard to problems in expression, reading, and writing (Daly & Burnett, 1996; Mensink-Ypma, 1990; St. Louis, 1992; St. Louis, Myers, Bakker, & Raphael, 2007; Tiger, Irvine, & Reis, 1980; Ward, 2006; Weiss, 1964). Daly outlines some co-occurring features between the two disorders, thus: 'Children with the following symptoms: impulsive, disorderly, inattentive, underachieving in school, specific reading problems and problems in language production, can easily belong to one of both categories' (1996, p. 54). Since the definition of cluttering was narrowed (St. Louis, Raphael, Myers, & Bakker, 2003; St. Louis et al., 2007), the differences and similarities between cluttering and learning disabilities have become clearer. St. Louis et al. (2007, pp. 299–300) use a description of symptoms in their working definition of cluttering:

> Cluttering is a fluency disorder characterized by a rate that is perceived to be abnormally rapid, irregular, or both for the speaker (although measured syllable rates may not exceed normal limits). These rate abnormalities further are manifest in one or more of the following symptoms: (a) an excessive number of disfluencies, the majority of which are not typical of people who stutter; (b) the frequent placement of pauses and use of prosodic patterns that do not conform to syntactic and semantic constraints; and (c) inappropriate (usually excessive) degrees of coarticulation among sounds, especially in multisyllabic words.

In an attempt to define cluttering from a more causal perspective, Van Zaalen defined cluttering as: 'a fluency disorder in which a person inadequately adjusts his or her speech rate to the linguistic or motor demands of the moment' (Van Zaalen & Winkelman, 2009, p. 21).

Conceptually, the term learning disabilities (LD) refers to children who evidence a marked disparity between their measured intelligence and their academic achievement. Put simply, these are children who despite normal intelligence have difficulty learning (Healey, Reid, & Donaher, 2005). Children are diagnosed with learning disabilities, if the ability to store, process, or reproduce information leads to academic and/or social problems due to a discontinuity in possibilities and achievements (Gettinger & Koscik, 2001; NCLD, 2002). Children with LD have, according to Prior (1996), an IQ above 80 and problems in at least one academic skill (reading, writing, or mathematics). Difficulties may be associated with problems in areas of cognition including short-term memory, auditory discrimination skills, and/or visual perception (Prior, 1996). Speech and language problems can co-occur with learning disabilities, but are not present in all children with learning disabilities.

The purpose of this chapter is to set objective norms for differential diagnosis of speech and language characteristics of cluttering and those of learning disabilities. In order to better understand differences in underlying neurolinguistic processes, similarities and differences will be discussed in relation to Levelt's (1989) language production model. In a recent study, Van Zaalen, Wijnen, and Dejonckere (2009b) concluded that while children with LD have problems in conceptualizing and formulation, language planning disturbances in children with cluttering (CWC) were considered to arise from insufficient time to complete the editing phase of grammatical or phonological encoding. A further goal of this chapter, therefore, is to test the hypothesis that CWC present with similar language and speech characteristics to children with LD, but differ from them in their response to speed rate variation. To investigate the viability of such a theory, both language and speech characteristics will be described as well as characteristics of disfluency.

It should be noted that most data on language production in CWC or children with LD mentioned in this chapter are based on analyses of retelling a memorized story. Liles (1993) stated that in retelling a story only the quantity and the accuracy of the content may differ across participants, whereas in spontaneous speech comparisons are difficult to make across participants due to the variability in topic selection. Analysis of a story retelling is therefore a better comparative measure than is spontaneous speech.

Aetiology

Before we begin to describe differences and similarities in speech and language production of people with cluttering (PWC) or LD, it is important to consider what is known about the aetiology of both disorders. The aetiology of cluttering has been conceptualized (but not yet proven) as a central imbalance in the language system (Weiss, 1964). There is some recent evidence that problems in language production may be due to disturbed activation of areas within the precentral gyrus in PWC (Van Zaalen et al., 2010). Alm (2005) suggested that dysfunctions of the basal ganglia in PWC lead to insufficient cortical inhibition (release of involuntary movements); these observations are supported by the findings of Van Zaalen (2009, pp. 99–124). Weiss (1964, 1968) postulated that cluttering is genetically based. This genetic base was supported by van Riper (1982) when he described his track II stuttering.

The aetiology of LD is believed to be correlated to disturbed neuropsychological processes (Gaddes, 1985; Knights & Bakker, 1976; Lyon, 1996; Stefani, 2004; Willes, Hooper, & Stone, 1992) or a change in brain structure (Elkins, 2007). Wong (1996) claims that LD is genetically based; however, many authors conclude LD is caused by problems during pregnancy or immediately after birth (Litt, Taylor, Klein, & Hack, 2005; NCLD, 2002; Strauss & Lehtinen, 1947). Whatever the cause of the problem, it is clear that disorders in the neuromotor system influence the learning process of the child (Kavale & Forness, 1992; Silver, 2006). Depending on what part of the cortex is affected, a student will have problems with learning, language, and/or motor function (Silver, 2006). These neurologically based processing difficulties might involve understanding or using language, spoken or written, resulting in a reduced ability to listen, think, speak, read, write, spell, or perform mathematical calculations.

In sum, both cluttering and learning disability have been hypothesized to be genetically based disorders. But where the problems in cluttering are hypothesized to be based on problems in language production, problems in children with learning disabilities seem to be mainly based on neurologically based processing difficulties.

Language

In recent years, many authors have described language production disorders in CWC or children with LD (Howell & Dworzynski, 2005; Messer and Dockrell, 2006; Prior, 1996; Richels & Conture, 2009; St. Louis & Hinzman, 1986; Van Zaalen & Winkelman, 2009; Ward, 2006; Weiss, 1964; Wigg & Semel, 1984). In this part of the chapter, we will summarize the relationship between the two disorders in relation to story-telling structure, lexical selection, and sentence structure. According to Levelt's language production model (Levelt, 1989), problems in organizing the story and adjusting the story to the listener (Levelt's conceptualizer phase) can be reflected by a frequent occurrence of sentence revisions and interjections. In the formulator, the grammatical encoding and lexical selection is done. While phonological encoding relates to the output from the formulator phase, programming the movements of the articulators takes place in the articulator phase. According to Ward (2006), CWC may experience problems at all three levels of speech production, that is, conceptualization, formulation, and articulation (see Figure 1, Levelt, 1989).

Weiss described cluttering as a result of a central language imbalance, and different authors have discussed the presence of language problems in fluency disorders (Damsté, 1984; Freund, 1952; Luchsinger, 1963; St. Louis, 1992; St. Louis et al., 2003, 2007; Scripture, 1912; Van Zaalen, Wijnen, & Dejonckere, 2009a; Voelker, 1935; Ward, 2004, 2006; Weiss, 1964, 1968). Further, language production disorders are mentioned in some descriptions of cluttering behaviour (Sick, 2004; Van Zaalen, 2009; Ward, 2006). However, many of these descriptions are limited to qualitative comments such as 'problems in story telling' or 'problems in sentence structure'.

Wigg and Semel (1984) studied the language production of children with LD, and observed a high frequency of nonstuttering-like disfluencies (NSLDs), such as interjections, fillers, pauses, and word and phrase repetitions. The same symptoms have been reported in cluttering (Daly, 1996; Damsté, 1984; Mensink-Ypma, 1990; Preus, 1992; St. Louis et al., 2007; Ward, 2006; Weiss, 1964). According to Ward (2006), CWC may experience problems at all three levels of language production, i.e. conceptualization, formulation and articulation (see Figure 1, Levelt, 1989).

In a qualitative and quantitative research project on language planning disturbances in CWC or children with LD, Van Zaalen et al. (2009b) hypothesized that differences in underlying processes of language disturbances between CWC and children with LD exist. In this study 103 Dutch-speaking children ranging in age between 10.6 and 12.11 years were divided into three groups: group 1: cluttering children (N = 11, mean age 11.5 years); group 2: children with learning disability (N = 37, mean age 11.6 years); and group 3: controls (N = 55, mean age 11.2 years). In the next paragraphs, we will describe some of the results of this product as they relate to language production in story telling, lexical selection, and sentence structure in cluttering and learning disabilities.

Story-telling structure

Jansonius-Schultheiss and Roelofs (2007) described a procedure to analyse story-telling skills of children using the Bus story by studying story elements.

Several authors (Daly & Cantrell, 2006; Myers, 1996; St. Louis et al., 2007; Teigland, 1996; Ward, 2006; Weiss, 1964) reported that PWC experience problems in organizing discourse information. In Van Zaalen et al.'s (2009) study, CWC did not experience story organization problems in reproducing a memorized story. To the contrary, CWC produced similar primary plot elements and secondary plot elements to age-matched controls. Primary plot elements are defined as 'the building stones of the story' and secondary plot elements as 'details' (Jansonius-Schultheiss & Roelofs, 2007). The finding in CWC may be attributed to the fact that the speech task restricted the language production options available to the speaker and provided a story organization. Results of Van Zaalen et al.'s (2009b) study also indicated that CWC can be differentiated from children with LD by the number of primary plot elements (N = 61; LD: M = 6.0; SD = 1.4; CWC: M = 9.2; SD = 0.8; controls M = 9.1; SD = 1.4; p = .001). Controls reproduced significantly more secondary plot elements compared with children with LD (controls: M = 4.4; SD = 1.1; LD: M = 2.8; SD = 1.6; CWC: M = 3.4; SD = 1.4; $p < .0001$), and less 'noise' in retelling 'The Wallet story' (Van Zaalen & Bochane, 2007). According to Jansonius-Schultheiss and Roelofs' (2007) story analysing structure, noise was indicated when a child added sentences or elements, or used fillers that did not belong to the story. Based on the content of the additional sentences, CWC and children with LD used 'noise' to cover up for language production problems.

Based on the findings in this study, Van Zaalen (2009) concluded that the underlying language production problems in CWC and children with LD are different. Van Zaalen (2009) hypothesizes that defective language automation is the basis of cluttering. While language production of children with LD was disturbed by problems in the conceptualizator and formulator stages, language planning disturbances in CWC were considered to arise due to insufficient time to complete the editing phase of sentence structuring (see paragraphs to follow on lexical selection and sentence structure).

Lexical selection

The lexicon contains, for each known word, its meaning characteristics, syntax, and phonological structure (Levelt, 1993). Lexical selection comprises the retrieval (or activation) of these three types of word properties, probably in succession (Levelt, 1993; Roelofs, 1992, 1997). Children with LD appear to experience difficulties in retrieving items from the lexicon, and such difficulties may pertain to specific classes of words. For example, Van Zaalen et al. (2009b), found that children with LD had three times more omissions of articles (article omission: N = 61; p = .03) compared with fluent controls and CWC. Surprisingly, CWC used neologisms five times more often compared with children with LD (p = .03) in retelling a memorized story (N = 61). Neologisms are often created by combining existing words or by giving words new and unique suffixes or prefixes. So, although CWC and children with LD use different strategies to cope with their encoding problems (CWC by inventing new words and children with LD by interjections or descriptions), both CWC and children with LD seem to gain time for encoding. This observation is consistent with findings by Messer and Dockrell (2006), who stated that children with LD appear to have difficulties in retrieving the necessary lemmas *within* the communication *time frame*, and by Ward (2006) and Van Zaalen and Winkelman (2009) who claim that PWC use repetitions to gain time for grammatical encoding.

It is important to note that we postulate that CWC experience problems in sentence structuring only when their speech rate is too fast (Van Zaalen & Winkelman, 2009; Ward, 2006). When CWC focus on speech production, the speech rate is lowered and problems in sentence structuring diminish. In a fast speech rate, CWC invent new words in order to continue speech at this rate. When children with LD focus on speech production, their speech rate is also lowered. But, in many children with LD, problems in lexical selection remain even at a slow rate. Words can only be reproduced in retelling a memorized story when the words are part of the lexicon.

Sentence structure

Lexical selection drives grammatical encoding. Lemmas are retrieved when their semantic conditions are met in the message. In their turn, they activate syntactic procedures that correspond to the syntactic specifications, resulting in correct sentence structures (Levelt, 1993, p. 7). Speakers need to gain extra time for planning whenever difficult material (e.g., a content word or sentence structure) is not ready. They can do this by pausing or fluently repeating one or more prior segments (Howell & Dworzynski, 2005). When word repetitions and sentence revisions are edited out from CWC's transcribed utterances, syntactically correct sentences appear that do not differ qualitatively from those produced by controls. It is conceivable that CWC's word repetitions serve to gain time for the formulation process (Ward, 2006). CWC seem to use the editing phase of the formulating process to produce grammatically correct sentence structures. In children with LD extending the editing phase did not result in correct structures comparable to controls and CWC. The authors speculate that CWC produce word and phrase repetitions when speaking at a rate that exceeds the limits of their encoding skills, and that this results in insufficient time to allow adequate sentence construction (grammatical encoding). When sentence structure is assessed in a transcribed language sample it is beneficial to consider the sentence structure in its final state (after revisions/repetitions have been edited out). CWC produce an amount of correct sentence structures comparable with fluent controls, while children with LD produce a higher than normal amount of incorrect sentence structures (Van Zaalen et al., 2009b). It is hypothesized that children with LD produce more syntactical errors in writing due to problems in lexical retrieval as well. In conclusion, a CWC is capable of producing correct sentences when there is enough time, while sentence production of children with LD is negatively influenced by problems in lexical retrieval.

Summary of language production issues in LD and cluttering

Children with cluttering can be differentiated from children with LD by both the primary and secondary story elements and by the percentage correct sentence structures. Although language production deficits were perceived to be present in CWC, when measured they are not. Persons with cluttering may experience disturbances in language production, but these are only expressed in (and perhaps ultimately result from) faster speech rate. Secondly, language production disturbances of CWC tend to disappear in writing and slower communication rate, while language production problems in children with LD remain in writing. Van Zaalen (2009) hypothesizes that defective language automation is the basis of cluttering. The hypothesis that CWC differ from children with LD in their response to speed rate variation has been described in relation to language production (on this subject also see Bakker, Myers, Raphael, & St. Louis, chapter 4 and Myers, chapter 10 this volume).

The articulator

The output of the formulator is a phonological representation of (parts of) the intended utterance (inner speech). This is input to two components of the system: the monitor and the articulator (Levelt, 1989). The monitor allows the speaker to evaluate the output of the formulator before it is articulated (Levelt, 1989). The articulator uses the phonological representation to programme a series of coordinated movements of the articulatory apparatus, which are subsequently executed.

Articulatory rate

According to St. Louis et al.'s (2003) working definition of cluttering, a high and/or irregular articulatory rate is a main characteristic in differential diagnostics between cluttering and stuttering; however, agreement on what defines abnormally fast and abnormally irregular articulatory rate is needed. It is hypothesized that there are PWC who maintain a high articulatory rate in a more demanding speaking situation, and their speech-language system (the formulator) cannot handle that fast speed. Due to speech motor or language planning problems in a high articulatory rate, intelligibility problems or disfluencies can occur (Daly, 1992). Van Zaalen et al. (2009b) found that articulatory rate (of a string of 10–20 consecutive syllables without pauses) measured in syllables per second in CWC and children with LD was comparable with fluent age-matched controls, $N = 103$; $M = 5.5$, $SD = 1.0$; $F(2, 102) = 1.036$; $p = .36$.

Phonetic and phonological errors

Many researchers and clinicians (Bezemer, Bouwen, & Winkelman, 2006; Daly, 1986; Eisenson, 1986; Luchsinger & Arnold, 1965; Shepherd, 1960; Simkins, 1973; St. Louis & Hinzman, 1986; St. Louis & Myers, 1997; Ward, 2006; Weiss, 1964; Wohl, 1970) report that PWC experience intelligibility problems due to exaggerated coarticulation (deletion of sounds or syllables in multisyllabic words) and indistinct articulation (substitution and/or distortion of sounds and/or syllables). Meanwhile, several researchers discuss the fact that although PWC experience intelligibility problems in running speech, they are able to produce correct syllable and word structures in controlled situations (Damsté, 1984; Van Zaalen & Winkelman, 2009; Ward, 2006; Weiss, 1964). In order to be able to produce correct syllable or word structures, speech motor control should be within normal limits (Van Zaalen et al., 2009a). Riley and Riley (1985) defined speech motor control as the ability to time laryngeal, articulatory, and respiratory movements that lead to fast and accurate syllable production.

In cluttering, encoding of complex low frequency words is disturbed at *high* speech rates, resulting in errors in word structure (Mooshammer & Hartinger, 2008; Van Zaalen et al., 2009a; Van Zaalen & Winkelman, 2009). In producing constraints of syllables at a fast rate, CWC produce sequencing errors and errors in rhythm and stress. Stefani (2004) hypothesized that children with LD experience moments of reduced speech intelligibility as a result of decreased focus on speech during moments of word retrieval problems.

Summary of speech production issues

The speech production of both CWC and children with LD is hypothesized to be influenced by disturbances in phonological encoding (Van Zaalen et al., 2009b; Ward, 2006). Speech production disturbances in children with LD are probably mainly influenced by problems in lexical retrieval and storage. As a result of storage problems in children with LD, errors in phonetic or phonological structures remain in slow speech. In contrast, phonetic and phonological problems in speech of CWC usually diminish in slow speech (Damsté, 1984; Van Zaalen & Winkelman, 2009).

Disfluency

According to Kolk and Postma (1997), the amount of disfluencies is usually connected to the number of speech revisions. Furthermore, the fluency of an utterance is influenced by pragmatic aspects. A language plan can be corrected during production in response to the nonverbal information of the listener. Fluency is also influenced by linguistic complexity. Finally, the number of disfluencies is influenced by speech rate. If speech rate is lowered, the amount of normal disfluencies is usually reduced and the intelligibility is heightened (Levelt, 1989). Levelt gives explanations for this phenomenon. First, in order to speak, one has to recall syllable structures (for instance CVC or CVCC) that, when combined, form a word or sentence. In order to recall these syllables, a certain amount of time is necessary. At a lower speech rate, more time is available to recall syllable structures and accordingly, fewer mistakes will be made. Second, the lowered speech rate will result in more attention to speech and language production resulting in a smaller amount of failures, because mistakes are detected before production (internal monitoring).

Type of disfluencies

Research on type and number of disfluencies in cluttering compared with learning disabilities is rare. Van Zaalen et al. (2009b) found that both CWC and children with LD produced more revisions compared with controls in retelling a memorized story: $F(2, 98) = 5.569$, $p = .005$; controls: $M = 2.0$, $SD = 1.4$; CWC: $M = 4.6$, $SD = 5.3$; LD: $M = 3.6$, $SD = 3.7$). While cluttering children produced more word and phrase repetitions compared with children with LD and controls, $F(2, 98) = 26.094$, $p < .0001$; CWC: $M = 5.8$, $SD = 3.2$; LD: $M = 2.0$, $SD = 2.4$; Controls: $M = 1.0$, $SD = 1.5$), children with LD produced more 'uh'-interjections compared with the CWC, $F(2, 98) = 6.143$; $p = .003$. More research projects on type and number of normal and stuttering-like disfluencies in cluttering and learning disabilities is required to confirm these results.

Ratio of disfluencies

Language production can be conceived as comprising separate planning and execution components (Levelt, 1989), and speakers can start an utterance before they have the complete plan, resulting in covert or overt repairs, postulated to be heard as disfluencies (Kolk & Postma, 1997). Both CWC and children with LD produce a high frequency of normal disfluencies (Van Zaalen et al., 2009b). The ratio between normal and stuttering-like disfluencies (RD) of children with LD is higher than in CWC or controls (Van Zaalen & Winkelman, 2009). The difference between the controls and CWC on the one hand and the children with LD on the other hand can be explained by the fact that in contrast to children with LD, CWC also produced a small number of part-word repetitions that, according to Campbell and Hill (1987), belong to the category of stuttering-like disfluencies.

Discussion

The purpose of this chapter was to set objective norms for differential diagnosis of speech and language characteristics of cluttering and those of learning disabilities. In order to better understand differences in underlying neurolinguistic processes, similarities and differences are discussed in relation to Levelt's (1989) language production model.

A second purpose of this chapter was to examine the hypothesis that CWC differ from children with LD in their response to speed rate variation. Some evidence is found to support the hypothesis for language production, speech production, and types of disfluencies, but not for the number of speech disfluencies. Both in cluttering and learning disability, language production disturbances occur. But where the problem in cluttering seems to be based on defective automation of language production, problems in children with learning disabilities seem to be based on both defective automation of language production and language processing disorders.

Both the group of children with cluttering characteristics in general and the group of children with LD are rather heterogeneous. Typology in children with learning disabilities described by Stefani (2004) divides children with LD into three categories: (1) learning disability characterized by a disorder in nonverbal functioning; (2) learning disability characterized by a disorder in output of all aspects of functioning; and (3) learning disability characterized by linguistic processing disorders. As in children with LD, some cluttering characteristics described (language problems or high frequency of disfluencies) are not found in all CWC. In 1984, Damsté described three different subtypes of cluttering behaviour: dysarthric, dysphasic, and dysrythmic cluttering. This typology was adjusted by Ward (2006) and Van Zaalen and Winkelman (2009) when they described two types of cluttering: linguistic cluttering and motoric cluttering. Van Zaalen (2009) conclude that children with linguistic/syntactic cluttering experience sentence structure problems (grammatical encoding), whereas children with phonological cluttering experience problems in word structures (phonological encoding). Combinations of both syntactic and phonological cluttering are rare. Future research on speech and language characteristics of cluttering and learning disability will be more efficient when children are included by both the disorder and the subtype of the disorder.

CWC could be differentiated from children with LD by both the number of main primary and secondary plot elements, the percentage correct sentence structures and the frequency of word- and phrase repetitions. Although language production deficits can be perceived to be present in CWC (Daly, 1996), when measured they can be within normal limits. It is hypothesized that the high number of phrase and word repetitions within a fast speech rate gives an impression of defective language automation, and leads to message comprehension problems for the listener. When a speech plan is not complete, the message cannot progress fluently. In this situation the speaker can retrieve the plan of a word or phrase that is recently used and execute it again (word or phrase repetition). In doing this the person gains time for encoding. Language production of children with LD is hypothesized to be mainly disturbed by problems in lexical selection, leading to errors in sentence structuring and a high frequency of normal disfluencies.

Both CWC and children with LD can experience problems in sentence structure, word, and story structure. The difference between CWC and children with LD is, however, that in CWC these problems diminish at a slower speech rate in verbal communication (both spontaneous and imitated) and in writing, while the problems in children with LD are basically not influenced by rate or language production style. For children with LD, expository writing is exceedingly difficult (Scott & Windsor, 2000), and as a result of that language production will not benefit from this nonverbal expression. In conclusion, we hypothesize that the theories of language production we have discussed and our preliminary data comparing CWC with children with LD provides initial support for the difference between these two groups in their response to speed rate variation.

Conclusion

Although speech and language production of PWC and people with LD have a number of similar characteristics, the underlying problems in language production seem to be different. Whereas CWC experience problems in the fluency of speech, especially in a situation in which they cannot adjust their speech rate to the linguistic or motoric demands of the speaking situation, speech rate seems to be of no critical influence in the number, type, or severity of speech and language problems in children with LD. Children with LD seem to experience problems in sentence or story organization mainly on the basis of problems in conceptualizing and/or lexical retrieval problems. Further research is needed to confirm or disconfirm the hypotheses proposed in this chapter in order to better understand speech and language characteristics of CWC.

Acknowledgements

Special thanks to Marloes Avenhuis, Loes Heijmans, Yvonne van Zoggel, Dirkje Scheenstra, Eva Strous, Carlijn Vermeer, Lieke Wijnen all speech language pathology students at Fontys University of applied sciences, Eindhoven, the Netherlands for their hard work in data collection and data analyzing.

References

Alm, P. (2005). *On the causal mechanisms of stuttering*. PhD thesis, University of Lund, Sweden.

Bezemer, B. W., Bouwen, J., & Winkelman, C. (2006). *Stotteren van theorie naar therapie*. Bussum: Uitgeverij Coutinho.

Campbell, J. H., & Hill, D. (1987). *Systematic disfluency analysis*. Paper presented at the annual convention of the American Speech Language and Hearing Association, New Orleans.

Daly, D. (1986). The clutterer. In K. St. Louis (Ed.), *The atypical stutterer: Principles and practice of rehabilitation* (pp. 155–192). New York: Academic Press.

Daly, D. (1992). Helping the clutterer: Therapy considerations. In F. Myers & K. St. Louis (Eds.). *Cluttering: A clinical perspective* (pp. 107–124). Leicester, UK: Far Communications. (Reissued in 1996 by Singular, San Diego, CA.)

Daly, D. (1996). *The source for stuttering and cluttering*. East Moline, IL: LinguiSystems.

Daly, D., & Burnett, M. (1996). Cluttering: Assessment, treatment planning, and case study illustration. *Journal of Fluency Disorders*, *21*, 239–244.

Daly, D. A., & Cantrell, R. P. (2006). *Cluttering characteristics identified as diagnostically significant by 60 fluency experts*. Proceedings of the Second World Congress on Fluency Disorders.

Damsté, P. H. (1984). *Stotteren*. Utrecht: Bohn, Scheltema & Holkema.

Eisenson, J. (1986). Dysfluency disorders: Cluttering and stuttering. In A. Goldstein, L. Krasner, & S. Garfield (Eds.), *Language and speech disorders in children* (pp. 57–75). New York: Pergamon Press.

Elkins, J. (2007). Learning disabilities: bringing fields and nations together. *Journal of Learning Disabilities*, *40*, 392–399.

Freund, H. (1952). Studies in the interrelationship between stuttering and cluttering. *Folia Phoniatrica*, *4*, 146–168.

Gaddes, W. H. (1985). *Learning disabilities and brain function: A neuropsychological approach* (2nd ed.). New York: Springer-Verlag.

Gettinger, M., & Koscik, R. (2001). Psychological services for children with disabilities. In J. N. Hughes & A. M. LaGreca (Eds.), *Handbook of psychological services for children and adolescents* (pp. 421–435). New York: Oxford Press.

Gregory, H. H. (1995). Analysis and commentary. *Language Speech and Hearing Services in the Schools*, *26*, 196–200.

Healey, E. C., Reid, R., & Donaher, J. (2005). Treatment of the child who stutters with co-existing learning, behavioral, and cognitive challenges. In R. Lees & C. Stark (Eds.), *Treatment of the school age child who stutters* (pp. 79–94). London: Whurr.

Howell, P., & Dworzynski, K. (2005). Planning and execution processes in speech control by fluent speakers and speakers who stutter. *Journal of Fluency Disorders*, *30*, 343–354.

Jansonius-Schultheiss, K., & Roelofs, M. (2007). Renfrew's Taalschalen Nederlandse Aanpassing (RTNA). Diagnostisch onderzoek en therapieopzet bij jonge taalgestoorde kinderen. *Logopedie en Fonatrie*, *11*, 21–26.

Kavale, A., & Forness, S. R. (1992). History, definition, and diagnosis. In N. N. Singh & I. L. Beale (Eds.), *Learning disabilities nature, theory and treatment. Disorders of human learning, behavior and communication* (pp. 3–43). New York: Springer-Verlag.

Knights, R. M., & Bakker, D. J. (Eds.). (1976). *The neuropsychology of learning disorders: Theoretical approaches*. Baltimore, MD: University Park Press.

Kolk, H., & Postma, A. (1997). Stuttering as a covert repair phenomenon. In R. F. Curlee & G. M. Siegel (Eds.), *Nature and treatment of stuttering: new directions* (pp. 182–203). Boston: Allyn & Bacon.

Levelt, W. J. M. (1989). *Speaking: From intention to articulation*. Cambridge, MA: MIT Press.

Levelt, W. J. M. (1993). Lexical selection, or how to bridge the major rift in language processing. In F. Beckmann & G. Heyer (Eds.), *Theorie und praxis des lexikons* (pp. 164–172). The Hague: De Gruyter.

Liles, B. Z. (1993). Narrative discourse in children with language disorders and children with normal language: A critical review of the literature. *Journal of Speech and Hearing Research*, *36*, 868–882.

Litt, J., Taylor, G., Klein, N., & Hack, M. (2005). Learning disabilities in children with very low birthweight: Prevalence, neuropsychological correlates, and educational interventions. *Journal of Learning Disabilities*, *38*, 130–139.

Luchsinger, R. (1963). *Poltern*. Berlin-Charlottenburg: Manhold Verlag.

Luchsinger, R., & Arnold, G. E. (1965). Cluttering: Tachyphemia. In *Voice-speech-language, clinical communicology: Its physiology and pathology* (pp. 598–618). Belmont, CA: Wadsworth.

Lyon, G. R. (1996). Learning disabilities. In E. J. Marsh & R. A. Barkley (Eds.), *Child psychopathology* (pp. 390–435). New York: Guilford Press.

Mensink-Ypma, M. (1990). *Broddelen en leerstoornissen*. Houten/Antwerpen: Bohn Stafleu van Loghum.

Messer, D., & Dockrell, J. E. (2006). Children's naming and word-finding difficulties: Descriptions and explanations. *Journal of Speech, Language, and Hearing Research*, *49*, 309–324.

Mooshammer, C., & Hartinger, M. (2008). Articulatory variability in cluttering. *Folia Phoniatrica Logopedia*, *60*, 64–72.

Myers, F. (1996). Annotations of research and clinical perspectives on cluttering since 1964. *Journal of Fluency Disorders*, *21*, 187–200.

NCLD: National Centre for Learning Disabilities. (2002). *LD basics and fast facts*. Retrieved June 3, 2002, from http://www.ncld.org/info/index.cfm

Preus, A. (1992). Cluttering or stuttering: Related, different or antagonistic disorders. In F. L. Myers & K. O. St. Louis (Eds.), *Cluttering: A clinical perspective* (pp. 55–70). Kibworth, UK: Far Communications.

Preus, A. (1996). Cluttering upgraded. *Journal of Fluency Disorders*, *21*, 349–358.

Prior, M. (1996). *Understanding specific learning difficulties*. Hove, UK: Psychology Press.

Richels, C., & Conture, E. (2009). Indirect treatment of childhood stuttering: Diagnostic predictors of treatment outcome. In B. Guitar & R. MacCauley (Eds.), *Treatment of Stuttering: Established and emerging approaches*. Baltimore, MD: Lippincott, Williams and Wilkins.

Riley, G. D., & Riley, J. (1985). *Oral motor assessment and treatment: Improving syllable production*. Austin, TX: Pro-Ed.

Roelofs, A. (1992). A spreading-activation theory of lemma retrieval in speaking. *Cognition*, *42*, 107–142.

Roelofs, A. (1997). The WEAVER model of word-form encoding in speech production. *Cognition*, *64*, 249–284.

Scott, C. M., & Windsor, J. (2000). General language performance measures in spoken and written narrative and expository discourse of school-age children with language learning disabilities. *Journal of Speech, Language, and Hearing Research, 43*, 324–339.

Scripture, E. W. (1912). *Stuttering and lisping*. New York: Macmillan.

Shepherd, G. (1960). Studies in tachyphemia: II. Phonetic description of cluttered speech. *Logos, 3*, 73–81.

Sick, U. (2004). *Poltern, theoretische grundlagen, diagnostik, therapie*. Stuttgart: Thieme.

Silver, L. (2006). *The misunderstood child: Understanding and coping with your child's learning disabilities* (4th ed.). New York: McGraw Hill.

Simkins, L. (1973). Cluttering. In B. B. Lahey (Ed.), *The modification of language behavior* (pp. 178–217). Springfield, IL: Charles C. Thomas.

Stefani, R. (2004). Neurological and neuropsychological aspects of learning and attention problems. In S. Burkhardt, F. E. Obiakor, & A. F. Rotatori (Eds.), *Current perspectives on learning disabilities* (pp. 65–93). Advances in special education. Oxford, UK: Elsevier.

St. Louis, K. O. (1992). On defining cluttering. In F. L. Myers & K. O. St Louis (Eds.), *Cluttering: A clinical perspective* (pp. 37–53). Kibworth, UK: Far Communications. (Reissued in 1996 by Singular, San Diego, CA.)

St. Louis, K. O., & Hinzman, A. R. (1986). Studies of cluttering: Perceptions of cluttering by speech-language pathologists and educators. *Journal of Fluency Disorders, 11*, 131–149.

St. Louis, K. O., & Myers, F. L. (1997). Management of cluttering and related fluency disorders. In R. Curlee & G. Siegel (Eds.), *Nature and treatment of stuttering: new directions* (pp. 313–332). New York: Allyn & Bacon.

St. Louis, K. O., Myers, F. L., Bakker, K., & Raphael, L. J. (2007). Understanding and treating cluttering. In E. G. Conture & R. F. Curlee (Eds.), *Stuttering and related disorders of fluency* (3rd ed., pp. 297–325). New York: Thieme.

St. Louis, K. O., Raphael, L. J., Myers, F. L., & Bakker, K. (2003, November 18). Cluttering updated. *The ASHA Leader*, 4–5, 20–22.

Strauss, A. A., & Lehtinen, L. E. (1947). *Psychopathology and education of the brain-injured child.* New York: Grune & Stratton.

Teigland, A. (1996). A study of pragmatic skills of clutterers and normal speakers. *Journal of Fluency Disorders, 21*, 201–214.

Tiger, R. J., Irvine, T. L., & Reis, R. P. (1980). Cluttering as a complex of learning disabilities. *Language, Speech and Hearing Services in Schools, 11*, 3–14.

van Riper, C. (1982). *The nature of stuttering* (2nd ed.). Englewood Cliffs, NJ: Prentice-Hall.

Van Zaalen, Y. (2009). *Cluttering identified.* Utrecht: Van Noordam.

Van Zaalen, Y., & Bochane, M. (2007). *The Wallet story.* 27th World congress of the International Association of Logopedics and Phoniatrics, Proceedings (p. 85).

Van Zaalen, Y., & Winkelman, C. (2009). *Broddelen, een (on) begrepen stoornis.* Bussum: Coutinho.

Van Zaalen, Y., Ward, D., Nederveen, A. J., Grolman, W., Wijnen, F., & Dejonckere, P. (2010, manuscript submitted for publication).

Van Zaalen, Y., Ward, D., Nederveen, A. J., Lameris, J. L., Wijnen, F., & Dejonckere, P. (2009). *Cluttering and stuttering: Different disorders and differing functional neurologies*. Presentation at Fifth International Fluency Association Congress, Rio de Janeiro.

Van Zaalen, Y., Wijnen, F., & Dejonckere, P. (2009a). A test on speech motor control on word level, the SPA test. *International Journal of Speech and Language Pathology*, *11*, 26–33.

Van Zaalen, Y., Wijnen, F., & Dejonckere, P. (2009b). Language planning disturbances in children who clutter or have learning disabilities. *International Journal of Speech and Language Pathology*, *11*, 496–508.

Van Zaalen, Y., Wijnen, F., Dejonckere, P. H. (2009c). Differential diagnostics between cluttering and stuttering, part one. *Journal of Fluency Disorders*, *34*, 137–154.

Van Zaalen, Y., Wijnen, F., Dejonckere, P. H. (2009d). Differential diagnostics between cluttering and stuttering, part two. *Journal of Fluency Disorders*, *34*, 137–154.

Voelker, C. H. (1935). The prevention of cluttering. *The English Journal*, *24*, 808–810.

Ward, D. (2004). Cluttering, speech rate and linguistic defect: a case report. In A. Packman, A. Meltzer, & H. F. M. Peters (Eds.), *Theory, research and therapy in fluency disorders* (pp. 511–516), Proceedings of the 4th World congress on fluency disorders, Montreal, Canada. Nijmegen: Nijmegen University Press.

Ward, D. (2006). *Stuttering and cluttering: Frameworks for understanding and treatment*. Hove, UK: Psychology Press.

Weiss, D. A. (1964). *Cluttering*. Englewood Cliffs, NJ: Prentice-Hall.

Weiss, D. A. (1968). Cluttering: Central language imbalance. *Pediatric Clinics of North America*, *15*, 705–720.

Wigg, E. H., & Semel, E. M. (1984). *Language assessment and intervention for the learning disabled* (2nd ed.). Columbus, OH: Charles E. Merrill.

Willes, W. G., Hooper, S. R., & Stone, B. H. (1992). Neuropsychological theories of learning disabilities. In N. N. Singh & I. L. Beale (Eds.), *Learning disabilities: Nature, theory and treatment*. Disorders of Human Learning, Behavior and Communication (pp. 201–245). New York: Springer-Verlag.

Wohl, M. T. (1970). The treatment of non-fluent utterance: A behavioural approach. *British Journal of Disorders of Communication*, *5*, 66–76.

Wong, B. Y. L. (1996). *The ABCs of learning disabilities*. New York: Academic Press.

8 Cluttering and autism spectrum disorders

Kathleen Scaler Scott

Introduction

Autism spectrum disorders (ASDs) are a group of disorders often diagnosed in childhood and characterized by impairments in communication, social interaction, and focused interests. The diagnoses of Autism, Pervasive Developmental Disorder Not Otherwise Specified, and Asperger's Disorder comprise the subgroups within the broader category of ASDs. Specific criteria distinguish these diagnoses from one another, and intelligence ranges from below to above average (American Psychiatric Association, 2000; Newschaffer et al., 2006). There is no definitive research regarding the etiological factors associated with ASDs.

Cluttering is often unidentified in many individuals, due at least in part to its definitional issues (see St. Louis & Schulte, chapter 14 this volume). Among the communication challenges experienced by some children and adults with ASDs are difficulties with speech production, including disorders in the areas of articulation, stress, resonance, phrasing, prosody, and fluency (Paul et al., 2005; Shriberg, Paul, McSweeny, Klin, Cohen, & Volkmar, 2001). If we examine the communication patterns of individuals on the autism spectrum, and compare them with the small number of studies that have been conducted regarding the speech fluency patterns in autism, we see the possibility that cluttering may have been missed in this population as well. Investigators have identified speech symptoms in individuals on the autism spectrum that match the symptoms outlined in the current working definition of cluttering. Additionally, underlying speech and language patterns are similar both for children with fluency disorders (stuttering and/or cluttering) and children with ASDs. Thus, both in terms of outward symptoms and underlying symptoms, the child with ASD presents with potential links to speech fluency disorders. Cluttering has been identified in small studies of individuals with autistic features (Thacker & Austen, 1996) and with Asperger's Disorder (Scaler Scott, 2008; Scott, Grossman, Abendroth, Tetnowski, & Damico, 2006). Results of these studies suggest that cluttering is a potential disorder speech-language therapists will need to consider when evaluating the communication patterns of individuals with ASDs.

The current working definition of cluttering has been proposed by St. Louis, Myers, Bakker, and Raphael (2007). The definition reads as follows:

> Cluttering is a fluency disorder characterized by a rate that is perceived to be abnormally rapid, irregular or both for the speaker (although measured syllable rates may not exceed normal limits). These rate abnormalities further are manifest in one or more of the following symptoms: a) an excessive number of disfluencies, the majority of which are not typical of people who stutter; b) the frequent placement of pauses and use of prosodic patterns that do not conform to syntactic and semantic constraints; and c) inappropriate (usually excessive) degrees of coarticulation among sounds, especially in multisyllabic words.
>
> (pp. 299–300)

Although the proposal has been made in this volume (St. Louis & Schulte, chapter 14) to update this definition, the symptoms remain the same in either case. We will first discuss how the symptoms of cluttering have presented themselves in varying combinations among individuals with ASDs. Next we will discuss how patterns of performance potentially underlying these symptoms are similar in both individuals with ASDs and individuals with fluency disorders. Finally, we will take these symptomatic and theoretical viewpoints and draw from them recommendations for future research and for evaluating and treating clients with ASDs and cluttered speech.

Common symptomatic links between cluttering and autism spectrum disorders

In examining the existing research on the speech patterns of individuals on the autism spectrum, cluttering has only been specifically identified in two studies. Thacker and Austin (1996) noted symptoms following the St. Louis, Hinzman, and Hull (1985) definition of cluttering in a 36-year-old man with a significant hearing impairment and 'autistic features'. Through analysis of the man's speech patterns, the authors concluded that the participant's symptoms of decreased intelligibility of speech, irregular speech rate and rhythm, syllable omissions, and word and phrase repetitions, were closest to a diagnosis of cluttering. A more recent study identified cluttering in three of a group of twelve children with Asperger's Disorder (AD), a diagnosis that is differentiated from those on the rest of the autism spectrum by lack of cognitive or language delay. Scaler Scott (2008) compared the speech fluency of 12 school-age children with AD to 12 age- and gender-matched children who stutter (CWS) and 12 age- and gender-matched children with no diagnosis. The investigator found three participants with AD whose speech met the criteria for the St. Louis et al. (2007) definition of cluttering (one for pure cluttering and two for cluttering-stuttering) during an expository discourse task.

Although these two studies are the only existing research that identifies the specific speech diagnosis of cluttering in ASDs, all of the symptoms in the St. Louis et al. definition have been identified in studies of speech patterns in ASDs. We examine each of these patterns in turn.

Rapid and/or irregular rate in autism spectrum disorders

There is little research on rate of speech in ASDs. In 1981, Baltaxe found that in comparison with typical speakers, speakers with higher functioning autism presented with more variability in the duration of their words, both in isolation and within sentences. Klin, Sparrow, Marans, Carter, and Volkmar suggest that the rate of speech of individuals with AD may be 'unusual (e.g. too fast)' (2000, p. 323). Shriberg et al. (2001) found that, based on a subjective rating scale, individuals with high-functioning autism (HFA; a diagnostic category described as including a history of a language delay and more severe social and communication deficits than those with AD; Klin et al., 2000; Volkmar & Klin, 2000) were more likely to receive ratings of slow articulation/pause time as compared with individuals with AD and individuals with no diagnosis. Ninety percent of the utterances of individuals with AD, HFA, and no diagnosis were subjectively rated as presenting with an appropriate speaking rate, although individual variability was noted within each of the groups. In a case study of a school-age child diagnosed with AD and cluttering-stuttering, Scaler Scott, Ward, and St. Louis (2010) found that although the child's perceived rate was rapid and/or irregular, the actual articulation rate was within normal limits for age. When the child decreased this rate to below average articulation rate via pausing, intelligibility increased significantly. Thus, the existing research on rate of speech in ASDs does not necessarily point to rapid rate of speech. Yet, two patterns of rate in ASDs described above seem congruent with explanations of rate regarding cluttering. First, variability observed in some studies of individuals with ASDs may point to the irregular rate of speech that St. Louis et al. (2007) proposed in their working definition of cluttering. Additionally, based on their findings that at a comfortable speaking rate individuals with cluttering produced diadochokinetic patterns and similar multisyllabic words at a slower rate than matched controls (Raphael, Bakker, Myers, St. Louis, & McRoy, 2004; Raphael et al., 2005), St. Louis et al. posit that individuals with cluttering may not speak at a rate that is faster than average, but rather, 'at a rate faster than they can easily, fluently, and accurately manage' (2007, p. 315). Certainly this seemed to be the case in the school-age boy with AD in the Scaler Scott et al. (2010) study. While subjective *perception* of speech rate may be rapid or irregular, actual speech rate may not be rapid. More objective measures of articulation rate are needed for both individuals with cluttering and individuals with ASDs, as well as subjective ratings of the articulation rates of individuals with ASDs.

Irregular rate could manifest as frequent stops and starts and/or bursts of rapid speech. In a synergistic framework of speech production (Myers & Bradley, 1992), the patterns observed in ASDs related to prosody and/or fluency (described in the next sections) could potentially combine to create the impression of irregular rate.

Disfluencies in autism spectrum disorders

General fluency patterns

Disfluency symptoms were more generally described as early as 1975, when Simmons and Baltaxe (1975) analyzed the language samples of seven adolescents (age range 14–21 years) diagnosed with autism and with at least an average intelligence quotient (IQ) score on the Weschler Adult Intelligence Scale (WAIS) (Weschler, 1955). Using the categories for 'speech and language faults' of Goldfarb, Goldfarb, Braunstein, and Scholl (1972), the investigators identified 'faults' in the category of fluency in four participants. Specific fluency issues identified were 'hesitations', 'repetitions', 'prolongations', and 'nonfluencies'. No participants were diagnosed with stuttering or cluttering. However, descriptively, Simmons and Baltaxe identified stuttering-like disfluencies (Ambrose & Yairi, 1999; Yairi & Ambrose, 1992) (SLDs; defined as part-word repetitions, single-syllable whole word repetitions with tension, prolongations, and blocks/tense pauses), including repetitions of sounds, syllables, and single-syllable whole words. Non-stuttering-like disfluencies (Ambrose & Yairi, 1999; Yairi & Ambrose, 1992) (NSLDs; defined as phrase repetitions, revisions, interjections, multi-syllable whole word repetitions, and single-syllable whole word repetitions without tension) including 'repetitions of whole utterances' were also described. Linguistically, the same four participants exhibited difficulties that were most commonly categorized as a 'disruption or disfluency' feature, such as repetitions of thought. These repetitions of thought are disruptions more like NSLDs than SLDs, as outlined in the St. Louis et al. (2007) definition. The analysis does not indicate whether the frequency of NSLDs exceeded the frequency of SLDs in this sample, but does indicate that the NSLDs were prominent enough to be coded as a disfluency disruption in the majority of cases. Likewise, Dobbinson, Perkins, and Boucher (1998) analyzed the conversational patterns of a 28-year-old woman diagnosed with autism and mental retardation. Through conversation analysis, the investigators identified a theme of repetitiveness in the woman's conversation. Although she did exhibit some part-word repetitions, the majority of the woman's repetitions were repetitions of syntactic structures and lexical items. Thus, the repetitions were again more characteristic of NSLDs, as outlined in the St. Louis et al. definition of cluttering.

In more recent years, studies regarding the speech patterns of children on the autism spectrum have become larger and more specific. Shriberg et al. (2001) and Paul et al. (2005) were among the first to study the speech patterns in a sample of 30 individuals with ASDs. These investigators compared the speech and voice-prosody profiles of 15 males with AD, 15 males with HFA, and 53 typically developing male speakers. Participants ranged in age from 10 to 50 years. Investigators identified that as compared with age-matched controls, 67 percent of the individuals with AD and 40 percent of the individuals with HFA had 'inappropriate or nonfluent phrasing' (authors defined as: sound, syllable, or word repetitions, and single-word revisions) on more than 20 percent of their utterances. There is not enough specific information to determine whether the majority of repetitions were more characteristic of SLDs or NSLDs.

Researchers have also examined more specific patterns of the finer details of speech disfluencies in ASDs. Hietella and Spillers (2005) observed patterns of disfluencies in two teens diagnosed within the category of ASDs. In speech samples, both teens exhibited what the authors termed 'abnormal disfluencies', defined as 'final-syllable repetitions' (e.g., 'football-ball'), rhyme repetitions (e.g., 'cat-at'), and disrhythmic phonation (authors defined as atypical pause within a word; also known in some categorization systems as 'broken words', e.g., 'mo—on'). In addition to the 'abnormal disfluencies', one participant also exhibited the more typically occurring patterns of disfluencies, including single-syllable whole word repetitions, revisions, and filler words. The ratio of NSDs to SLDs in this study is unknown.

Descriptive studies of the specific disorder of AD are beginning to identify similar trends in speech fluency as those identified within the broader category of ASDs. Sisskin (2006) described two cases of students with AD, one age 7 and the other age 17, who both exhibited SLDs, including part and whole word repetitions and blocks; and NSLDs, including phrase repetitions, revisions, and interjections. In addition to these more typically occurring categories of disfluencies, 50 percent of the 7-year-old's disfluencies included types less typically seen among CWS or children who do not stutter (CWNS), including mid-syllable insertions (defined by Sisskin as 'a short exhalation resembling the production of /h/', e.g., 'way-*h*ay'; 2006, p. 13) and word-final disfluencies (WFDs; e.g., 'train-ain'). In the case of the 17-year-old, 90 percent of his disfluencies consisted of these latter two types. Neither demonstrated awareness of their disfluency patterns. Such patterns of disfluencies have been noted more in populations of children within a diagnostic category other than stuttering, such as children and adults with neurological insults (Ardila & Lopez, 1986; Bijleveld, Lebrun, & Van Dongen, 1994; Lebrun & Leleux, 1985; Lebrun & Van Borsel, 1990; Rosenfield, Viswananth, Callis-Landrum, Didanato, & Nudelman, 1991; Stansfield, 1995; Van Borsel, Geirnaert, & Van Coster, 2005; Van Borsel, Van Coster, & Van Lierd, 1996). More typical SLDs, including part word repetitions and blocks, as well as NSLDs including phrase repetitions and interjections, were also identified in two cases of young adults with AD (Scott et al., 2006). Both participants demonstrated at least some awareness of their disfluencies. Again, the ratio of NSLDs to SLDs is unknown. Table 8.1 summarizes the existing literature on occurrence of SLDs in ASDs.

NSLDs

As mentioned, Scaler Scott (2008) compared the patterns of speech fluency in 12 children with AD with those of 12 children with no diagnosis and 12 CWS during an expository discourse task. In the AD group, 33 percent met the diagnostic criteria for a speech fluency disorder (i.e. stuttering and/or cluttering). As a group, the children with AD appeared to exhibit more of a tendency toward disfluent speech than the children with no diagnosis. This disfluency presented differently than for CWS. Specifically, although 67 percent of the children with AD qualified as stuttering on the Stuttering Severity Instrument (SSI-3; Riley, 1994), the overall stuttering severity ratings were less severe than for the CWS, with the average severity ratings

Table 8.1 Literature identifying types of stuttering-like-disfluencies in conversation samples in autism spectrum disorders

Reference	*SSWWR*[a]	*PWR*[a]	*PR*[a]	*TP*[a]	*BW*[a]
Simmons and Baltaxe (1975) (*n* = 7) Higher-functioning autism	X	X	X	?	
Thacker and Austin (1986) (*n* = 1) Autistic features		X			
Dobbinson et al. (1998) (*n* = 1) Autism/retardation		X			
Shriberg et al. (2001)[b]; Paul et al. (2005) (*n* = 15)[b] AD/HFA	?	X	X	X	
Hietella and Spillers (2005) (*n* = 2) ASD	X				X
Scott et al. (2006) (*n* = 2) AD	?	X		X	
Sisskin (2006) (*n* = 2) AD 70–90% of SLDs were word-final disfluencies (e.g., 'train-ain'), or mid-syllable insertions (e.g., 'see-hee')	X	X		X	
Scaler Scott (2008) (*n* = 12) AD	X	X	X	X	X

a SSWWR = single syllable whole word repetition; PWR = part word repetition; PR = prolongation; TP = tense pause; BW = broken word.
b These two studies represent the same sample of individuals with AD.
? = unclear from data description whether these disfluencies were present, but possible.

for the AD group falling in the 'very mild' range. Additionally, while 8 of 12 participants with AD qualified as stuttering on the SSI-3, only 3 of these 8 had been identified as having stuttering issues by their parents or other professionals. The remaining 63 percent exhibited enough disfluent speech to be classified as mild stuttering on the SSI-3, but in 4 out of 5 of these children, the percentage of words that contained NSLDs was greater than the percentage of words containing SLDs. Again, these children on the autism spectrum presented with more of the type of disfluencies proposed by St. Louis et al. (2007) in their working definition of cluttering. The participants also presented with an irregular rate of speech at times, which seemed to be related to tense pauses between words and/or phrases that seemed similar to very mild stuttering blocks. It is unclear whether these blocks were truly SLDs or a different kind of increased tension in speech.

Overall, studies are beginning to identify disfluent speech in ASDs that may consist of some combination of: (1) SLDs, as comprise the majority of disfluencies in stuttering; (2) NSLDs, as comprise the majority of disfluencies in cluttering; and (3) other types of atypical disfluencies including word-final disfluencies, which have been identified in isolation, or in conjunction with stuttering or cluttering (Scott et al., 2006). The presence of excessive NSLDs is most relevant to the St. Louis et al. (2007) definition of cluttered speech, and requires further exploration within the ASD population. Table 8.2 summarizes the existing literature on occurrence of NSLDs in ASDs.

Table 8.2 Literature identifying types of non-stuttering-like disfluencies in conversation samples in autism spectrum disorders

Reference	*MSWWR*[a]	*PHR*[a]	*REV*[a]	*INT*[a]
Simmons and Baltaxe (1975) (n = 7)		X		
Higher-functioning autism				
Thacker and Austin (1986) (n = 1)	?	X		
Autistic features Dobbinson, Perkins, and Boucher (1998) (n = 1)		X		
Autism/retardation Shriberg et al. (2001)[b]; Paul et al. (2005)[b] (n = 15)	?		X	
AD/HFA Hietella and Spillers (2005) (n = 2)			X	X
ASD Scott et al. (2006) (n = 2)	?	X		X
AD Sisskin (2006) (n = 2)		X	X	X
AD Scaler Scott (2008) (n = 12)	X	X	X	X
AD				

a MSWWR = multi-syllable whole word repetitions; PHR = phrase repetitions; REV = revisions; INT = interjections.
b These two studies represent the same sample of individuals with AD.
? = unclear from data description whether these disfluencies were present, but possible.

Pausing and prosodic patterns in autism spectrum disorders

Atypical prosody is often associated as a core feature of the speech of individuals with ASDs. Prosody is divided into pragmatic, grammatical, and affective functions (for a review, see Shriberg et al., 2001). Grammatical prosody includes such features as word stress, which signals syntactic information (i.e. a noun versus a verb). Pragmatic prosody includes such features as emphatic stress (e.g. 'I meant *her*, not her'), which conveys the social information of a sentence. Affective prosody includes features that convey the feelings of the message, such as use of a worried or angry tone. Based on prior studies and hypotheses regarding the intact grammatical skills of many on the autism spectrum, it was proposed that prosodic differences in ASDs were related to the pragmatic and affective rather than to the grammatical functions of prosody. However, Shriberg et al. (2001) found that the previously described inappropriate or nonfluent phrasing exhibited by individuals with AD and HFA was best explained by increased speaking demands that exceeded the individuals' capacities for fluent phrasing. Given that a positive relationship was found between length of utterance and number of phrasing errors, the authors proposed this explanation of phrasing errors was most consistent with deficits in grammatical prosody. These differences in prosody are most consistent with the manner in which St. Louis et al. indicate that rate issues in cluttering may manifest themselves: 'the frequent placement of pauses and use of prosodic patterns that do not conform to syntactic and semantic constraints' (2007, p. 300). This type of prosodic pattern relates at least in part to the stop and start nature that the listener may perceive as cluttered speech (St. Louis, Myers, Faragasso, Townsend, & Gallaher, 2004).

In a prior study of cluttered speech, frequency of pausing was found to be less for an individual with cluttering (Scaler Scott & Tetnowski, 2006) as compared with age-established norms. If pausing is in fact exhibited less by individuals with cluttering, this would result in a perception of overall increased rate. Similarly, longer pauses could result in perception of the irregular rate sometimes characteristic of cluttering. As compared with age-matched typical speakers, pauses have been found to be longer in some individuals with ASDs (Shriberg et al., 2001) and in some individuals with cluttering (Teigland, 1996). Based on the limited findings thus far regarding pausing and prosody in ASDs as they relate to a diagnosis of cluttering, it appears that difficulties in grammatical prosody and/or increased pause time could result in a perception of cluttered speech among some individuals with ASDs. Those with ASDs who are highly verbal may exhibit more difficulties with grammatical prosody, as Shriberg et al. indicate, 'the longer the utterance the greater the opportunities for a revision or repetition on one or more words' (2001, p. 1106). Thus, those with higher verbal skills and ASDs may also exhibit more signs of the prosodic breakdowns observed in cluttered speech. It is interesting to note that in the Shriberg et al. study, those with

HFA, whose language skills are thought to be less developed than those with AD, exhibited longer pause time than those with AD and age-matched typical speakers. It is reasonable to propose that while those with greater verbal skills and ASDs may exhibit more signs of the atypical prosodic aspect of cluttered speech, those with less verbal skills and ASDs may exhibit more signs of the atypical pausing aspect of cluttered speech.

Excessive coarticulation in autism spectrum disorders

There has been minimal work done examining articulation patterns in ASDs. Shriberg et al. found that individuals with AD and HFA ages 10–50 years exhibited 'a high prevalence of residual articulation errors' (2001, p. 1111). These included distortions of sibilants, liquids, and rhotocized vowels. Based upon Paul's (1992) findings of increased disfluency and articulation errors in the narratives of young children whose language is still developing and in late talkers, and Shriberg et al.'s finding of increased phrasing errors with increased utterance length in individuals with ASDs, Shriberg et al. hypothesized that children with ASDs may have difficulty allocating the necessary resources for speech production. Consequently, the investigators submit that disfluencies and articulation errors may increase within an individual with an ASD in contexts that involve high linguistic complexity and/or social knowledge.

Occurrences of excessive coarticulation have only been reported in studies in which those with an ASD were diagnosed with cluttering or cluttering-stuttering (Scaler Scott, 2008; Scaler Scott et al., 2010; Thacker & Austen, 1996). In the Scaler Scott study of 12 school-age children with AD, all three participants with AD who presented with cluttering presented with excessive coarticulation (particularly of word endings), resulting in decreased intelligibility of speech. More research needs to be done to confirm that this symptom of cluttered speech occurs not in isolation (as in an overall motor weakness) in ASDs, but in combination with other symptoms that match the criteria for a cluttering diagnosis.

Cluttered speech does not equal an ASD . . . but the opposite can be true

The limited research that has explored speech patterns in ASDs demonstrates that cluttered speech is not a symptom in all individuals with an ASD. Following the preliminary data that we do have on cluttering, we might expect to find higher incidence of symptoms of cluttering in the ASD population than in a comparison population with no diagnosis. There is not yet conclusive evidence to determine why the speech of those with an ASD may be more prone to cluttering than the speech of those with no diagnosis. However, the current theories regarding what underlies specific cluttering symptoms may also apply to individuals with ASDs. These theoretical factors may then combine to create a reasonable explanation for increased potential for cluttered speech in individuals with ASDs.

Theoretical explanations for rapid and/or irregular rate

As previously mentioned, St. Louis et al. (2007) submit that those with cluttering may speak rapidly relative to themselves, suggesting difficulties with self-monitoring or self-regulation of rate. In individuals with ASDs, difficulties with self-regulation as it relates to social interaction and behavior is a hallmark feature of the disorder (American Psychiatric Association, 2000). Shriberg et al. suggest that increased articulation errors in individuals with HFA and AD 'may reflect a speaker's failure to attend to and/or allocate resources for fine-tuning speech production to match the model of the ambient linguistic community' (2001, p. 1109). Adults with cluttering have reported that when they monitor their speech, slowing down and focusing on producing all syllables, they have limited to no problems with intelligibility. Yet they also report that maintaining such levels of self-regulation is difficult (see Scaler Scott & St. Louis, chapter 13 this volume). Perhaps difficulties in maintaining a speech rate that allows for intelligible speech are related to difficulties with auditory and/or proprioceptive feedback. Difficulties with such systems in individuals with ASDs have been proposed to be related to 'loud, slow, high-pitched, and/or nasal speech' (Shriberg et al., 2001). Adults with cluttering have reported that feedback at times needs to be explicit for them to realize they need to monitor their speech rate (see Scaler Scott & St. Louis, chapter 13 this volume). Similarly, individuals on the autism spectrum have been found to require exaggerated nonverbal cues to elicit appropriate responses (Landa, 2000). In both cluttering and ASDs, decreased awareness of feedback may result in difficulties with regulation of appropriate rate for effective conversational interaction.

Theoretical explanations for excessive disfluencies

Given the fact that both are fluency disorders that have been found to co-occur, it is not unreasonable to assume that the disfluencies in both cluttering and stuttering may have similar origins. However, the fluency symptom that distinguishes cluttering from stuttering is that of excessive NSLDs in relation to frequency of SLDs. Investigators have identified a common link between an increased number of NSLDs in preschool and young school-age CWNS and linguistic patterns relative to each child's mean length of utterance (MLU). Namely, Zackheim and Conture (2003) found that among these children, the relationship between disfluency and utterance length and/or complexity is not always linear. Rather, Zackheim and Conture contend that disfluency results from individual dissociations between the length and/or complexity of an utterance a child is trying to produce relative to his or her mean length of utterance. The CWNS produced more NSLDs on both complex and non-complex utterances above their MLU. The investigators concluded that the disfluencies seemed to be related to the mismatch or dissociation between the utterance produced and the child's MLU rather than to absolute length or complexity of utterance alone. This analogy is similar to that of individuals with cluttering speaking fast relative to themselves, one of the results of which may be excess NSLDs.

An important similarity between children on the higher functioning end of the autism spectrum and CWS is that in both populations, language disorders are not part of the diagnostic criteria. Although some CWS may also have identifiable co-occurring language disorders (Van Borsel & Tetnowski, 2007), the majority of CWS do not (Anderson & Conture, 2000; Anderson, Pellowski, & Conture, 2005; Bernstein Ratner, 1997; Westby, 1974; Yairi, Ambrose, Paden, & Throneburg, 1996). Yet investigators have found linguistic differences (rather than deviations) in skill development between two or more areas of language in both CWS (Anderson & Conture, 2000; Anderson et al., 2005) and in ASDs (Tager-Flusberg, 1994), suggesting asynchronous language development. As stuttering and cluttering have often been found to co-occur, these linguistic dissociations may add to the recipe for disfluent speech in ASDs, which may manifest itself as stuttering and/or cluttering.

Theoretical explanations for atypical pausing and prosodic patterns

As mentioned, difficulties with all functions of prosody (grammatical, pragmatic, and affective) have been identified in ASDs. Difficulties with fluent phrasing identified in AD and HFA have been attributed to difficulties with the grammatical aspect of prosody (Shriberg et al., 2001). Aside from the association between pragmatic deficits as a core issue in ASDs and this area serving as one of the key functions of prosody, there are no known studies that have identified the root of prosodic difficulties. Future study of prosodic patterns in individuals with cluttering and individuals with ASDs is needed before any conclusions can be drawn between what factors may underlie symptoms in these two populations.

In terms of pausing, Teigland found that when giving directions to a peer, students in junior high with cluttering had more 'breaks in form of empty pauses of 4 seconds or more' (1996, p. 210) than the age- and gender-matched typical speakers. Teigland theorized that these pauses were related to difficulties with speech fluency in dialogues. Shriberg et al. (2001) also found difficulties with fluent phrasing in individuals with HFA and AD. From this perspective, disfluent speech would be the root of atypical pausing rather than atypical pausing resulting in disfluent speech. The relation between pausing and speech fluency in both individuals with ASDs and individuals with cluttering requires further study.

Theoretical explanations for excessive coarticulation

Shriberg et al. (2001) found a significantly higher presence of speech sound distortion in their participants with HFA and AD than is estimated in the neurotypical adult population. Higher prevalence of articulation disorders have also been noted in both stuttering (Blood, Ridenour, Qualls, & Hammer, 2003) and cluttering (St. Louis et al., 2007). One of the proposed factors in the development of speech sound disorders of otherwise unknown origin are delays in phonological development (Flipsen, Bankson, & Bernthal, 2009). These delays have also been found in preschoolers who stutter. Watkins, Yairi, and Ambrose (1999) completed a longitudinal study of 84 children between the ages of 2 and 5 years. Spontaneous language samples were taken from each child at the time of entrance to the study. Participants were followed for a minimum of 4 years, at the end of which time 62 were classified as recovered from stuttering and 22 were classified as persistent stutterers. Language skills at the time of entry into the study were compared with a normative sample. Results revealed that regardless of their eventual grouping, all children scored at least within the average range of performance on the language variables of mean length of utterance, number of different words, number of total words and syntactic and morphological analyses. Children who entered the study at earlier ages tended to score 1 year above their peers entering the study at later ages. Dissociations were suggested when it was noted that no such precocious findings were identified for these children in the area of phonological/articulation development. Thus, although this subgroup of children exhibited precocious expressive language skills, these skills were disassociated from their phonological development. Children who persisted in stuttering exhibited phonological development that progressed in the same sequence as their recovered peers and used the same substitution patterns as their peers. However, the persistent group tended to score lower than their recovered peers on all formal testing measures of phonological development. The investigators concluded that CWS who exhibit delays in phonological development are at increased risk for persistent stuttering (Paden, Yairi, & Ambrose, 1999). Given delays in phonological development and at least average expressive language skills, dissociations between different areas of speech and language are suggested early on in the development of persistent stuttering.

Despite overlap in articulation delays in stuttering, cluttering, and ASD populations, such delays alone would not result in excessive coarticulation, but rather would result in speech sound errors. Additionally, rapid rate alone should not result in excessive coarticulation. It is probable, however, that a rapid rate combined with phonological/articulatory difficulties could result in excessive coarticulation. Since it is proposed that the rate of speech for those with cluttering is not necessarily excessively rapid but too rapid for themselves, the excessive coarticulation again may be a combination of issues with phonological/articulatory delays and/or deviances, and self-monitoring related to difficulties with auditory or proprioceptive feedback. However, given that articulation disorders are not present in all individuals with cluttering, this recipe for excessive coarticulation may relate only to subgroups of individuals with cluttering and/or ASDs.

Although it is unlikely that phonological delays and/or deviances cause disfluent speech, if one is prone to disfluent speech in preschool and has delayed and/or deviant phonological development, it stands to reason that one's system is taxed more and that the likelihood disfluencies will persist is increased. The fact that phonological delays/deviances and disfluencies have both been more likely to occur in ASDs than in undiagnosed comparison groups may place individuals with ASDs at increased risk for communication disorders such as cluttering.

Evaluation of cluttered speech in autism spectrum disorders

Matching speech symptoms in ASDs to the current working definition of cluttered speech makes diagnosis of cluttering a straightforward process. Too often speech, language, and learning characteristics that may commonly co-occur with cluttering are mistakenly taken as evidence for diagnosis of cluttering. It is important to keep in mind that to engage in evidence-based practice, we must differentiate the symptoms of cluttered speech from those symptoms that may commonly co-occur with cluttered speech, but for which we currently lack evidence that these are more than features commonly *associated* with cluttering. By following the current working definition of cluttered speech, speech-language therapists can determine whether a child with an ASD fits the diagnostic criteria for cluttered speech. The speech-language therapist should still treat any other associated speech and language symptoms outside of this definition. The diagnosis of cluttering is just not made based on these associated symptoms. For example, if the child's speech symptoms match the diagnostic definition of cluttered speech, and the child also has pragmatic language issues such as failure to maintain topic, this symptom must be taken into consideration in determining a holistic treatment plan. If a child is veering off topic in the middle of a conversation, this may make the child just as unintelligible (in terms of content) as if they were speaking too quickly and over co-articulating syllables. In this case, both cluttered speech and topic maintenance skills would be addressed in treatment.

Treatment of cluttered speech in autism spectrum disorders

Because few treatment studies have been completed for cases of cluttering, we are sorely lacking in evidence to support treatment methods for cluttered speech. However, we can focus on the aspects of cluttered speech (according to the working definition) that present themselves in each client, and treat these according to the existing evidence that we have for each aspect (Bernstein Ratner, 2005). There is preliminary evidence for the successful impact of pausing on rate control in two school-age children matching the current working definition of cluttering (Scaler Scott et al., 2010; Simkins, Kingery, & Bradley, 1970). Investigators in the area of voice therapy have demonstrated preliminary success with pacing boards for monitoring rate, and with the Lee Silverman Voice Therapy treatments for increasing speech intelligibility (Helm, 1979; Ramig, Countryman, Thompson, & Horii, 1995; and Yorkston, 1996, which includes a review of speech treatments to address such factors as prosody, rate, articulation, intelligibility, self-monitoring).

Certain considerations must be taken into account when treating cluttering in the ASD population. First, self-regulation is a key component of treatment for both cluttered speech and for ASDs in general. Prizant and Meyer (1993) propose that children on the autism spectrum tend to have difficulties with engagement with others. This lack of engagement leads to difficulties in the development of self-regulation, which also leads to difficulties with effective communication. This is a circular pattern whereby failure in self-regulation leads to communication failure, which leads to failure to develop self-regulation. The ability to self-regulate is therefore crucial for clients with ASDs, and becomes even more important when the client needs to also monitor cluttered speech. Therefore, it is critical that clients with ASDs be actively engaged in therapy activities. It can be difficult to sustain an ongoing interaction with a client on the autism spectrum when they have difficulty establishing eye contact that is so necessary to keep a communicative exchange going. In addition, to repair cluttered speech, the client needs to examine the listener's face for clues that there has been a communication breakdown. Often individuals with ASDs are not aware of: (1) their listener's perspective that they haven't been understood and (2) the breakdowns in their speech. A way to address this lack of awareness is to work on giving the client a purpose for eye contact. Higher functioning clients can be taught that by looking at someone while talking to them, they can be a 'detective', identifying and repairing communication breakdowns as they occur. Use of ongoing conversations on topics of the child's interest provides a constantly changing and therefore challenging but interesting and purposeful context for practice. For lower functioning individuals, more work may need to be done to maintain active engagement (see Greenspan, 2001). Once engaged, children can imitate models of clearer speech, focusing on pausing (if needed to reduce speed), and precise articulation of syllables and word endings.

Where do we go from here?

Clearly there is much work to be done in studying the speech fluency patterns in ASDs and as concerns this reader, specifically, cluttering within this population. But given what has been found to this point, it is also certainly warranted that speech-language therapists be aware that cluttered speech can be found within this population, and should be ruled out during a speech and language evaluation. If cluttering is identified in a client, treatment methods should take into account what is known about evidence-based treatment of these symptoms. Additionally, treatment should take into account the best treatment practices for individuals with ASDs. Such consideration involves combining best practice of cluttering treatment with best practice of treatment principles in the ASD population. It is not enough to treat cluttering symptoms within the ASD population. Cluttering treatment must not only be presented, but must actually *reach* an individual with an ASD. In order to reach the individual, treatment must be presented with consideration for the unique needs of the autism spectrum population (see also Scaler Scott et al., 2010).

A small start has been made toward understanding patterns of cluttered speech in the ASD population. Continued work in research and treatment is greatly needed. To expedite this work toward development of best practice, evaluation data should be gathered to track the co-occurrence of cluttered speech and ASDs. Additionally, treatment efficacy data should be gathered to objectively measure cluttering treatment outcomes within this specific population. If we focus on identifying symptoms of the current working definition of cluttering within the ASD population, and on identifying effectiveness of treatments to change these specific symptoms, we can better understand the link between cluttering and ASDs. Given the fact that the number of individuals diagnosed with ASDs is continually increasing (Newschaffer et al., 2006), working toward these changes could go a long way toward helping individuals with ASDs become more effective communicators.

References

Ambrose, N. G., & Yairi, E. (1999). Normative disfluency data for early childhood stuttering. *Journal of Speech, Language, and Hearing Research*, *42*, 895–909.

American Psychiatric Association. (2000). *Diagnostic and statistical manual of mental disorders* (4th ed., text revision). Washington, DC: American Psychiatric Association.

Anderson, J. D., & Conture, E. G. (2000). Language abilities of children who stutter: A preliminary study. *Journal of Fluency Disorders*, *25*, 283–304.

Anderson, J. D., Pellowski, M. W., & Conture, E. G. (2005). Childhood stuttering and dissociations across linguistic domains. *Journal of Fluency Disorders*, *30*, 219–253.

Ardila, A., & Lopez, M. V. (1986). Severe stuttering associated with right hemisphere lesion. *Brain and Language*, *27*, 239–246.

Baltaxe, C. (1981). Acoustic characteristics of prosody in autism. In P. Mittler (Ed.), *Frontier of knowledge in mental retardation* (pp. 223–233). Baltimore, MD: University Park Press.

Bernstein Ratner, N. (1997). Stuttering: A psycholinguistic perspective. In R. F. Curlee & G. M. Siegel (Eds.). *Nature and treatment of stuttering: New directions* (pp. 97–127). Boston, MA: Allyn & Bacon.

Bernstein Ratner, N. (2005). Evidence-based practice in stuttering: Some questions to consider. *Journal of Fluency Disorders*, *30*, 163–188.

Bijleveld, H., Lebrun, Y., & Van Dongen, H. (1994). A case of acquired stuttering. *Folia Phoniatrica et Logopaedica*, *46*, 250–253.

Blood, G. W., Ridenour Jr., V. J., Qualls, C. D., & Hammer, C. S. (2003). Co-occurring disorders in children who stutter. *Journal of Communication Disorders*, *36*, 427–448.

Dobbinson, S., Perkins, M. R., & Boucher, J. (1998). Structural patterns in conversations with a woman who has autism. *Journal of Communication Disorders*, *31*, 113–134.

Flipsen Jr., P., Bankson, N. W., & Bernthal, J. E. (2009). Classification and factors related to speech sound disorders. In J. E. Bernthal, N. W. Bankson, & P. Flipsen Jr. (Eds.), *Articulation and phonological disorders: Speech sound disorders in children* (pp. 121–186). New York: Pearson.

Goldfarb, W., Goldfarb, N., Braunstein, P., & Scholl, N. (1972). Speech and language faults in schizophrenic children. *Journal of Autism and Childhood Schizophrenia*, *2*, 219–233.

Greenspan, S. I. (2001). *The affect diathesis hypothesis: The role of emotions in the core deficit in autism and in the development of intelligence and social skills.* Retrieved August 31, 2007, from www.floortime.org/downloads/affect_diathesis_hypothesis.pdf

Helm, N. A. (1979). Management of palilalia with a pacing board. *Journal of Speech and Hearing Disorders*, *44*, 350–353.

Hietella, A., & Spillers, C. (2005, November). *Disfluency patterns in children with autism spectrum disorders.* Poster session presented at the Annual ASHA Convention, San Diego, CA.

Klin, A., Sparrow, S. S., Marans, W. D., Carter, A., & Volkmar, F. R. (2000). Assessment issues in children and adolescents with Asperger syndrome. In A. Klin, F. R. Volkmar, & S. S. Sparrow (Eds.), *Asperger syndrome* (pp. 309–339). New York: The Guilford Press.

Landa, R. (2000). Pragmatic language intervention for children with autism spectrum disorders. In P. J. Accardo, C. Magnusen, & A. J. Capute (Eds.), *Autism: Clinical and research issues* (pp. 163–192). Baltimore: York Press.

Lebrun, Y., & Leleux, C. (1985). Acquired stuttering following right-brain damage in dextrals. *Journal of Fluency Disorders*, *10*, 137–141.

Lebrun, Y., & Van Borsel, J. (1990). Final sound repetitions. *Journal of Fluency Disorders*, *15*, 107–113.

Myers, F. L., & Bradley, C. L. (1992). Clinical management of cluttering from a synergistic framework. In F. L. Myers & K. O. St. Louis (Eds.), *Cluttering: A clinical perspective* (pp. 85–105). Kibworth, UK: Far Communications. (Reissued in 1996 by Singular, San Diego, CA.)

Newschaffer, C. J., Croen, L. A., Daniels, J., Giarelli, E., Grether, J. K., Levy, S. E., et al. (2006). The epidemiology of autism spectrum disorders. *Annual Reviews of Public Health, 305*, 28:21.1–28:21.24.

Paden, E. P., Yairi, E., & Ambrose, N. G. (1999). Early childhood stuttering II: Initial status of phonological abilities. *Journal of Speech, Language, and Hearing Research, 42*, 1113–1124.

Paul, R. (1992). Speech-language interactions in the talk of young children. In R. S. Chapman (Ed.), *Processes in language acquisition and disorders* (pp. 235–254). Boston, MA: Mosby Year Book.

Paul, R., Shriberg, L. D., McSweeny, J., Cicchetti, D., Klin, A., & Volkmar, F. (2005). Brief report: Relations between prosody performance and communication and socialization ratings in high functioning speakers with autism spectrum disorders. *Journal of Autism and Developmental Disorders, 35*, 861–869.

Prizant, B. M., & Meyer, E. C. (1993, September). Socioemotional aspects of language and social-communication disorders in young children and their families. *American Journal of Speech-Language Pathology*, 56–71.

Ramig, L. O., Countryman, S., Thompson, L. L., & Horii, Y. (1995). Comparison of two forms of intensive speech treatment for Parkinson disease. *Journal of Speech and Hearing Research, 38*, 1232–1251.

Raphael, L. J., Bakker, K., Myers, F. L., St. Louis, K. O., Fichtner, V., & Kostel, M. (2005). *An update on diadochokinetic rates of cluttered and normal speech.* Poster presented at the Annual Convention of the American Speech-Language-Hearing Association. San Diego, CA.

Raphael, L. J., Bakker, K., Myers, F. L., St. Louis, K. O., & MacRoy, M. (2004). *Diadochokinetic rates of cluttered and normal speech.* Paper presented at the Annual Convention of the American Speech-Language-Hearing Association. Philadelphia, PA.

Riley, G. D. (1994). *Stuttering severity instrument for children and adults* (3rd ed.). Austin, TX: Pro-Ed.

Rosenfield, D. B., Viswanath, N. S., Callis-Landrum, L., Didanato, R., & Nudelman, H. B. (1991). Patients with acquired dysfluencies: What they tell us about developmental stuttering. In H. F. M. Peters, W. Hulstijn, & C. W. Starkweather (Eds.), *Speech motor control and stuttering* (pp. 277–284). Amsterdam: Elsevier.

Scaler Scott, K. (2008). *A comparison of disfluency and language in matched children with Asperger's disorder, children who stutter, and controls during an expository discourse task.* Doctoral dissertation, University of Louisiana at Lafayette.

Scott, K. S., Grossman, H. L., Abendroth, K. J., Tetnowski, J. A., & Damico, J. S. (2007). Asperger syndrome and attention deficit disorder: Clinical disfluency analysis. In J. Au-Yeung & M. M. Leahy (Eds.), *Research, treatment, and self-help in fluency disorders: New Horizons. Proceedings of the Fifth World Congress on Fluency Disorders* (pp. 273–278). Dublin: International Fluency Association.

Scaler Scott, K., & Tetnowski, J. (2006, November). *Analysis of the physical correlates of cluttering: A case study*. A technical presentation at the annual convention of the American Speech-Language-Hearing Association, Miami, FL.

Scaler Scott, K., Ward, D., & St. Louis, K. O. (2010). Cluttering in a school-aged child. In S. Chabon & E. Cohn (Eds.), *Communication disorders: A case-based approach* (pp. 261–272). Boston, MA: Pearson/Allyn & Bacon.

Shriberg, L. D., Paul, R., McSweeny, J. L., Klin, A., Cohen, D. J., & Volkmar, F. R. (2001). Speech and prosody characteristics of adolescents and adults with high-functioning autism and Asperger syndrome. *Journal of Speech, Language, and Hearing Research*, *44*, 1097–1115.

Simkins, L., Kingery, M., & Bradley, P. (1970). Modification of cluttered speech in an emotionally disturbed child. *The Journal of Special Education*, *4*, 81–88.

Simmons, J. Q., & Baltaxe, C. (1975). Language patterns of adolescent autistics. *Journal of Autism and Childhood Schizophrenia*, *5*, 333–351.

Sisskin, V. (2006). Speech disfluency in Asperger's syndrome: Two cases of interest. *Perspectives on Fluency and Fluency Disorders*, *16*, 12–14.

Stansfield, J. (1995).Word-final disfluencies in adults with learning difficulties. *Journal of Fluency Disorders*, *20*, 1–10.

St. Louis, K. O., Hinzman, A. R., & Hull, F. M. (1985). Studies of cluttering: Disfluency and language measures in young possible clutterers and stutterers. *Journal of Fluency Disorders*, *10*, 151–172.

St. Louis, K., Myers, F., Bakker, K., & Raphael, L. (2007). Understanding and treating cluttering. In E. G. Conture & R. F. Curlee (Eds.), *Stuttering and related disorders of fluency* (3rd ed., pp. 297–325). New York: Thieme.

St. Louis, K. O., Myers, F. L., Faragasso, K., Townsend, P. S., & Gallaher, A. J. (2004). Perceptual aspects of cluttered speech. *Journal of Fluency Disorders*, *29*, 213–235.

Tager-Flusberg, H. (1994). Dissociation in form and function in the acquisition of language by autistic children. In H. Tager-Flusberg (Ed.), *Constraints on language acquisition: Studies of atypical children* (pp. 175–194). Hillsdale, NJ: Lawrence Erlbaum Associates Inc.

Teigland, A. (1996). A study of pragmatic skills of clutterers and normal speakers. *Journal of Fluency Disorders*, *21*, 201–214.

Thacker, A. J., & Austen, S. (1996). Cluttered communication in a deafened adult with autistic features. *Journal of Fluency Disorders*, *21*, 271–279.

Van Borsel, J., Geirnaert, E., & Van Coster, R. (2005). Another case of word-final disfluencies. *Folia Phoniatrica et Logopaedica*, *57*, 148–162.

Van Borsel, J., & Tetnowski, J. A. (2007). Stuttering in genetic syndromes. *Journal of Fluency Disorders*, *32*, 279–296.

Van Borsel, J., Van Coster, R., & Van Lierd, K. (1996). Repetitions in final position in a nine-year-old boy with focal brain damage. *Journal of Fluency Disorders*, *21*, 137–146.

Volkmar, F. R., & Klin, A. (2000). Diagnostic issues in Asperger syndrome. In A. Klin, F. R. Volkmar, & S. S. Sparrow (Eds.), *Asperger syndrome* (pp. 309–339). New York: The Guilford Press.

Watkins, R. V., Yairi, E., & Ambrose, N. G. (1999). Early childhood stuttering III: Initial status of expressive language abilities. *Journal of Speech, Language, and Hearing Research*, *42*, 1125–1135.

Weschler, D. (1955). *Weschler Adult Intelligence Scale*. New York: Psychological Corporation.

Westby, C. E. (1974). Language performance of stuttering and nonstuttering children. *Journal of Communications Disorders*, *12*, 133–145.

Yairi, E., & Ambrose, N. (1992). A longitudinal study of stuttering in children: A preliminary report. *Journal of Speech and Hearing Research*, *35*, 755–760.

Yairi, E., Ambrose, N., Paden, E., & Throneburg, R. (1996). Predictive factors of persistence and recovery: Pathways of childhood stuttering. *Journal of Communication Disorders*, *29*, 51–77.

Yorkston, K. M. (1996). Treatment efficacy: Dysarthria. *Journal of Speech and Hearing Research*, *39*, S46–S57.

Zackheim, C. T., & Conture, E. G. (2003). Childhood stuttering and speech disfluencies in relation to children's mean length of utterance: A preliminary study. *Journal of Fluency Disorders*, *28*, 115–142.

Part III

Assessment and treatment of cluttering

9 The assessment of cluttering: rationale, tasks, and interpretation

Yvonne van Zaalen, Frank Wijnen, and Philipe Dejonckere

Introduction

As Ward (2006) has stated, no one speaks 100 percent fluently. Even the most eloquent speakers have occasional speech failures. In all likelihood, Ward continues, most of us make these mistakes more often than we actually want to. Ward notes that different kinds of speech failures exist. For instance, we can add words or sounds to gain time, such as 'uh', or 'well'. It is also possible to reconstruct a sentence during speech when we notice that the formulated sentence does not have the effect we wanted. Word repetitions or stumbling over one's words are common speech failures. In response to failures like this, the layperson may say, 'Oh, I am stuttering again.' Such fluency failures, Ward contends, are not typically characteristic of stuttering but are common in another fluency disorder known as cluttering. When a person produces a *high frequency* of these slips of the tongue, that happen in *different* speech situations and *often* (Ward, 2006), and they are produced in conjunction with irregularities of speech rate, prosody, and/or intelligibility, it may be called cluttering (Ward, 2006).

After the German Kussmaul (1887) and the Austrian Weiss (1964) pointed attention to this remarkable phenomenon, cluttering appeared to be a recognized disorder in Europe in particular. In other parts of the world, however, cluttering did not fit in any other nosological disorder area and remained misunderstood until the end of the last century.

In the last several decades, a diversity of difficult-to-measure symptoms were attributed to cluttering, which made it difficult to clarify what cluttering is. From the late 1980s, more North American publications began to be written on cluttering (St. Louis, Myers, Bakker, & Raphael, 2007). Because of the contributions of authors such as St. Louis, Daly, Myers, Raphael, Bakker, and Preus, the disorder began to have increased recognition around the world.

Definition and subtyping of cluttering

St. Louis et al. (2007) defined cluttering as a fluency disorder in which a person's speech has either a (too) fast or (too) irregular speech rate combined with one or more of the following characteristics: a high frequency of normal disfluencies; inadequate word or sentence structures; or inadequate use of pausing (too often, not enough, or in linguistically incorrect places). Van Zaalen hypothesized that cluttering is based on defective language automation (Van Zaalen, 2009).

Pure cluttering is rare, whereas specific cluttering symptoms or behaviours occur much more frequently. Ward (2006) divides cluttering into two different types: linguistic cluttering and motoric cluttering. Van Zaalen's (2009) subtyping is comparable to Ward's (2006) subtyping, but is more linguistically based. Phonological cluttering, diagnosed when speech rate is insufficiently adjusted to the phonological encoding skills, results in reduced intelligibility due to telescoping, coarticulation, and syllable sequencing errors (see also Myers, chapter 10 this volume; Van Zaalen, 2009). Syntactical cluttering, diagnosed when speech rate is insufficiently adjusted to the grammatical encoding skills and linguistic complexity of the message, results in sentence revisions ('I went, walked home.'), phrase repetitions ('I went, I went . . . I went to the cinema this weekend.'), interjections ('I, uh, I don't know, uh, I went home.'), and semantic paraphasias (Van Zaalen, 2009). In semantic paraphasias, the speaker uses an unintended word, but of the same semantic category as the intended word. For example, the speaker might say 'When I was ten *days* old' when 'When I was ten *years* old' was meant.

Age and diagnosis

According to Weiss (1964), cluttering has its origin in difficulties with central language abilities, and most persons are troubled by their cluttered speech at the earliest in late childhood and often not earlier than in adolescence or early adulthood. Daly (2008, July), Mensink-Ypma (1990), and Ward (2006) stated that cluttering manifests itself when language development is in a far advanced stage, and the person has a high urgency to speak. Cluttering is often difficult to diagnose before the age of 8 years. Two explanations for this point can be given: first, speech rate of young children as a group (e.g., Walker et al., 1991) is too slow (although there certainly are exceptions) to have a major influence on speech intelligibility and speech fluency. Secondly, mistakes in story, word, and sentence structures in children who clutter are difficult to differentiate from those of children with developmental language disorders (van Zaalen, Wijnen, & Dejonckere, 2009b, 2009d).

Differential diagnosis

In this chapter, we attempt to clarify the assessment and differential diagnosis of cluttering and other disorders of speech fluency, based on recent scientific knowledge (evidence-based practice) and clinical reports (practice-based evidence). One of the problems in diagnosis and treatment of cluttering is that cluttering often co-occurs with other disorders. Some of these disorders are speech-based, such as stuttering, and others are language-based, such as learning disabilities (Ward, 2006). As Gregory (1995) concluded, the disorder of cluttering provides us with an obvious example of how much speech, language, and learning disabilities have in common.

In pure stuttering, a high frequency of involuntary disruptions in the fluency of speech appears. People who stutter often experience a sense of loss of control (Guitar, 2006; Quesal, 2004; Shapiro, 1998; St. Louis et al., 2007; Ward, 2006). The interruptions in stuttering usually have the form of: (tensed) repetitions of sounds, syllables or one-syllable words; prolongations of sounds; and/or blocks of breathing or speech voicing. As mentioned, the interruptions in cluttering more often take the form of non-stuttering like disfluencies (Ambrose & Yairi, 1999; Yairi & Ambrose, 1992) including interjections, revisions, or repetitions of multisyllabic words and/or phrases.

For Preus (1996), cluttering has more in common with learning disabilities than with stuttering. Many researchers contend that the coherence of problems in cluttering and learning disabilities exists mainly with regard to problems in expression, reading, and writing (see also Van Zaalen et al., Chapter 7, this volume). In learning disabilities, speech rate is usually comparable with that of fluent controls, while language production is disturbed by incomplete sentences, word-finding problems, incorrect sentence structures, and reading disorders (Van Zaalen et al., 2009b).

In some cases, a person with cluttering (PWC) can become afraid of speaking. Speech fear can develop through negative responses from listeners ('What did you say?', 'I did not catch what you said', 'I do not understand you') or by a tensed nonverbal reaction. In these listener responses, the speech symptoms are not specified, reactions can confuse the speaker (Winkelman, 1990). The listener responses make clear that the PWC is doing something wrong, but what it is remains unmentioned. In the end, the PWC can become apprehensive of speaking because of this uncertainty.

Speech tasks

In order to distinguish cluttering from other disorders of speech fluency, cluttering assessment should focus on different aspects of communication and cognition. Assessment includes oral reading, spontaneous speech, retelling a memorized story, a test of speech motor coordination, and questionnaires. Digital video and audio recording of the client are taken in a variety of speaking tasks for subsequent analyses of fluency, rate, articulation, language, and voice. Comparing the client's and the clinician's perspective at baseline assessment can be enlightening.

Oral reading

Because the level of reading material may influence the degree of cluttering, the clinician should present clients with appropriate reading material that varies in levels of difficulty. The more difficult passages, containing more multisyllabic words and linguistically more complex sentences, may produce more cluttering behaviours compared with the less difficult passages (i.e., short sentences with one- or two-syllable words). It is also suggested that the client reads one passage with and one passage without preparation, to compare the results of the prepared and unprepared readings (Van Zaalen, Myers, Ward, & Bennett, 2008).

Language

As cluttering is considered to be an expression of a defective language automation (Van Zaalen, 2009), cluttering assessment should be focused on different linguistic levels and within different speech rates. People who clutter commonly experience breakdowns in communication at a high level of language production (i.e. narrative (re)telling). They also exhibit difficulties with pragmatic aspects of language, such as not taking into account the listener's viewpoint or knowledge, or frequent interruption of the communicative partner (Daly, 1986; Myers & Bradley, 1992; Teigland, 1996; Van Zaalen & Winkelman, 2009; Ward, 2006).

In order to assess these potentially difficult areas of language, the clinician should engage the client in a more relaxed exchange on a subject that is of high interest to the client. This can include explaining a videogame, talking about their favourite sport or leisure activity, or telling a story about a recent exciting event that the client experienced. The clinician should record at least 10 minutes of this language sample. The language sample should consist of a narrative rather than iterations of events as in a list (Van Zaalen et al., 2008; Ward, 2006).

Phonological tasks ranging from short and structured tasks to longer and less structured tasks are also of importance. Examples of the former include rote tasks such as counting (e.g., the client has to count backwards from 100 in 3s). Older clients should read some words that are difficult to pronounce (e.g., 'statistical', 'chrysanthemum', 'tyrannosaurus') and produce these words three times in succession, first at a comfortable rate and then at a faster speech rate (see also Bakker et al., chapter 4 this volume). Older clients should also read some words with changing stress pattern sequences, such as 'apply, application, applicable' (a_ply' / a_pli_ca'_tion / a_pli'_ca_ble). Younger children should name pictures (four different pictures of one- or two-syllable word pictures) within/without the same semantic category that are presented in a dysrythmic order (see Figure 9.1).

As mentioned, story retelling is an important component of assessment, as it is at this high level that communication may break down. The 'Wallet story' (Van Zaalen et al., 2009b) can be used for adolescents or adults, and the 'Bus story' for young children (Renfrew, 1997). The clinician should observe the following as the client retells the story: (1) ability to paraphrase the story with the major points of the narrative in logical sequence and with intact story grammar; (2) ability to maintain syllable, word, and sentence structure; (3) appropriate pausing; (4) adequate speech intelligibility; and (5) appropriate pragmatics.

Another component of assessment is imitation of sentences of increasing length (up to 20-word sentences for adults and adolescents, up to 14 words for 10-year-olds and up to 10 words for 8-year-olds). This task provides information on auditory memory skills and on the level of language

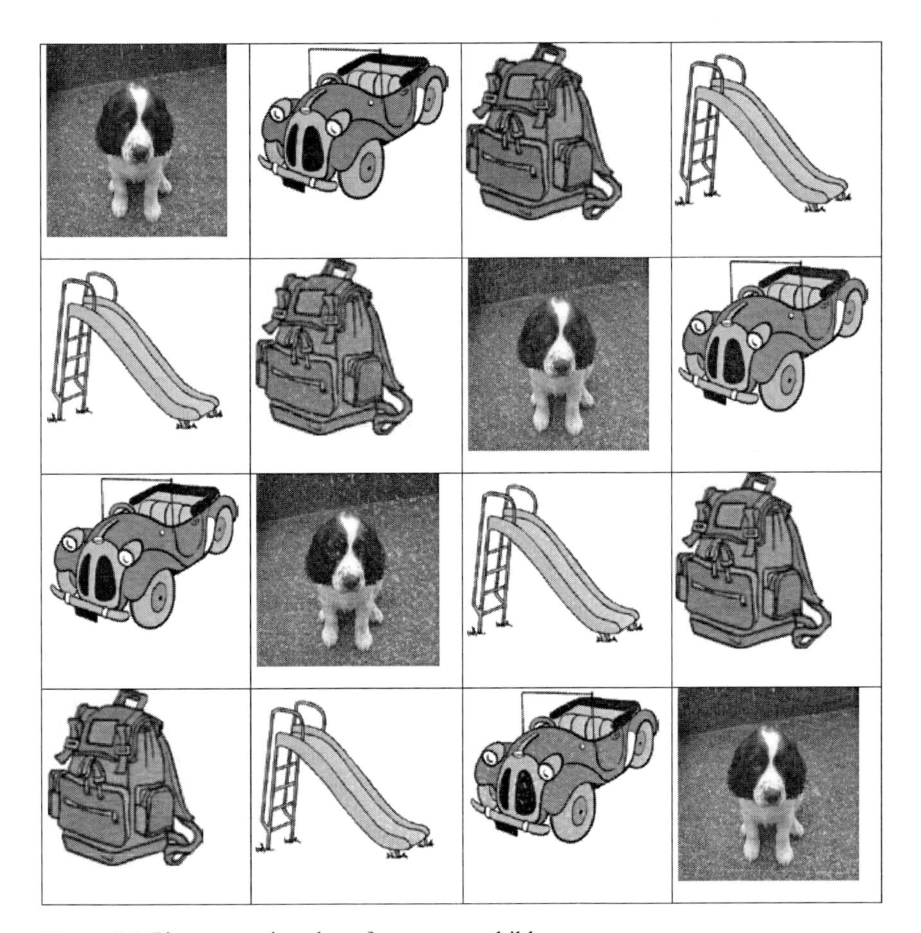

Figure 9.1 Picture naming sheet for younger children.

complexity where the client's communication breaks down (Van Zaalen et al., 2008).

Self-assessment

The emotional component of cluttering includes the effect of the speech on the speaker himself. As mentioned, when a person has not been understood several times, he can develop communication fear. A client who has little awareness of his symptoms judges his speech positively and blames the listener for not listening well enough. Communicative apprehension may develop when no connection is made between one's own speech production and the listener's reaction. Communication fear can develop unconsciously, and may occur as a hidden problem in cluttering. Speech-language therapists should be aware that a positive self-image could change when a PWC connects the listener's response to his speech. A person's attitude towards communication can be assessed with the Communication Attitude Test (CAT, Behaviour Assessment Battery; Brutten & Vanrijckegem, 2006).

Cluttering checklists and self-assessment

In 2006, Daly and Cantrell developed the Predictive Cluttering Inventory (PCI) on the basis of a worldwide survey amongst fluency specialists. The PCI contains 33 symptoms associated with cluttering, in four domains: (1) pragmatics; (2) speech motor; (3) language and cognition; and (4) motor coordination and writing problems. Every symptom can be ranked with a score on a 7-point scale (0 = not present, 6 = always present) in order to predict possible cluttering. In two independent research projects by Van Zaalen et al. (2009d) and Van Borsel and vanderMeulen (2008), it was concluded that the PCI in its early form (Daly & Burnett, 1996) was not sensitive and not specific enough to differentially diagnose possible cluttering. In a recent study results on the Dutch translation of the PCI of PWC, people who stutter (PWS), and controls were studied in connection to the subjective and objective measurements made by specialized SLTs (van Zaalen et al., 2009c). In this study, 137 Dutch-speaking participants ranging in age from 10.6 to 12.11 years were tested with the PCI by eight different SLTs. The PCI was completed based on observation of spontaneous speech, retelling a memorized story, reading aloud, and parental information. Pearson correlations were used to determine relationships between subjective and objective clinical judgement and the checklist norm studied. It was found that the PCI was not sensitive and specific enough to detect cluttering. A factor analysis was performed to determine factors that may explain the variance present in the basic variables: 'speech production, language production, alertness and other behaviours'. Results of the factor analysis were compared with results of a cluster analysis. Based on the significantly different items, a revised PCI was conducted. The interpretation of item scores in the revised PCI heightened the sensitivity to a low but acceptable score and was specific enough to detect possible cluttering behaviour (van Zaalen et al., 2009c).

Computer-based cluttering assessment tool

Because of the multidimensional nature of cluttering, supplementary assessment of individual dimensions such as rate and fluency, with a means to rate the overall severity of cluttering, is valuable. The Cluttering Assessment Program (CLASP), a freeware assessment tool developed to determine the percentage talking time cluttered, can be used to determine severity of cluttering (Bakker, 2005).

Differential diagnosis

As mentioned, pure cluttering is rare. Although solid numbers are missing, it is hypothesized by different authors that pure cluttering occurs in 5–16 percent of disfluent children (Bakker, 2005; St. Louis & McCaffrey, 2005). Weiss (1964) mentioned a ratio of 7 percent pure cluttering compared with 21 percent pure stuttering. In 1992, Preus analysed the results from seven research projects in which cluttering-stuttering was diagnosed from among a group of stutterers (Dalton & Hardcastle, 1989; Daly, 1986; Freund, 1952; Langová & Morávek, 1970; Preus, 1981; Seeman, 1974; Van Riper, 1982). The mean prevalence of cluttering-stuttering was 35 percent (range 18–67 percent). This means that in one of three stuttering clients, a cluttering component was present.

We hypothesize that the percentage of cluttering persons increases during adolescence. Influenced by a natural growth of speech rate, adolescents lose their prior speech control and become less intelligible as a result. Cluttering is often not identified until early adolescence (around 10 years of age), when the demands on communication become great enough for communication to break down in those who may have the predisposition to clutter. In other words, the demands on communication change, and this is when cluttering symptoms appear in those who are prone to clutter. Normally, in early adulthood speech rate decreases (Boey, 2000). A number of affected people will continue to experience problems in adjusting their speech rate to the motor and linguistic demands, and will remain cluttering (Van Zaalen & Winkelman, 2009).

In the following sections, we describe the assessment of the cluttering component. In this description, we make use of normative data collected in a cluttering sample of children, adolescents, and adults. Assessments took place between January 2006 and August 2009 in two centres of fluency therapy in the Netherlands. Additional assessment on co-occurring disorders should be done according to international standards. Furthermore, assessment has a temporal worth; repetition of the assessment after a period is important to discuss possible changes in time and to adjust the therapy plan (Van Zaalen et al., 2008).

Mean articulatory rate

Although a PWC often sounds as if he is speaking at a fast rate, when measured, this rate may not be as fast as the listener perceives. Pindzola, Jenkins, and Lokken (1989) and Hall, Amir, and Yairi (1999) stated that articulatory rate measures are intended to reflect how quickly sound segments are produced in stretches of speech that have no pauses. In order to measure the mean articulatory rate of speech, five at-random selected measures were taken within a sample of a recorded speech task. In stretches of 10–20 fluent syllables without pauses, the number of syllables produced per second was determined. Van Zaalen (2009) chose to use the linguistic word form instead of speech motor output in determining the number of syllables. Van Zaalen, Wijnen, and Dejonckere (2009c) defined fast articulatory rate as a rate ≥1.0 *SD* above the mean articulatory rate (MAR) of a sample of 54 disfluent speakers. In this research project with children, adolescents, and adults, Van Zaalen et al. (2009c) determined a fast articulatory rate of young children to be > 5.1 SPS (syllables per second), > 5.4 SPS for adolescents, and > 5.6 SPS for adults. Although these values were replicated in a later project with 99 participants (van Zaalen, Wijnen, & Dejonckere, 2009a), fast articulatory rate cannot serve as a sole differentiating characteristic. In both research projects, a small group (for monologue: 55.6 percent; reading: 33 percent; retelling: 25 percent) of PWC fit the description of fast articulatory rate. Daly and Burnett support this finding, stating, ‘in cluttering accelerated speech is not always present, but impairment in formulating language usually is’ (1996, p. 239). In their working definition of cluttering, St. Louis et al. (2007) contend that although perceived as fast, the actual articulatory rate of PWC can be normal when measured. The perception of the listener is possibly disturbed by, for instance, telescoping, coarticulation, or a high frequency of normal disfluencies. Therefore, when assessing clients for potential cluttering, the clinician should bear in mind that speech rate may not exceed that of those without communication disorders (see Table 9.1).

Ratio disfluencies

The ratio of disfluencies describes the relationship between the number of nonstuttering-like disfluencies (NSLDs) and the number of stuttering-like disfluencies (SLDs). A number of authors describe the high frequency of normal disfluencies in cluttered speech (Damsté, 1984; Myers & Bradley, 1992; St. Louis et al., 2007; van Zaalen & Winkelman, 2009; Ward, 2006; Weiss, 1964). Myers and Bradley (1992) suggested that PWC divided themselves from normal speakers by a higher frequency of nonstuttering-like disfluencies. St. Louis (1992) confirmed this observation and described

Table 9.1 Communication features described for cluttering. (For communication features for stuttering and learning disabilities, see Van Zaalen & Winkelman, 2009.)

Communication feature	*Description*
1. Mean articulatory rate (over 5 random measures)	Rapid and/or irregular rate
2. Ratio disfluencies (NSLDs to SLDs) in monologue or retelling	High in favour of NSLDs
3. SSI severity rating	No stuttering; very mild stuttering
4. Errors in word structure	Possible
5. Possible cause of errors in sentence structures	Phrase or word repetitions or revisions
6. Pauses	Too few, too short, or in linguistically inappropriate places
7. Attention makes speech:	Better
8. Relaxation makes speech:	Worse
9. Speaking a foreign language is:	Better
10. Reading out loud of a known text is:	Worse
11. Reading out loud of a unknown text is:	Better
12. Communication or speech fear	Possible
13. Awareness of symptoms	Mostly not
14. Awareness of speech disorder	Often
15. Word fear mainly in case of . . .	Multi-syllabic words
16. Sound fear	Absent

cluttering as a speech-language disorder with an increased frequency of disfluency different from stuttering.

In order to find a normative standard for possible differential diagnosis, Van Zaalen et al. (2009c) examined the relationship between the nonstuttering-like and stuttering-like disfluencies between PWC, PWS, and controls (children and adults; PWC, N = 47, PWS, N = 68; Controls, N = 397). The ratio was determined by dividing the nonstuttering-like disfluencies by the stuttering-like disfluencies. Van Zaalen et al. (2009c) found significant difference between the PWC and the PWS in terms of ratio of disfluencies in monologue and story retelling, but not in reading. A ratio disfluencies (the percentage nonstuttering-like disfluencies divided through the percentage stuttering-like disfluencies) of 1.7 or higher was found to be an indicator of possible cluttering behaviour in this sample. This number can be used as a guideline in assessing potential cluttering, but should not be used as a sole differential characteristic.

Stuttering Severity Instrument

Little research data on the Stuttering Severity Instrument (SSI-4; Riley, 2008) has been conducted with PWC. A person receives a high score on the SSI-3 when they produce SLDs with tension and a relatively long (> 1 second) duration. In pure cluttering, SLDs are rare, and thus a score on the SSI-3 will be low, with severity ranging from no stuttering to very mild stuttering. Regarding the fact that cluttering and stuttering can occur in one person (Craig, 1996; Damsté, 1984; Van Zaalen & Winkelman, 2009; Ward, 2006), it is possible for persons who clutter-stutter (PWCS) to score according to PWS (i.e., severity ratings ranging from very mild stuttering to very severe stuttering).

Errors in word structure

In order to diagnose cluttering accurately, it is important to accentuate that the articulation errors in cluttering are hypothesized to be caused by planning problems and not by articulation defects (St. Louis, 1992, 1996; St. Louis et al., 2003, 2007; Van Zaalen & Winkelman, 2009; Ward, 2006). Words are built from syllable strings. Syllable order determines word meaning. It may be speculated that when a speaker reduces the time for planning, it is possible that word structure errors occur due to incorrect sequencing or telescoping effects (e.g., 'Many thinkle peep so' for 'Many people think so'). In cluttering, word structure errors have been noted especially when speaking at a fast rate or when producing complex low-frequency multisyllabic word strings (e.g., 'possibilities'). The errors in production may appear as errors of syllable structure or syllable sequencing.

The Screening Pittige Articulatie (SPA; Van Zaalen et al., 2009a) is an assessment tool to assess speech motor control at the word level. The SPA assesses speech motor planning by asking clients to repeat multisyllabic words at a fast rate. People with cluttering may produce a higher than normal number of errors in flow (correct rhythm and accentuation), coarticulation (telescoping), and sequencing (syllable order), whereas PWS will produce a higher number of coarticulation errors that are related to pausing rather than telescoping.

Assessment of word structure at a fast rate (speech motor control on word level) cannot easily be done using spontaneous speech or reading. Spontaneous speech is difficult to compare between participants, and articulatory rate effect on word structure in reading is often less, due to the lack of need for language formulation in reading. In order to assess word structure in spontaneous speech, preparing a written sample of monologue, dialogue, or reading recordings is necessary. Within the written sample, the SLT looks for errors in coarticulation or syllable sequencing. Errors in coarticulation can be recognised when the number of the produced syllables is compared with the number of syllables in the citation form of the words. Errors in syllable sequencing can be recognised when the order of the produced syllables is compared with the order of syllables in the citation form of the words.

Cause of errors in sentence structures

Some researchers (e.g. St. Louis et al., 2003, 2007) do not include a language component in their definition of cluttering because there are some PWC who exhibit no language-based symptoms. Although there is acknowledgement that language planning difficulties may be implicated in cluttering (Ward, 2006), we do not yet have definitive data to draw this conclusion for cluttering in general.

Communication breakdowns among PWC have often been observed to be less likely in a controlled (test) situation. Therefore, it has been speculated that disturbances of sentence production occur because the PWC does not take enough time to complete the editing phase of sentence planning (Van Zaalen et al., 2009b; Ward, 2004, 2006), resulting in a high level of NSLDs. Following this logic, when a PWC takes an accurate amount of time (e.g., in a controlled situation or in writing), no communication breakdowns will be expected.

Assessment of sentence structure production should be conducted in controlled situations inside the clinic (e.g., retelling a story; van Zaalen & Bochane, 2007), and less controlled situations outside the clinic. A written transcript of each speech situation can be analysed for sentence structure production. When a correct sentence structure is produced immediately, or after reformulating in reaction to internal monitoring, the sentence is scored as a grammatically correct sentence structure on first attempt (after deletion of word and phrase repetitions) or at second attempt (after deletion of normal disfluencies including revisions and false starts) (see VanZaalen et al., 2009d).

Extra or non-linguistic pauses

Many researchers in the field of cluttering mention PWC as experiencing problems in planning accurate linguistic pauses (Daly & Cantrell, 2006). The mean duration of a pause is between 0.5 and 1.0 seconds (Van Zaalen & Winkelman, 2009). This pause time is essential for breath taking and language formulation of the speaker and language comprehension of the listener. A fast speech rate is directly correlated to shorter and/or fewer pauses (Levelt, 1989). Cluttered speech is characterized by a high variability in pause duration (i.e., too few or too short; Sick, 2004).

Attention and speech monitoring

Cluttering behaviours become more evident the more informal, spontaneous, and extensive the talk (Van Zaalen et al., 2008). Parents or partners of PWC often tell clinicians that the PWC's speech inside the clinic is much better than when in a relaxed speaking situation (e.g., talking with friends) (Daly, 1996; Op 't Hof & Uys, 1974; Van Zaalen & Winkelman, 2009; Weiss, 1964). The clinician is most likely to record 'uncontrolled' cluttering when the client is unaware of being recorded. Such speech may also be observed when recording the interaction between, for instance, the parent and the child, or the adult and partner while the clinician leaves the room.

Reading aloud an unknown text or speaking a foreign language requires a high level of attention. In such linguistic contexts, the level of focus on speech is heightened. Conversely, reading the same story repeatedly lowers the level of alertness to speech, resulting in more cluttering errors. This outcome is different from stuttering, where repeated readings often result in a decreased frequency of stuttering. Because stuttering and cluttering often co-occur, the clinician will need to closely examine linguistic contexts in which errors increase or decrease in individual clients. Comparison of the number of reading errors, coarticulation, or telescoping words in contexts that do and do not require a high level of focus on speech can provide information on the effect of concentration on the PWC's speech.

Communication, speech, sound, or word fear

As mentioned, people with cluttering can develop communication fear. In response to this communication fear, some PWC may avoid speaking in certain situations. In using a speech situation checklist (SSC in Behavior Assessment Battery; Brutten & Vanryckeghem, 2006), the clinician can determine which words or situations are more or less difficult for the PWC. Specific sound fear is not common in PWC, but can be present in PWCS.

Awareness of symptoms or speech disorder

People with cluttering are often aware of their speech problems in general, but often not at the moment symptoms occur. Most commonly, PWC are aware of their fast rate, disfluencies, unintelligibility, and pausing problems when listening to their recorded speech. The reason why they do not respond to these problems in running speech may be related to the fact that the pace of such speaking situations do not afford the time for reflection that listening to a recording of one's speech does.

When assessing cluttering, it is useful to ask the client to critique his own speech during various recorded tasks. The clinician and the client can use a 5-point rating scale to simultaneously judge the recorded samples on each of the major dimensions of the client's speech and language. Comparison of the client's and the clinician's ratings allows the clinician to get a good idea about the client's symptom awareness.

Conclusion

Cluttering assessment involves the careful analysis and comparison of speech rate, fluency, and intelligibility in various speaking contexts. In order to diagnose a person's speech as cluttering, the main characteristic of a (too) fast or (too) irregular rate must be present. When a person does not fit the main characteristics of cluttering, but expresses some communicative features of the disorder, he may be diagnosed as having cluttering behaviour. Additionally, in order to gain a picture of all of the client's symptoms, assessment of awareness of speech and possible coexisting communication disorders should be conducted. As with all clients in the field of communication disorders, the general principles of assessment presented in this chapter apply, but must be tailored to each client's individual presentation of symptoms.

References

Ambrose, N. G., & Yairi, E. (1999). Normative disfluency data for early childhood stuttering. *Journal of Speech, Language, and Hearing Research*, *42*, 895–909.

Bakker, K., St. Louis, K. O., Myers, F., & Raphael, L. (2005). *A freeware software tool for determining aspects of cluttering severity*. Annual National Convention of the American Speech Language and Hearing Association, San Diego, CA.

Boey, R. (2000). *Stotteren detecteren en meten*. Leuven-Apeldoorn: Uitgeverij Garant.

Brutten, G., & Vanryckeghem, M. (2006). *Behavior Assessment Battery for school-age children who stutter*. San Diego, CA: Plural Publishing.

Craig, A. (1996). Long-term effects of intensive treatment for a client with both a cluttering and stuttering disorder. *Journal of Fluency Disorders*, *21*, 329–336.

Dalton, P., & Hardcastle, W. (1989). *Disorders of fluency and their effects on communication*. London: Elsevier North Holland.

Daly, D. (1986). The clutterer. In K. St. Louis (Ed.), *The atypical stutterer: Principles and practice of rehabilitation* (pp. 155–192). New York: Academic Press.

Daly, D. (1996). *The source for stuttering and cluttering*. East Moline, IL: LinguiSystems.

Daly, D. (2008, July). *Strategies for identifying and working with Difficult-to-treat cluttering clients*. Paper presented at the Oxford Dysfluency Conference, 2008, Oxford, UK.

Daly, D., & Burnett, M. (1996). Cluttering: Assessment, treatment planning, and case study illustration. *Journal of Fluency Disorders*, *21*, 239–244.

Daly, D. A., & Cantrell, R. P. (2006, July). *Cluttering: Characteristics labelled as diagnostically significant by 60 fluency experts*. Paper presented at the 6th IFA World Congress on disorders of fluency, Dublin, Ireland.

Damste, P. H. (1984). *Stotteren*. Utrecht: Bohn, Scheltema & Holkema.

Freund, H. (1952). Studies in the interrelationship between stuttering and cluttering. *Folia Phoniatrica*, *4*, 146–168.

Gregory, H. H. (1995). Analysis and commentary. *Language Speech and Hearing Services in the Schools*, *26*, 196–200.

Guitar, B. (2006). *Stuttering: An integrated approach to its nature and treatment* (3rd ed.). Baltimore, MD: Lippincott Williams & Wilkins.

Hall, K. D., Amir, O., & Yairi, E. (1999). A longitudinal investigation of speaking rate in preschool children who stutter. *Journal of Speech Language and Hearing Research*, *42*, 1367–1377.

Kussmaul, A. (1887). Speech disorders. *Encyclopedia of the practice of medicine, XIV*. New York.

Levelt, W. J. M. (1989). *Speaking: From intention to articulation*. Cambridge, MA: MIT Press.

Mensink-Ypma, M. (1990). *Broddelen en leerstoornissen*. Houten/Antwerpen: Bohn Stafleu van Loghum.

Myers, F. L., & Bradley, C. L. (1992). Clinical management of cluttering from a synergistic framework. In F. L. Myers & K. O. St. Louis (Eds.), *Cluttering: A clinical perspective* (pp. 85–105). Kibworth, UK: Far Communications. (Reissued in 1996 by Singular, San Diego, CA.)

Op 't Hof, J., & Uys, I. (1974). A clinical delineation of tachyphemia (cluttering): A case of dominant inheritance. *South African Medical Journal*, *48*, 1624–1628.

Pindzola, R. H., Jenkins, M. M., & Lokken, K. J. (1989). Speaking rates of young children. *Language, Speech, and Hearing Services in Schools*, *20*, 133–138.

Preus, A. (1981). *Identifying subgroups of stuttering*. Oslo: Universitetsforlaget.

Preus, A. (1992). Cluttering or stuttering: Related, different or antagonistic disorders. In F. L. Myers & K. O. St. Louis (Eds.), *Cluttering: A clinical perspective*. Kibworth, UK: Far Communications.

Preus, A. (1996). Cluttering upgraded. *Journal of Fluency Disorders*, *21*, 349–358.

Quesal, B. (2004). *Fluency and fluency disorders*. Stuttering course. Retrieved June 1, 2007, from http://www.mnsu.edu/comdis/kuster/StutteringCourseSyllabi/Quesal.html

Renfrew, C. (1997). *The Renfrew language scales: Bus story test, a test of narrative speech*. Bicester, UK: Speechmark.

Riley, G. D. (2008). *SSI-4, Stuttering severity instrument for children and adults*. Austin, TX: Pro Ed.

Seeman, M. (1974). *Sprachstorungen bei Kindern*. Berlin: VEB Verlag Volk und Gesundheit.

Shapiro, D. (1998). *Stuttering intervention: A collaborative journey to fluency freedom*. Austin, TX: Pro Ed.

Sick, U. (2004). *Poltern, theoretische grundlagen, diagnostik, therapie*. Stuttgart: Thieme.

St. Louis, K. O. (1992). On defining cluttering. In F. L. Myers & K. O. St. Louis (Eds.), *Cluttering: A clinical perspective* (pp. 37–53). Kibworth, UK: Far Communications. (Reissued in 1996 by Singular, San Diego, CA.)

St. Louis, K. O. (Ed.). (1996). Research and opinion on cluttering: State of the art and science [special issue]. *Journal of Fluency Disorders*, *21*, 171–371.

St. Louis, K. O., & McCaffrey, E. (2005, November 18). *Public awareness of cluttering and stuttering: Preliminary results*. Poster Presented at the 2005 ASHA Convention, San Diego, CA.

St. Louis, K. O., Myers, F. L., Bakker, K., & Raphael, L. J. (2007). Understanding and treating cluttering. In E. G. Conture & R. F. Curlee (Eds.), *Stuttering and related disorders of fluency* (3rd ed., pp. 297–325). New York: Thieme.

St. Louis, K. O., Raphael, L. J., Myers, F. L., & Bakker, K. (2003, November 18). Cluttering updated. *The ASHA Leader*, 4–5, 20–22.

Teigland, A. (1996). A study of pragmatic skills of clutterers and normal speakers. *Journal of Fluency Disorders, 21*, 201–214.

Van Borsel, J., & vanderMeulen, A. (2008). Cluttering in Down syndrome. *Folia Phoniatrica, 60*, 312–317.

Van Riper, C. (1982). *The nature of stuttering*. San Diego, CA: College Hill Press.

Van Zaalen, Y. (2009). *Cluttering identified. Differential diagnostics between cluttering, stuttering and speech impairment in learning disabilities*. PhD thesis, Utrecht University.

Van Zaalen, Y., & Bochane, M. (2007). *The Wallet story*. 27th World congress of the International Association of Logopedics and Phoniatrics, Proceedings (p. 85). Copenhagen: Kandrup.

Van Zaalen, Y., Myers, F., Ward, D., & Bennett, E. (2008). *The cluttering assessment protocol*. http://associations.missouristate.edu/ICA/

Van Zaalen, Y., Wijnen, F., & Dejonckere, P. (2009a). A test on speech motor control on word level: The SPA test. *International Journal of Speech and Language Pathology, 11*, 26–33.

Van Zaalen, Y., Wijnen, F., & Dejonckere, P. (2009b). Language planning disturbances in children who clutter or have learning disabilities. *International Journal of Speech and Language Pathology, 11*, 496–508.

Van Zaalen, Y., Wijnen, F., & Dejonckere, P. (2009c). Differential diagnostics between cluttering and stuttering, part one. *Journal of Fluency Disorders, 34*, 137–146.

Van Zaalen, Y., Wijnen, F., & Dejonckere, P. (2009d). Differential diagnostics between cluttering and stuttering, part two. *Journal of Fluency Disorders, 34*, 146–154.

Van Zaalen, Y., & Winkelman, C. (2009). *Broddelen, een (on) begrepen stoornis*. Bussum: Coutinho.

Walker, J. F., Archibald, L. M. D., Cherniak, S. R., & Fish, V. G. (1992). Articulation rate in 3 and 5 year old children. *Journal of Speech and Hearing Research, 35*, 4–13.

Ward, D. (2004). Cluttering, speech rate and linguistic defect: a case report. In A. Packman, A. Meltzer, & H. F. M. Peters (Eds.), *Theory, research and therapy in fluency disorders* (pp. 511–516). Proceedings of the 4th World congress on fluency disorders, Montreal, Canada. Nijmegen: Nijmegen University Press.

Ward, D. (2006). *Stuttering and cluttering: Frameworks for understanding and treatment*. Hove, UK: Psychology Press.

Weiss, D. A. (1964). *Cluttering*. Englewood Cliffs, NJ: Prentice-Hall.

Winkelman, C. L. (1990). Broddelen. In M. Mensink-Ypma, *Broddelen en Leerstoornissen* (pp. 142–167). Utrecht: Bohn, Scheltema & Holkema.

Yairi, E., & Ambrose, N. (1992). A longitudinal study of stuttering in children: A preliminary report. *Journal of Speech and Hearing Research, 35*, 755–760.

10 Treatment of cluttering: a cognitive-behavioral[1] approach centered on rate control

Florence L. Myers

> I thought that cluttering was only a speech problem, but now I know it is really a communication problem that affects the whole person and can chart out the rest of their life, has [sic] it has done mine . . .
>
> (Kissagizlis, 2007)

Introduction

Cluttering has been referred to as an 'orphan' in the family of communication disorders (Daly, 1986). Fortunately this is no longer the case, as this orphan has been adopted by the world community and is now a thriving toddler. Evidence of this adoption is exemplified by the contributions to this text by authors worldwide, as well as the founding of the International Cluttering Association (ICA) (http://associations.missouristate.edu/ICA) at the First World Conference on Cluttering in 2007. For comprehensive reviews of recent efforts to understand this enigmatic and complex disorder, see the reference list on the ICA website as well as citations in this volume. These efforts represent only the beginnings of growth and development of the field, much like the beginning steps taken during toddlerhood.

The study and treatment of cluttering is immensely challenging. This challenge emanates largely from the fact that cluttering is a multifaceted disorder. A critical issue in need of deliberation and research is to what extent the multifaceted symptoms of cluttering are inclusive—or exclusive—of the disorder itself. Weiss (1964), for example, viewed cluttering as a 'central language imbalance' that influences nearly all facets of communication. Daly (1992) and Daly and Burnett (1999) grounded their conception of cluttering in multiple domains including disfluencies, poorly organized thinking, and language anomalies. According to Daly, 'Accelerated speech is not always present, but an impairment in formulating language almost always is' (1992, p. 107). Ward (2006, 2007) frames cluttering as a spectrum disorder to be inclusive of both motoric as well as linguistic behaviors, and posits a continuum between people with cluttering (hereafter referred to as 'PWC') and typical speakers. A widely acknowledged working definition by St. Louis,

Myers, Bakker, and Raphael (2007) culls out the dimensions of rate/rhythm, fluency, articulation, and prosody to comprise the 'common denominator' elements of cluttering.

A significant footnote associated with the above working definition (see St. Louis et al., 2007, p. 300), however, indicates that Myers' own clinical views of cluttering include the linguistic encoding process as part of the complex of symptoms comprising cluttering. This framework differs somewhat from the so-called 'common denominator' working definition (see also St. Louis & Schulte, chapter 14 this volume), and will be explained under the two constructs below. An oft-said adage is that we are in need of empirical research to gain a better understanding of cluttering. Ongoing research by this author and colleagues has evolved to examine PWC's speech disfluency (Myers & St. Louis, 1996, 2006; Myers, St. Louis, Bakker, Raphael, & Frangis, 2004; Myers, St. Louis, Lwowski et al., 2004; Myers, St. Louis, Raphael, Bakker, & Lwowski, 2003); speech rate control (Bakker, Raphael, Myers, St. Louis, & MacRoy, 2004; Raphael, Bakker, Myers, & St. Louis, 2007; Raphael, Bakker, Myers, St. Louis, & MacRoy, 2001, 2004; Raphael et al., 2005); and self-awareness of rate and clarity (Myers, Bakker, Raphael, & St. Louis, 2005). Results on rate behaviors for a subset of PWC for whom data have been collected, compared with age- and gender-matched speakers with exceptionally rapid speech (ERS) and controls, are summarized and discussed by Bakker, Myers, Raphael, and St. Louis (chapter 4 this volume).

The present chapter will (1) set forth key constructs that undergird an integrated therapy approach to cluttering and (2) discuss therapy principles and strategies that address these constructs. Due to space limitations in the present volume, the reader is referred to previously published references as well as other chapters in the present volume for pertinent reviews of the literature on treatment as well as assessment considerations.

Construct #1: The treatment of cluttering can be viewed from a systems approach

A *systems approach* implies that the various parts of the speech and language system need to be considered as a unified whole. This notion is especially pertinent to the treatment of cluttering given its multifaceted, interactive, and complex nature. The upside of this notion is that therapy addressing one dimension, especially rate control, will benefit the other dimensions. As will be discussed in greater detail under construct #2, rate—including the means to monitor, moderate, and modulate rate—may be a suprastructure that influences how well this system functions (Myers, 1992; Myers & Bradley, 1992; St. Louis et al., 2007).

Construct #2: Rate relative to one's encoding ability is an overarching variable that governs the synchrony and synergy with which the various parts of the communication system function

In this construct, encoding refers to the formulation of speech and language functions, with the corollary of decoding referring to the receiving end of the communication chain. As Kent (2000, p. 393) has stated:

> The production of spoken language includes: prelinguistic aspects (intentions, preverbal message), discourse regulation (such as a discourse record mutually maintained by a speaker and listener), language formulation (lexical selection and syntactic construction), phonologic operations, phonetic specifications, and the motor control of the speech production system to generate acoustic patterns.

At this point in the study of cluttering, no one is equipped to speculate—much less confirm with data on PWC—which specific aspect(s) of the formulation or 'encoding' process is amiss (e.g., storage, retrieval, matching the preverbal intention to the motoric gestures and language units of the message). However, given the clinical and theoretical information we have at this point both about cluttering specifically and communication in general, this author proposes a relationship between rate and encoding ability, and elaborates on this relationship pertaining to cluttering.

Starkweather (1987) reported that most people speak at or close to their maximum rate. People with cluttering have often been perceived to speak too rapidly or with a spurty cadence (St. Louis et al., 2007). If we speak faster than we can handle, it stands to reason that some kind of disorganization will surface. This disorganization can manifest itself in the temporal domain (i.e., dissynchrony) and/or the content domain (i.e., dissynergy or disorganization in the motoric and/or linguistic encoding of messages). Accordingly, Myers (1992) advocated the therapy principle of moderating one's speaking rate as antidote to reduce cluttering symptoms.[2]

'Synchrony' has to do with the timing of events. Dissynchrony, or anomalies in the timing of speaking events, can be observed in the speech of PWC when they speak with a rate that is too rapid or irregular. For example, dissynchrony occurs when filled or unfilled pauses disrupt the flow or timing of a message as in 'What (pause) a beau- (well, sort of) beautiful (um) day this is.' We know that the speaker intends to say, 'What a beautiful day this is,' but the utterance does not flow smoothly in time due to the insertions of pauses and fillers. We also need to take note that speaking rate varies as a function of the type of talk being engaged and the degree of motoric and linguistic constraints associated with that speaking task. Sentence repetition, for example, is a relatively simple and constrained task that does not require much motoric or linguistic formulation (that is, the speaker has only to replicate a sentence syllable-for-syllable and word-for-word), compared with discussing one's vacation plans for next year in the face of uncertainties. It has been my clinical experience that a PWC is more likely to clutter when speaking with less discourse constraints, such as when chatting informally with friends. In these informal contexts, the PWC (as well as typical speakers) speak with somewhat less monitoring and modulation of rate and clarity of communicative output.

Presently, evidence for rate control as a therapy principle for cluttering comes primarily from clinical observations: the efficacy of rate control treatment through Delayed Auditory Feedback to increase speech intelligibility in a case study of a client with severe cluttering (St. Louis et al., 1996); the self-awareness statements made by PWC (Scaler Scott & St. Louis, chapter 13 this volume); and the observation that when 'normalizing' (that is, speaking in a more self-monitored manner as when being recorded), PWC exhibit a striking co-occurrence of heightened speech/language clarity as they talk in a more deliberate manner. This synergistic interaction brought about at least in part by rate control should not come as a surprise to clinicians, as rate control has been demonstrated to be a pivotal ingredient in the treatment efficacy for stuttering as well (O'Brian, Onslow, Cream, & Packman, 2003).

In addition to the moderation or tempering of speaking rate, treatment for cluttering needs also to consider the degree of motoric and linguistic loading inherent in the speaking task, to bring about increased cohesiveness—or synergy—of speech and language output. As discussed elsewhere in this and other chapters in this volume, the more complex, extemporaneous, and/or propositional the speaking task, the greater the motoric and linguistic loading. Greater loading, coupled with a fast rate, can influence the degree of motoric and/or linguistic synergy of the message output. PWC indicate that they often have difficulty organizing their preverbal intentions or formulating their thoughts into language (see Scaler Scott & St. Louis, chapter 13 this volume).

Symptoms reflecting dissynergy at the motoric level include sound and syllable deletions, as well as phonemic distortions due to insufficient or nonspecific excursion of articulatory gestures (i.e., mumbling). Indistinct articulation, in turn, can also lead to distorted resonance, as when non-neutral vowels such as /i/ or /u/ are neutralized, thus changing the size and shape of the oral cavity. Prosody can be affected as well, as when speaking in a monotone or when trailing off at the end of utterances. Speaking at a rate beyond one's means does not allow for sufficient time to modulate the articulatory gestures for speech clarity, nor the prosodic elements such as rate and inflections that accentuate and embellish the meaning of an utterance (for example, accentuating or not accentuating the third word in 'I like that one.').

Dissynergy can also be reflected by inappropriate mid-phrase revisions or when one's overall narrative contains 'revisions' such as going off on tangents. Examples of revision behaviors are seen in the following: 'I think I'll have the choc-, no, the vanilla, well, actually, come to think of it, I had such a big lunch I think I'll not, I think I'll, if you don't mind, I think I'll skip dessert but thanks anyway.' These disfluencies reflect disorganization in the formulation of the message itself (LaSalle & Conture, 1995; Logan & LaSalle, 1999; Myers, St. Louis, & Faragasso, 2008; Ward, 2010). Parents I have worked with often report that their youngster with cluttering 'is all over the place' when telling stories because the narratives lack focus, cohesion, coherence, efficiency, and succinctness of expression. Discourse management may also lack synchrony and synergy. Some PWC show inappropriate timing by interrupting someone else's conversational turns, or are inattentive to listener feedback reflective of communication breakdowns, or may simply talk about offshoots of the main conversational agenda, thereby reducing the cohesiveness of discourse. In sum, as pointed by Peter Kissagizlis' quote at the beginning of this chapter as well as by others (see also chapter by Scaler Scott & St. Louis, chapter 13 this volume), the disorganization of output can occur at multiple levels of the communication exchange. According to Myers (in St. Louis et al., 2007, p. 300), cluttering may be viewed:

> as a spectrum disorder with resultant 'subgroups,' depending on where 'derailment' occurs along the communication chain as a function of attempting to speak faster than the speaker is capable. One subgroup may have excessive disfluencies, another may produce excessive disfluencies with articulatory anomalies, and another may manifest non-cohesive linguistic output.

Treatment for cluttering: constructing an A-frame to house therapy principles and approaches using a cognitive-behavioral approach

Therapy for cluttering is challenging for both the client and the clinician. This challenge stems from the 'deep-rooted' and multidimensional nature of the disorder. The reader is referred to Alm (chapter 1 this volume) to gain an appreciation of the proposed systemic nature of the disorder; that is, its etiology may be embedded 'higher up' in the basal ganglia and the 'executive hub' of the cortex that govern the synchrony and synergy of message output. Cluttering is not comprised of a simple [w/r] substitution; the latter is unidimensional, more isolatable, more circumscribed, and more peripheral in nature compared with cluttering. Moreover, not every PWC manifests the same degree of impairment in the various domains of communication behaviors, nor do they necessarily share the same set of symptoms. Individual differences need to be acknowledged in the treatment of cluttering. These insights lead some to posit a cluttering spectrum disorder to account for the range and variations of cluttering-like symptoms, giving rise to subgroups within the cluttering syndrome (as in the above quote from Myers; see also

Alm, chapter 1 this volume) as well as overlaps between PWC and typical speakers (Ward, 2006, 2010). Given the multiplicity of symptoms, a well-reasoned treatment approach needs first and foremost to prioritize therapy goals to arrive at a hierarchy of objectives. Beginning clinicians, as well as their clients, are often bewildered by the multiplicity of symptoms and do not know which symptom(s) to work on first or which goals have greater impact on communication.

We will use the building of an A-frame home as a metaphor for constructing a *cognitive-behavioral therapy approach* to cluttering, as depicted in Figure 10.1. Some of the therapy techniques described below have been discussed by this author in St. Louis et al. (2007) and elsewhere, as well as by other authors (see Bennett Lanouette, chapter 11 and Miyamoto chapter 12 this volume; Daly, 1996). Additional techniques are included, contextualized with rationale, organized by communication domain, and bonded by therapy principles.

- The *foundation*: developing meta-awareness and understanding of the nature, and associated behaviors, of cluttering.
- The *insulation*: developing the skills for monitoring, moderating, and modulating behaviors.
- The *central beam*: developing skills in rate control to support the *motoric* and *linguistic* elements of noncluttered communication.

Increasing meta-awareness of cluttering: building the foundation

The foundation of effective therapy rests on the client's understanding of the underlying nature of cluttering and its influences on the speaker's communication output. Importantly, the client must also realize the burden cluttered communication has on the listener who is trying to process what is being said. As speech is a highly automatic act for most speakers, but perhaps 'too automatic' for clutterers, we take talking for granted. Nonetheless, clinicians need to do whatever is necessary and possible to heighten their client's self-awareness skills (Myers et al., 2006). Analogies to illustrate the nature and impact of cluttering can be very useful, as a mainstay to increase meta-awareness. The analogies listed below address: (1) the nature of different encoding rates and how they influence cluttering severity; (2) the impact of cluttering on one's communication and on the processing load assumed by the listener; and (3) the nature of temperament and its influence on behaviors, including cluttering. For each of the analogies and exemplars listed below, discuss with the client the degree to which these analogies apply (or do not apply) to his own cluttering-related behaviors and inclinations.

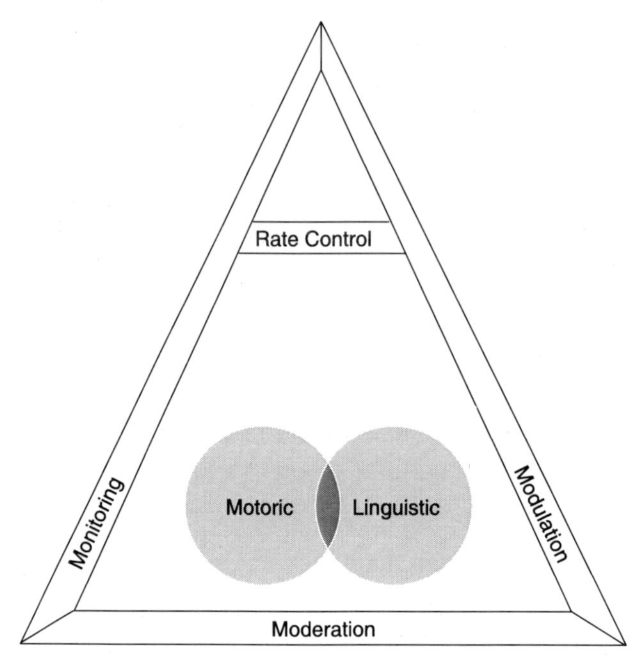

Figure 10.1 A schematic framework to house therapy strategies for a cognitive-behavioral approach to cluttering therapy, with rate control as a central beam.

For younger children

Auditory analogies and exemplars of rate variations:

- Listening to radio commercials that have extremely fast speech (especially toward the end when disclaimers are listed) that impede listener processing.
- Listening to different types of music (e.g., smooth, gentle lullaby compared with rock music); talk about the influence of rate and the beat of music as analogies of the influence of speech rate variations on our listeners.

Movement analogies for rate:

- Train that is going too fast and jumps the tracks, derailing at curves and getting 'all jumbled up'.
- Movements of animals:
  - Fast and smooth movements: racehorses, cheetahs, dolphins.

  - Fast but less smooth movements: jackrabbits, squirrels.
  - Slow and smooth movements: turtle.
  - Slow and less smooth movements: duck, penguin.

Analogies for the need to coordinate parts of a system:

- The inexperienced juggler who juggles too many pins too fast, resulting in: (1) movements that are jerky, inefficient, erratic and (2) occasional dropping of pins (analogous to dropping sounds and syllables in cluttered speech); this is in contrast to the experienced juggler whose movements are smooth and well synchronized.

For older children, adolescents, and adults

- Driving habits: learning to monitor, moderate, and modulate speed:
  - the skillful driver who knows how to modulate rate by slowing down to take the curves in the road
  - the driver who brakes erratically (to illustrate irregular speech rate as when pausing at inappropriate linguistic junctures such as in the middle of a phrase).
- Different types of music (listening to the tempo and harmony vs. dissonance of different types of music): erratic tempo and dissonance of a composition by Stravinsky vs. lyric opera by Puccini; presto vs. andante, legato vs. staccato; pitch and loudness variations of music contrasted with speech that is monotone and 'robotic'.
- Trained athlete: the 'coarticulated' (or coordinated) limb movements of the Olympic runner are fluent, efficient, accurate, and graceful.
- Tai-chi movements (slow, smooth, and blended) contrasted with boxing movements (fast, erratic, intense).
- Difficulties in finding things in a cluttered and disorganized closet, chest of drawers, or pile of paper (analogous to following someone whose narratives and discourse are hard to follow because of poor focus and organization).
- Variations in temperament: yin/yang (aim for a balance so that one's talking is neither 'boring' nor 'too fast and intense'); volatility of volcanoes (what's going on inside the mountain to cause it to erupt and 'blow its top'); contrast between how we feel when we come home from school or work and want to tell our family all the things that went wrong during the day as opposed to waking up with serenity after a good night's sleep on a family trip to the country.
- Synergy:
  - braids or rope whose strands are cohesively woven with good sequencing and proper tension

- a sweater that is knitted with even stitches (with even tension and no holes because of dropped stitches, as in dropped syllables)
- a Porsche engine (all the parts run smoothly, in synchrony and synergy).

In addition to analogies, the clinician may also partner with the client to come up with terminologies that are user-friendly to get at aspects of cluttering behaviors: talk which is 'all over the place' to refer to cluttered language; 'mumble jumble' to refer to low intelligibility speech; 'nice and crisp' to refer to precise articulation; 'news broadcasting speech' to refer to fluent and clear speech and language that gets to the main points efficiently and fluently. Additionally, as part of understanding the nature and impact of one's cluttering on communication, clinicians may need to do some counseling regarding the influence of cluttered communication on quality of life issues such as making and keeping friends, giving oral reports at school or at work, getting that promotion to be a top salesperson. By addressing such functional life concerns, the clinician can be sensitive to quality of life issues based on the dictates of the World Health Organization in defining severity of disorders (Yaruss, 1998).

Increasing skills to monitor, moderate and modulate: putting in the insulation for successful therapy

Treatment of cluttering requires the development of insight and strategies needed to **m**onitor, **m**oderate and **m**odulate behaviors (see Figure 10.1). Such insight provides, as it were, the *insulation* for successful therapy by providing rationale for clinical strategies. If a client understands the nature of his communication disorder and the rationale for treatment approaches, his motivation for behavioral changes will increase. In essence, this *cognitive-behavioral approach* to the treatment of cluttering incorporates appreciation of the intricate and telltale dissynchronous interplay between one's speaking rate and the encoding of multiple thoughts during extended discourse or monologue.

Additionally, the client needs to come to the realization that one is particularly vulnerable to speaking fast when the pragmatic context is informal, extemporaneous, exciting, or when speaking in an unguarded fashion. In such contexts, the clutterer is likely to find it effortful to maintain vigilance.

Monitoring

Many, though not all, individuals with cluttering have difficulty in *monitoring* signals that come from internal as well as external sources. (It should be noted that some PWC can normalize their speech patterns, thus reflecting ability to monitor at least for short durations; see Bakker, Myers, Raphael, & St. Louis, chapter 4 this volume.). By and large, most PWC are not fully aware that others have difficulty understanding *what* they have to say because of *how* they say it. Some PWC may even deny that there is any problem with their communication, even when given feedback that their messages are difficult to follow. Perhaps the most important therapy goal for the treatment of cluttering is to sharpen the client's monitoring skills, as these skills have great implications for transfer and maintenance. One reason self-monitoring is challenging is that the process requires sustained vigilance at *multiple* levels of the communication system. In order to take steps to adjust or modulate the message output, the client needs *first* to develop a sensitivity to the following: (a) the integrity of one's speech and language output; (b) the verbal and nonverbal reactions of the listener; and (c) the appropriateness of one's responses (e.g., to repair the conversational breakdown) relative to the listener's verbal and nonverbal reactions.

Techniques to increase monitoring skills

MONITORING OF ONE'S OWN SPEECH AND LANGUAGE

- Heightening one's sensory feedback associated with variations in rate by attending to the sensations associated with a very fast vs. typical vs. very slow rate of talking (using a hierarchy of utterances with increasing length and complexity).
- Using another physical activity that client enjoys or is good at (e.g., swimming, running, tennis, playing the piano, drumming) and deliberating on the sensory feedback and effectiveness of the movements accompanying variations in rate.
- Negative practice (contrasting the sensory feedback associated with the production of words first said in a cluttered manner immediately followed by noncluttered manner).
- Using rating scales (informal 3- or 5-point rating scales, or the Cluttering Severity Instrument being developed by Bakker & Myers, 2008) to assess one's taped or live speech.
- Transcribing one's speech and language sample to recognize points in the transcript that are disjointed, disfluent, unclear.

MONITORING THE IMPACT OF ONE'S COMMUNICATION ON THE LISTENER

Monitoring verbal and nonverbal feedback from one's listener reflective of:

- not understanding what one said and/or
- misunderstanding what one said:
  - asking for clarification (What? Do you mean. . . .?)
  - frowns, quizzical look
  - signs of disinterest or frustration.

MONITORING OTHERS' SPEECH

Using drama and rhetoric as a means to increase monitoring skills:

- Watching videos to analyze gifted actors' verbal and nonverbal behaviors that contribute to effective communication.
- Role playing of different characters to bring forth intended meanings in the lines of various characters in a skit; then monitor/critique the success with which client(s) convey(s) these meanings and intents.
- Listening and critiquing how rate is effectively modulated by famous orators (such as Presidents Kennedy and Obama; Prime Minister Churchill; Martin Luther King, Jr.) through appropriate variations of rate and phrasing, as well as getting to the point efficiently and effectively.
- Clinician simulating cluttered communication so client realizes impact of unclear and incoherent messages on the listener; have client specify what motoric and linguistic/communicative behaviors rendered the message unclear. Work with the client who is unaware or denies that the communication breakdown emanates from his end, including some counseling. One PWC said to me, 'I don't talk too fast; you just have to listen faster.'

Moderation

A top priority for the treatment of cluttering is to facilitate moderation; that is, to develop skills toward a slower rate of output so that the motoric and linguistic encoding does not exceed one's ability (Myers, 1992). According to Starkweather (1987), we speak at or near our maximum rate capacity. Most of us have an internal sense of our maximum ability and 'instinctively' do not cross that threshold. Some PWC indicate that they cannot as readily detect their threshold, or have difficulty in moderating and modifying their communication output so as not to exceed this threshold. Other PWC have said they have a tendency to want to 'talk fast, walk fast, do just about everything fast'. Given this type of feedback from clients, experts in treating cluttering agree that the tempering of rate serves as a powerful antidote to harness or moderate the system (Bennett, 2006; Myers, 2010; St. Louis et al., 2007). Some PWC convey an impression of heightened intensity in temperament. We all exhibit behaviors reflecting (or at least experience an internal sense of) occasional moments of compulsivity, impulsivity, and propulsivity (CIP). These moments occur when we have the urge to exceed the posted speed limit, when taking a chance in passing another car on a two-lane road, or when we experience and succumb to an impulse to buy an outfit that we don't really need just because it is on sale. We might speculate that clutterers, given a tendency toward intensity of temperament, are more vulnerable to these impulses when talking. We might also speculate that people with different brain functions of the basal ganglia need greater stimuli to feel that they are functioning in their 'comfort zone'. Based on an extensive review of the literature on the neurological bases of behaviors using EEG and responses to drugs, for example, Alm (2004, 2010 and Alm, chapter 1 this volume) posits that a primary mechanism responsible for cluttering behaviors is 'hyperactivation and dysregulation of the medial frontal cortex. This may be secondary to disinhibition of the basal ganglia circuits, for example as a result of a hyperactive dopamine system' (p. 331). Interestingly, the basal ganglia has been found to influence both motor as well as cognitive functions, including those related to language processing (Middleton & Strick, 2000). Given this information, it is reasonable to speculate that the rapidity of speech movements may be due in part to an impaired ability of the so-called supplementary motor area (SMA) of the cortex to time the motor gestures so that successive motor gestures are initiated prematurely. What we perceive as 'overcoarticulation' (Dalton & Hardcastle, 1989), such as deletion of sounds and syllables, may be the perceptual byproduct of these neurological activities.

Individuals with cluttering may also have difficulty recognizing or acknowledging their tendencies to rush, so there is little attempt to avoid disintegrations when experiencing the drive toward moments of CIP disintegrations. This drive may be sporadic, leading, for example, to the impression of rate irregularity—that is, speeding ahead with spurts of words only to pause or use fillers at inappropriate linguistic junctures. The drive may be more sustained, leading to the impression of a more steady-state rapid rate with various speech and language disintegrations. Such behaviors detract from the intelligibility and predictability—as occurs when there is an incomplete phrase followed by revisions—of the flow of information in one's message. Reduced intelligibility and predictability of the message exact a cost by imposing a burden on the listener's attempts to process what is being said.

Approaches to moderation: 'change through tempering'

(This section relates to changes through moderation of rate. The next section continues to talk about changes, or modulation, but of other aspects of the communication system.)

MODERATION OF RATE

Clinicians need to realize that simply asking the PWC to 'slow down' rarely works. The clinician needs to give the client more concrete, circumscribed strategies, such as those listed below.

Moderating the rate at which one encodes output:

- Using pauses and appropriate phrasing:
  - between phrases and clauses
  - at punctuation marks during oral reading

  - between thoughts
  - between breath groups.

- Finger tapping for successive syllables.
- Arm gestures, such as pretending to be a symphony conductor (to pace oneself using visual and kinesthetic feedback to regulate rate); or have the client be the conductor to regulate the rate of others' speech during an automatic speech task (e.g., reciting the alphabet, then nursery rhymes).
- Using devices that provide feedback to help moderate rate:

  - Visipitch
  - delayed auditory feedback
  - pacing boards
  - video games that give feedback of 'crashing' if one drives too fast.

- Issuing of speeding tickets using a pretend speedometer; reverse role and client issues speeding tickets to clinician's fast rate; anchor a rate associated with typical 60 mph, then clinician dictates which speed to go (e.g., give me 70 mph, 40 mph) and focus on sensory feedback associated with the variations in rate.
- Prolonging syllables and vowels.
- Accentuating stressed syllables.
- Role playing of situations where slower, more incisive, and clearer communication is paramount (e.g., emergency room receptionist, pilot to airport controller).
- Shadowing the slower speech of the clinician during a reading or recitation task.
- Negative practice (purposely speeding to be immediately followed by markedly slower rate to contrast the associated sensory feedback).

Moderation when experiencing moments of CIP (compulsive, impulsive, propulsive)

- Recognizing that PWC can have moments of CIP and need to learn to anticipate and harness these tendencies.
- Recognizing the importance of equilibrium in temperament (e.g., balance of yin/yang; implications of hyper vs. hypo functions for our general well-functioning being, including the function of communication).
- Recognizing the contrast in feelings associated with inner states that are relatively more vs. less CIP.
- Recognizing that cluttering may be aggravated when talking about a complex and emotional topic; or when speaking informally, extemporaneously, spontaneously, in an unguarded fashion.
- Developing a client-specific hierarchy of situations that incur moments

of CIP and trying to desensitize oneself to these moments of heightened intensity; reassure the client that this may take effort, analogous to persuading a driver who is a chronic speeder to drive more slowly.
- Enrollment in programs that facilitate ways to calm the mind and relax the body (Rustin, Cook, & Spence, 1995); consider the benefits of yoga and the use of imagery (Daly, 1992, 1996) and counseling.

Modulation: adjusting the system

Along with strategies to monitor and moderate one's rate as discussed above, the client also needs to develop skills in *modulating* or behaviorally changing other aspects of his communication output. The *Oxford English Dictionary* (Soanes & Stevenson, 2006) defines modulation as:

> exert(ing) a modifying influence on; (to) regulate; (to) vary the strength, tone, or pitch of one's voice; (to) alter the amplitude or frequency of (an oscillation or signal) in accordance with the variations of a second signal; (to) change from one key to another (in music).

Modulation during speech refers to our ability to change or adjust in keeping with: (a) the pragmatic and semantic context of the message output and (b) the feedback one is receiving from internal sources—such as from our kinesthetic sense or a 'sense of being' related to our inherent disposition—as well as external sources such as listener feedback. As is also the case for typical speakers, the client needs first to learn how to harness or moderate underlying inclinations to 'charge ahead' (using suggested approaches in the previous section), before learning to modulate other aspects of communication. In keeping with the 'synergistic approach' to therapy discussed at the beginning of the chapter, it is important to note that modulation or change in one facet of communication influences another facet (Myers, 1992). For example, better organization of prelinguistic intentions is likely to facilitate positive change in fluency and language output.

The Cluttering Severity Instrument (CSI; Bakker & Myers, 2008) specifies major dimensions of communication that need to be assessed in cluttering. Besides the dimensions of rate and rate regularity, the other dimensions include: prosody, fluency, clarity of speech (including precision of articulatory gestures and overall speech intelligibility), language organization, and management of discourse. Means to change or moderate rate, as the 'central beam' for this cognitive-behavioral program, has already been discussed. The techniques below aim to change or modulate other behaviors of cluttering, such as those assessed by the CSI.

Approaches to improve articulation and overall speech clarity and intelligibility

- Using more precise and definitive approximation of the articulators: just as in the shutting off of the kitchen faucet so that water does not drip, the 'valving' function of our articulators needs to be complete; using the term 'crisp vs. sloppy articulation' helps some clients to gauge the adequacy of their articulation ('Was that nice and crisp, or was that mushy and mumbled?'). This author has found that activities such as pretending to be a plumber working on valves can be fun and helpful for youths to appreciate the need for precise articulatory gestures.
- Using wider excursion of the articulatory gestures: use exaggerated movements and excursions at first to register the sensory feedback associated with precise and firm articulatory posturing.
- Attending to word endings, unstressed syllables in multisyllabic words, and consonant clusters, as these phonological contexts often result in cluttered behaviors.
- Emphasizing stressed syllables (linguistic stress adds duration to the stressed syllable to provide greater opportunity for improved articulation and greater prosodic variations).

Approaches to improve language organization: appealing to the executive functions

Executive functions refer to brain activities that help us organize and regulate emotions and behaviors to achieve context-appropriate goals (Westby & Watson, 2004). At a special double miniseminar at the American Speech-Language-Hearing Association, Wiig (Myers et al., 2002a, 2002b) alluded to the role of executive functions in PWC. Examples of these functions include abilities to inhibit impulses, shift, monitor, plan, and organize responses so that main ideas receive priority during communication. While executive functions have most commonly been applied to disorders such as attention deficit hyperactivity disorder (ADHD) (Barkley, 1997), they appear to have relevance to cluttering as well. See Alm (chapter 1 this volume) for a discussion of the 'executive hub' of our cortex that is presumed to govern the organization of speech and language behaviors. We do not yet have the research to fathom prelinguistic processing; however, clinically speaking, PWC speak of difficulties in organizing (or even slowing down) the multiple thoughts that come seemingly simultaneously. Peter Kissagizlis, a leading advocate for individuals who clutter and who himself was a person with severe cluttering, recently shared with me his insights about the difficulty with which he organizes his thoughts and language:

> The first thoughts are relevant but further thoughts may not be relevant to an [sic] given strategy in respect of [sic] the original thought. Whilst

speaking, or even thinking my mind can and does wander off to other totally unrelated subjects. Although I try hard to stabilise my thoughts, words etc and to project them, they may not be projected in the same way that it was planed [sic] and the resulting sentenc [sic] can be out of context.

(Kizzagizlis, personal communication, 15 May 2009)

- Be acquainted with the essential parts of story grammar in order to organize thoughts into extended talk:
  - Have visuals of the major parts that need to be included in story grammar (e.g., index cards that represent 'setting', 'problem', 'problem resolution', 'punch line of the story').
  - Learn to identify the different parts of story grammar as someone else tells a story.
  - Learn to put the cards in proper sequence to tell a cohesive story.
  - Client purposely tells a story with cards in wrong sequence (e.g., telling about the problem without telling the listener the setting and main characters) and reflect on the 'oddity' or dissynergistic nature of such stories.
  - Clinician purposely tells a story that is not organized, and in which the different parts of grammar are not in appropriate sequence; client discusses why the narrative lacks coherence and cohesion.
  - Grammar Markers Program (Moreau & Fidrych, 2007).
- Facilitate presuppositional skills: develop the ability to encode information pertinent to the viewpoint and needs of the listener (i.e., information that is new, essential, salient, relevant, topic-focused rather than tangential, succinct yet with sufficient embellishment of ideas).
- Develop the outline of a presentation so that the monologue is focused, sequenced and organized; realize that when thought and language are organized, talk is more fluent and easier to process for the listener:
  - conveying important points subsuming the related subpoints of a topic
  - sequencing the important points in a logical order
  - learning to leave out unrelated or irrelevant details
  - practicing the talk using a PowerPoint with key ideas from the outline (the process of developing PowerPoints itself will be helpful to facilitate organization).
- Record and transcribe one's own talk using the Systematic Disfluency Analysis: the intended parts of the message (i.e., the parts that convey information) are underlined; all other parts such as maze behaviors (e.g., interjections, incomplete phrases) are not underlined; the act of listening and analyzing one's own speech helps to sensitize the client to the overall informativeness, clarity, and efficiency of one's language.

The analysis provides a visual of the degree to which the message contains nonessential, unintended, unsorted, revision-laden, nonfluent verbiage.

- Increase word-finding skills through activities that facilitate semantic categorization: synonyms, antonyms, denotation and connotation of words; semantic mapping exercises.
- Increase cohesion and coherence of extended talk through appropriate use of relational terms such as 'however' and 'nonetheless', which signal the logical relationship between utterances; these connecting words provide powerful and efficient means to cement propositions together cohesively and coherently.

Approaches to improve prosody (for rate control techniques see also section above on 'Moderation')

A 'systems' approach implies that there is interconnectedness among the different parts of communication. For example, therapy to promote greater prosodic variations by enhancing stressed syllables will also improve rate by increasing duration of the stressed syllable, as well as speech clarity by providing greater modulation of the articulators with increased volume. This multi-fold benefit of prosodic variations through linguistic stress will in turn enhance the semantic and pragmatic contours of an utterance. The following are activities that lend themselves to prosodic variations:

- Poetry reading.
- Accentuate stressed syllables.
- Reading of plays.
- Variations of saying a sentence, such as 'It's great to see you.', to convey different emotions or pragmatic intents (e.g., sincerity, sarcasm, anger, wit, humor, sadness).
- Negative practice: contrasting saying something in monotone vs. with greater prosodic variations; listen to recordings and critique why speech with appropriate prosodic variations sounds more interesting.

Approaches to improve fluency

Differential diagnosis of disfluencies associated with stuttering and cluttering has been discussed elsewhere in this volume; many clients exhibit both cluttering and stuttering. The clinician needs to differentially diagnose when the disruptions in the flow of speech are due to motoric struggles, to the disruptions in language formulation, and when it might be the result of both. It has been my experience that clients themselves are keen on making this differential diagnosis of their disfluencies once they understand the difference. One stutterer-clutterer told me the following: 'I know what I want to say when I stutter but just can't get the sounds out. When I clutter, I don't know what I want to say but keep on talking anyway. When I clutter, I have SO many thoughts coming at me all at once.'

- Differentiate disfluencies associated with cluttering (nonstuttering disfluencies such as interjections and revisions) vs. stutterering-like disfluencies such as prolongations.
- Transcribe one's own speech: this gives the client both the auditory as well as the written fluency samplings of one's communication and allows the client to self-critique the degree to which the message is disrupted or interrupted by interjections, incomplete phrases, and revisions. Discuss how such disfluencies detract from the 'ongoingness' and overall effectiveness of the speech. Ask the client to repeat or paraphrase what was said but using fewer disfluencies.
- Focus on words and phrases that are essential to the information base of the message with *conscious effort to inhibit* the nonessential such as the interjections of 'um' and 'uh' (as even typical speakers need to do). It should be noted that incomplete phrases followed by revisions exact a greater toll on the flow of the message compared with interjections (Fox Tree, 2001).
- Discuss with the client that there is a synergistic interaction between fluency and language processing skills; improvement in one area will have a beneficial effect in the other area.

Approaches to discourse management

With some clients, therapy may need to focus on discourse management to maximize the adjacency as well as contingency effects of conversational turns. Interruptions of someone else's turn violate the 'adjacency' or timing of successive (adjacent) turns by the conversational partners. Going off on a tangent violates the semantic relatedness (contingency) of the conversation. Saying too much, especially of information that the listener already knows, violates the presuppositional aspects of pragmatic contingency. These types of violations influence the organization of conversation.

- Discuss the idea that conversations need *reciprocity*, a give and take; this reciprocity requires *the monitoring* and *modulation* of what and when one says something and how much to say in a given turn. Use the analogy of an unbalanced seesaw that cannot go up and down (no reciprocity) if one side is too 'heavy' (i.e., talking too much, especially if going off on a tangent, or too intensely) compared with the other side. Learn to modulate the quantity and quality of talk during one's turn.
- Become aware of one's own discourse patterns and count the number of interruptions or going off on tangents, then modulate these pragmatic violations.

- Clinician simulates the client's discourse behaviors and client reflects on how such behaviors detract from the momentum, balance, and cohesion of the interaction.
- Role play a conversation that requires the slowing down of rate, as when one's best friend is in deep sorrow or when visiting an ailing person in hospital.
- Desensitize to pragmatic situations that are exciting, emotional, or extemporaneous so that one does not succumb to cluttering due to moments of CIP.
- Watch for listener feedback.
- Learn to respond to the other speaker in a semantically contingent and pragmatically appropriate fashion (e.g., not going off on a tangent).
- Appreciate the degree of effort required by the listener to process what one is saying. Think about the impact of cluttering on the listener that results in: misinterpreting a message; feeling frustrated in not being able to understand you (but sometimes not wanting to 'hurt your feelings' by pointing out the conversational *faux pas*); having to listen to a message with jerky rate (pauses at unexpected places), or a message that lacks predictability because of maze behaviors; feeling frustrated because the message is inefficiently coded (aborts, false starts, revisions).

Therapy activities that aim to bring the entire communication system into synchrony and synergy

The following therapy activities serve well as culminating group activities or as activities for transfer and maintenance of skills learned. Focus on transfer and maintenance is especially critical for cluttering, as PWC may find it difficult to maintain vigilance to attend to and monitor the sensory feedback associated with improved communication (see Alm, chapter 1 this volume).

- Skits and plays: increase awareness of different speakers' turns; reduce likelihood to interrupt someone if lines of the skit are read or recited when performing a skit; pauses imposed by lines from different speakers automatically stop the clutterer from perseverating or festinating.
- Poetry: poems are meant to be read and recited with feeling, interpretation, and 'drama'; different lines from the poem impose a certain pacing and cadence to cultivate prosodic variations.
- Conducting of music: client dictates tempo of a song for the group members to sing; client chooses which music to play to illustrate variations of rate.
- Group effort to write and perform a play: incorporate story grammar to the drama; appreciate how different roles are projected through variations in rate and prosody by reviewing a videotaping of the performance.

- Classroom presentations: accentuate need to make one's talk clear, coherent, and cohesive; opportunity to take into consideration the nonverbal feedback from the audience to modulate one's delivery.
- Videotape client's monologues or dialogues and have client self-analyze the clarity, coherence, and cohesion of his discourse; point out instances where the speech and language was effective, as well as how other instances can be improved.
- Have members rank order several client-specific speaking situations (e.g., summer job interview, giving reports) that mandate noncluttered speech; practice with the group first and then in a real-life situation.
- Finally, PWC can benefit from various support groups or counseling, to deal with quality of life issues emanating from the impact of cluttering on one's sense of wellbeing in social, academic, and work settings. These group sessions can also serve to enable clients to maintain and transfer their newly-learned knowledge and skills related to cluttering to a wider variety of communication settings.

Notes

1 Cognitive-behavioral therapy emanated from clinical psychology (Beck, 1995). A major premise is that one's thoughts have a direct impact on feelings and behaviors. While the treatment approach discussed in this chapter does not constitute psychotherapy, it does emphasize the need to *understand* the underlying nature of cluttering (hence, 'cognitive') to facilitate behavioral changes.

2 It should be noted that while the symptoms of cluttering can be ameliorated by rate control, the etiology of cluttering may be due to factors specific to certain neurological dynamics such as those discussed by Alm (chapter 1 this volume).

References

Alm, P. A. (2004). Stuttering and the basal ganglia circuits: A critical review of possible relations. *Journal of Communication Disorders*, *37*, 325–369.

Alm, P. A. (2010). The dual premotor model of cluttering and stuttering: A neurological framework. In K. Bakker, L. J. Raphael, & F. L. Myers (Eds.), *Proceedings of the First World Conference on Cluttering* (pp. 207–210). Katarino, Bulgaria. http://associations.missouristate.edu/ICA

Bakker, K., & Myers, F. L. (2008). *The development of a quantifiable measure of cluttering severity*. Paper presented at the annual convention of the American Speech-Language-Hearing Association, Chicago, IL.

Bakker, K., Raphael, L. J., Myers, F. L., St. Louis, K. O., & MacRoy, M. (2004). *DDK production variability in cluttered speech*. Poster session presented at the annual convention of the American Speech-Language-Hearing Association, Philadelphia, PA.

Barkley, R. A. (1997). Behavioral inhibition, sustained attention, and executive functions: Constructing a unifying theory of ADHD. *Psychological Bulletin*, *121*, 65–94.

Beck, J. S. (1995). *Cognitive therapy: Basics and beyond*. New York: Guilford Press.

Bennett, E. M. (2006). *Working with people who stutter: A lifespan approach*. Upper Saddle River, NJ: Pearson Merrill Prentice Hall.

Dalton, P., & Hardcastle, W. (1989). *Disorders of fluency and their effects on communication*. London: Elsevier, North-Holland.

Daly, D. A. (1986). The clutterer. In K. O. St. Louis (Ed.), *The atypical stutterer* (pp. 155–192). New York: Academic Press.

Daly, D. A. (1992). Helping the clutterer: Therapy considerations. In F. L. Myers & K. O. St. Louis (Eds.), *Cluttering: A clinical perspective* (pp. 107–124). Leicester, UK: FAR Communications. (Reissued in 1996 by Singular, San Diego, CA.)

Daly, D. A. (1996). *The source for stuttering and cluttering*. East Moline, IL: LinguiSystems.

Daly, D. A., & Burnett, M. (1999). Cluttering: Traditional views and new perspectives. In R. F. Curlee (Ed.), *Stuttering and related disorders of fluency* (2nd ed., pp. 222–254). New York: Thieme.

Fox Tree, J. E. (2001). Listeners' uses of um and uh in speech comprehension. *Memory and Cognition*, *29*, 320–326.

Kent, R. D. (2000). Research on speech motor control and its disorders: A review and prospective. *Journal of Communication Disorders*, *33*, 391–428.

Kissagizlis, P. (2007, October 2). *Re: The sound of cluttering*. [Msg 2]. Message posted http://cahn.mnsu.edu/10myers/disc59/00000006.htm

LaSalle, L. R., & Conture, E. G. (1995). Disfluency clusters of children who stutter: Relation of stutterings to self-repairs. *Journal of Speech and Hearing Research*, *38*, 965–977.

Logan, K. J., & LaSalle, L. R. (1999). Grammatical characteristics of children's conversational utterances that contain disfluency clusters. *Journal of Speech, Language, and Hearing Research*, *42*, 80–91.

Middleton, F. A., & Strick, P. L. (2000). Basal ganglia output and cognition: Evidence from anatomical, behavioral, and clinical studies. *Brain and Cognition*, *42*, 183–200.

Moreau, M. R., & Fidrych, H. (2007). *Theme maker: A teachers' manual for comprehension, critical thinking and writing of expository text*. Springfield, MA: MindWing Concepts.

Myers, F. L. (1992). Cluttering: A synergistic framework. In F. L. Myers & K. O. St. Louis (Eds.), *Cluttering: A clinical perspective* (pp. 71–84). Leicester, UK: FAR Communications. (Reissued in 1996 by Singular, San Diego, CA.)

Myers, F. L. (2010). Primacy of self-awareness and the modulation of rate in the treatment of cluttering. In K. Bakker, L. J. Raphael, & F. L. Myers (Eds.), *Proceedings of the First World Conference on Cluttering* (pp. 108–114). Katarino, Bulgaria. http://associations.missouristate.edu/ICA

Myers, F. L., Bakker, K., Raphael, L. J., & St. Louis, K. O. (2005). *Self-ratings of speaking rate and clarity by clutterers following DDK*. Poster session presented at the annual convention of the American Speech-Language-Hearing Association, San Diego, CA.

Myers, F. L., Bakker, K., Raphael, L. J., St. Louis, K. O., Dycka, D., Lawson, S., & Hencken, C. (2006). *Self-awareness of communication behaviors in clutterers and nonclutterers*. Poster session presented at the annual convention of the American Speech-Language-Hearing Association, Miami Beach, FL.

Myers, F. L., & Bradley, C. L. (1992). Clinical management of cluttering from a synergistic framework. In F. L. Myers & K. O. St. Louis (Eds.), *Cluttering: A clinical perspective* (pp. 85–106). Leicester, UK: FAR Communications. (Reissued in 1996 by Singular, San Diego, CA.)

Myers, F. L., & St. Louis, K. O. (1996). Two youths who clutter, but is that the only similarity? *Journal of Fluency Disorders, 21*, 297–304.

Myers, F. L, & St. Louis, K. O. (2006). Disfluency and speaking rate in cluttering: Perceptual judgments versus counts. *Bulgarian Journal of Communication Disorders, 1*, 28–35.

Myers, F. L., St. Louis, K. O., Bakker, K., Raphael, L. J., Wiig, E. K., Katz, J., et al. (2002a). *Putting cluttering on the map: Looking back*. Invited double seminar presented at the annual convention of the American Speech-Language-Hearing Association, Atlanta, GA.

Myers, F. L., St. Louis, K. O., Bakker, K., Raphael, L. J., Wiig, E. K., Katz, J., et al. (2002b). *Putting cluttering on the map: Looking ahead*. Invited double seminar presented at the annual convention of the American Speech-Language-Hearing Association, Atlanta, GA.

Myers, F. L., St. Louis, K. O., Bakker, K., Raphael, L. J., & Frangis, G. (2004). *Disfluencies of cluttered and excessively rapid speech*. Poster presented at the annual convention of the American Speech-Language-Hearing Association, Philadelphia, PA.

Myers, F. L., St. Louis, K. O., & Faragasso, K. A. (2008). Disfluency clusters associated with cluttering. *Bulgarian Journal of Communication Disorders, 2*, 1–19.

Myers, F. L., St. Louis, K. O., Lwowski, A., Bakker, K., Raphael, L. J., & Frangis, G. (2004). *Disfluencies of cluttered and excessively rapid speech*. Poster session presented at the annual convention of the American Speech-Language-Hearing Association, Philadelphia, PA.

Myers, F. L., St. Louis, K. O., Raphael, L. J., Bakker, K., & Lwowski, A. (2003). *Patterns of disfluencies in cluttered speech*. Poster session presented at the annual convention of the American Speech-Language-Hearing Association, Chicago, IL.

O'Brian, S., Onslow, M., Cream, A., & Packman, A. (2003). The Camperdown Program: Outcomes of a new prolonged-speech treatment model. *Journal of Speech, Language, and Hearing Research, 46*, 933–946.

Raphael, L. J., Bakker, K., Myers, F. L., & St. Louis, K. O. (2007). *Syllable rates in the speech of clutterers and controls*. Poster session presented at the annual convention of the American Speech-Language-Hearing Association, Boston, MA.

Raphael, L. J., Bakker, K., Myers, F. L., St. Louis, K. O., Fichtner, V., & Kostel, M.(2005). *An update on diadochokinetic rates of cluttered and normal speech*. Poster session presented at the annual convention of the American Speech-Language-Hearing Association, San Diego, CA.

Raphael, L. J., Bakker, K., Myers, F. L., St. Louis, K. O., & MacRoy, M. (2001). *Articulatory/acoustic features of DDKs in cluttered, tachylalic, and normal speech*. Poster session presented at the annual convention of the American Speech-Language-Hearing Association, New Orleans, LA.

Raphael, L. J., Bakker, K., Myers, F. L., St. Louis, K. O., & MacRoy, M. (2004). *Diadochokinetic rates of cluttered and normal speech*. Poster session presented at the annual convention of the American Speech-Language-Hearing Association, Philadelphia, PA.

Rustin, L., Cook, F., & Spence, R. (1995). *The management of stuttering in adolescence: A communication skills approach*. London: Whurr.

Soanes, C., & Stevenson, A. (2006). *Concise Oxford English dictionary* (11th ed.). Oxford, UK: Oxford University Press.

Starkweather, C. W. (1987). *Fluency and stuttering*. Englewood Cliffs, NJ: Prentice-Hall.

St. Louis, K. O., Myers, F. L., Bakker, K., & Raphael, L. J. (2007). Understanding and treating cluttering. In E. G. Conture & R. F. Curlee (Eds.), *Stuttering and related disorders of fluency* (3rd ed., pp. 297–325). New York: Thieme.

St. Louis, K. O., Myers, F. L., Cassidy, L. J., Michael, A. J., Penrod, S. M., Litton, B. A., et al. (1996). Efficacy of delayed auditory feedback for treating cluttering: Two case studies. *Journal of Fluency Disorders*, *21*, 305–314.

Ward, D. (2006). *Stuttering and cluttering: Frameworks for understanding and treatment*. Hove, UK: Psychology Press.

Ward, D. (2010). Stuttering and normal nonfluency: Cluttering spectrum behaviour as a functional descriptor of abnormal nonfluency. In K. Bakker, L. J. Raphael, & F. L. Myers (Eds.), *Proceedings of the First World Conference on Cluttering* (pp. 261–266). Katarino, Bulgaria. http://associations.missouristate.edu/ICA/

Weiss, D. A. (1964). *Cluttering*. Englewood Cliffs, NJ: Prentice-Hall.

Westby, C., & Watson, S. (2004). Perspectives on attention deficit hyperactivity disorder: Executive functions, working memory and language disabilities. *Seminars in Speech and Language*, *25*, 241–254.

Yaruss, J. S. (1998). Describing the consequences of disorders: Stuttering and the international classification of impairments, disabilities, and handicaps. *Journal of Speech, Language, and Hearing Research*, *41*, 249–257.

11 Intervention strategies for cluttering disorders

Ellen Bennett Lanouette

Cluttering is an intriguing, yet fairly unknown fluency disorder. The early writing of Weiss (1964) outlined cluttering as a central language imbalance exhibiting deficits in the areas of cognition, language, pragmatics, speech, and motor skills. More recently, St. Louis, Myers, Bakker, and Raphael (2007) defined cluttering as a fluency disorder characterized by abnormally rapid and/or irregular speech rate. The authors contend that:

> rate abnormalities further are manifest in one or more of the following symptoms: an excessive number of disfluencies, the majority of which are not typical of people who stutter; frequent placement of pauses and use of prosodic patterns that do not conform to syntactic and semantic constraints; and inappropriate (usually excessive) degrees of coarticulation among sounds, especially in multisyllabic words.
>
> (St. Louis et al., 2007, pp. 299–300)

Ward (2006) postulated the concept of 'Cluttering Spectrum Behavior' (CSB) for individuals who exhibit *some* cluttering features, yet do not have enough of these features to warrant a diagnosis of cluttering, or where cluttering-like symptoms might equally be considered features of a coexisting diagnosis. Regardless of which definition the clinician prescribes to, the specific difficulties of this group of people is interesting. Table 11.1 outlines possible target areas of change in people with cluttering (PWC) and possibly those identified with CSB. The reader is reminded that this list of deficits is not all inclusive, as every client exhibits his/her own profile of strengths and weaknesses that must be addressed during the treatment process.

Principles of intervention

Therapy for cluttering, following the above definitions and parameters set forth in the previous chapters of this book, is multidimensional. Treatment must follow a comprehensive evaluation as outlined by Van Zaalen, Wijnen, and Dejonckere (chapter 9 this volume). Goals should be set in each of the

Table 11.1 Parameters of cluttering that might require intervention in people who clutter based on the definitions of Weiss (1964) and St. Louis et al. (2007)

Domain	*Areas of weakness*
Cognition	• Awareness including listener perception and self-monitoring • Thought organization (including sequencing and categorization) • Memory • Impulsivity
Language	Expressive language domain • Poor storytelling • Language formulation difficulties • Frequent revisions and repetitions • Improper linguistic structure • Syllabic or verbal transpositions • Improper pronoun use • Word-finding difficulties • Frequent filler words, empty words • Sentence fragments Written language domain • Run-on sentences in written text • Omissions and transpositions of letters, syllables, and words in written text • Reading disorders
Pragmatics	Conversations • Inappropriate topic maintenance and termination • Inappropriate turn taking • Poor listening skills • Impulsive responses • Lack of consideration of listener perspective • Verbose or tangential responses Nonverbal communication • Poor eye contact • Inadequate processing of nonverbal signals
Speech	Speech disfluency • Excessive repetition of words/phrases • Silent gaps/hesitations in breathing Rate/prosody • Rapid or irregular • Poor rhythm • Loud, trails off • Lacks pauses between words • Vocal monotony Slurred articulation • Omits sounds • Omits syllables • Difficulty with complex sounds (i.e., blends, affricates, and fricatives) • Syllabic or verbal transpositions
Motor	• Poor speech motor control • Disrhythmic breathing • Clumsy and uncoordinated • Poor penmanship

domains based on the client's presenting symptoms. However, there are several overarching principles of treatment that must be incorporated into the treatment plans for PWC (see Table 11.2). First, the client must understand the *language of fluency*, i.e., the major components that contribute to the production of fluent speech. Starkweather (1987) defined fluency as the interaction between rate, effort, and continuity. *Rate* refers to the amount of information given within a certain period of time. Rate of speech is faster for longer utterances and impacts speech comprehension when it exceeds 275 words per minute (Starkweather, 1987). Rate is also influenced by a combination of linguistic and speech factors, i.e., word length, word familiarity, message significance, situational concerns, coarticulation, phoneme sequences, stress, and prosody (for a discussion of these parameters, see Bennett, 2006b).

The *effort* portion of Starkweather's definition refers to the degree of muscular exertion required for speech production. The effortless flow of speech produces the perception of light articulatory contacts, regular breathing patterns, and easy vocal fold vibration. Increased effort may be perceived as tense articulatory contacts, breathstream irregularities, and/or glottal fry. Effort is the equivalent of increased tension in the vocal mechanism. The third component of fluency is *continuity*, defined as smooth-flowing speech void of excessive or inappropriately placed pauses. Starkweather wrote that there is predictability and usefulness of 'conventional pauses . . . that a competent speaker makes for emphasis or to signal something linguistically important, while idiosyncratic pauses are an aspect of performance reflecting hesitations or uncertainty over word choice, style, or syntax' (1987, p. 21). An understanding of these concepts related to fluency will assist clients in their understanding of the nature of their difficulties.

Secondly, therapy must help the client understand the dimensions of his/her own *cluttering profile*. Understanding the theoretical foundations of cluttering and the various parameters associated with the disorder will provide the client with a core set of terms used to describe his behavior. The

Table 11.2 Principles of intervention for cluttering that help clients understand the therapy process

Principles of intervention for cluttering
1. Therapy must teach clients the language of fluency.
2. Therapy must help the client understand the dimensions of his/her own cluttering profile.
3. Therapy must encourage and teach the client to self-monitor.
4. Therapy activities must be initiated with a clear rationale for each task.
5. Therapy should follow a strict routine and sequence of practice.
6. Therapy should incorporate repetitive practice of stimuli through an assortment of therapy tasks.
7. Therapy should incorporate activities that are concrete and conceptually based.

following are just a few terms the PWC can learn: cadence, cluttering, co-articulation, disfluencies, dysrhythmic, maze behaviors, narratives, phrasing, pragmatics, rate, restarts, revisions, semantics, sound/syllable elisions, speed, and syntax. Through the process of discussing these terms and providing examples, the client should develop the next principle of treatment, self-monitoring.

The third principle of intervention focuses on the development of *self-monitoring skills*. The ability of the client to self-monitor is essential to treating cluttering (Bennett, 2006a; Daly, 1992, 1996; Myers & St. Louis, 1992; St. Louis & Myers, 1997; St. Louis, Raphael, Myers, & Bakker, 2003; St. Louis et al., 2007; Ward, 2006). The ability to identify behaviors that need modification is critical to any change process. However, for PWC, this is a particular area of weakness. Ward acknowledges that once cluttering symptoms are pointed out to a client, awareness can range from great awareness ('Wow, I never knew I talked so fast!') to gross indifference ('I can't see much wrong there') (2006, p. 365). Clinicians can use audio and video segments to help clients develop this skill (Mosheim, 2004), but this may take several sessions.

The fourth principle of intervention focuses on providing clear *rationales* for therapy tasks. Clients need to know why they are being asked to perform various behaviors. A complete understanding of the learning process does not occur without this knowledge. One of this author's adult clients, at the end of his therapy program, indicated that the one feature of treatment he appreciated most was the clear explanation of why a particular strategy was important to learn. He reported that by learning the 'why' of therapy, he was more likely to comply with the assignments. Daly (1992) emphasized the role of repetition in discussing therapy rationales and procedures. He wrote the following words of advice when working with people who clutter: 'First, tell them what you are going to tell them, tell them, then tell them what you just told them. Finally, the importance of repetition and persistence when working with cluttering clients cannot be overstated' (1992, p. 121).

Following a strict *routine and sequence* of practice is the fifth principle of intervention. There is a subgroup of PWC who exhibit attention deficits and short-term memory difficulties (Daly, 1992; Daly & Burnett, 1999; Scaler Scott & Ward, 2008; St. Louis & Myers, 1997). Therapy that is consistent in its structure will help the client retain skills taught and maintain focus. Each therapy session might be structured accordingly:

1 Begin with a check-in regarding speech assignments and speech status.
2 Review previous therapy session and check for recall.
3 Start with an easier, motor task as a form of warm-up.
4 Challenge the client with an activity that is more difficult.
5 Return to a simpler task that the client will have a high degree of success.

6 Close with a discussion of how the client can apply this knowledge outside the therapy setting, being specific with assignment details (who, what, when, where, and why).

Next, therapy should incorporate *repetitive practice of stimuli* through an assortment of therapy activities. Keeping the stimulus pictures/words the same across therapy activities and sessions facilitates the development of automaticity, i.e., the use of a skill without mental effort (Bennett, 2006b). Overtraining skills assists in the transfer component of therapy and contributes to the replacement of old habits with new habits (Gregory, 2003; Prins, 1997). Motor learning theory suggests that multiple practice sessions, grouped closely together, that provide the learner hundreds of trials within the session are necessary for change to occur (Marshall & Karow, 2002). Clinicians must remember that change is a gradual process that can be positively influenced through the careful planning of therapy activities. Based on the client's cluttering profile, the clinician selects stimuli for practice based on the following criteria:

1 Stimuli should be relevant to and maintain the interest level of each client.
2 Stimuli should be selected based on the coarticulatory patterns of each client.
3 Stimuli should be incorporated into linguistic structures that are manipulated for length and complexity.

The last principle of intervention maintains that therapy should incorporate activities that are *concrete and conceptually based*. Particularly with children with cluttering (CWC), therapy tasks should consider the child's current knowledge-base to ensure comprehension. For example, the clinician may discuss baseball with an elementary-age student to help with catching cluttering moments. The following is an example of such an analogy: The center fielder's job is to catch any balls coming in his direction and throw it toward home base to get the runner out. If he misses the ball or drops the ball, the team gets an error and loses the opportunity to get the player out. However, if he catches the ball and throws it toward home plate, he increases the likelihood that his team will get the player out. The goal of catching one's cluttering is to develop the self-monitoring skills to be able to change that moment before it is over (not drop the ball or miss it). Most clients will understand this concept through discussions and become better able to apply this knowledge.

Overview of the literature on treatment

Resources available on the treatment of cluttering are limited to short chapters in textbooks on stuttering disorders, a few articles in professional journals, and two textbooks specifically devoted to this topic. The paucity of systematic research involving controlled studies is troubling to those interested in cluttering disorders. The field of speech pathology has been challenged to remedy this situation. With the creation of the International Cluttering Association in 2007, consumers and professionals have banned together to collaborate in research efforts to gather more information on this presumably low-incidence disorder. The future holds promise for greater insights into this disorder and methods of treatment. Until then, treatment suggestions are based on the clinical judgment of the practitioner utilizing the theoretical beliefs set forth by those who have published their ideas, i.e., Bennett (2006a), Bennett Lanouette (2007), Daly and Burnett (1999), Myers (1992), Myers and Bradley (1992), Myers and St. Louis (1992), St. Louis and Myers (1995, 1997), St. Louis et al. (2007), and Ward (2006). It is acknowledged that there is much overlap in the following information due to the similarities in treatment approaches among this small group of clinicians. However, each program approaches cluttering from slightly different theoretical orientations.

Bennett Lanouette (2007) approaches cluttering treatment from a cognitive-linguistic approach oriented towards older CWC. Utilizing methods taken from language disorders, this author incorporates verbal elaboration and mental mapping strategies to assist CWC with organizing their thought processes. Daly and Burnett (1999) presented a rate control model for the treatment of cluttering with the treatment goal of teaching the client to produce a slower, more deliberate speech rate. Myers and Bradley (1992) discussed a tri-fold approach to the treatment of cluttering incorporating the dimensions of rate/articulation, language, and awareness. Myers (1992) described a synergistic treatment approach that includes improvement in the domains of rate and rhythm, articulation, language functioning, self-monitoring, and fluency (Myers, 2010; Myers & St. Louis, 1992; St. Louis & Myers, 1995, 1997; St. Louis et al., 2007). Synergistic is defined as 'parts of the communication system working together in a highly coordinated and well timed or synchronous manner' (St. Louis & Myers, 1997, p. 324) (see Figure 11.1). The underlying belief driving treatment is that failure in any one domain impacts the remaining components of communication. For example, as the client increases rate of speech, articulatory proficiency and/or language formulation becomes compromised. The goal of therapy is to establish a pattern of clear, meaningful, and fluent communication through rate modulation and self-monitoring. Ward (2006) outlined his interrelated treatment orientation incorporating information gathered from a number of sources (i.e., client, parent/significant other, school, and other professionals). Ward's treatment protocol begins with the identification of the client's concerns,

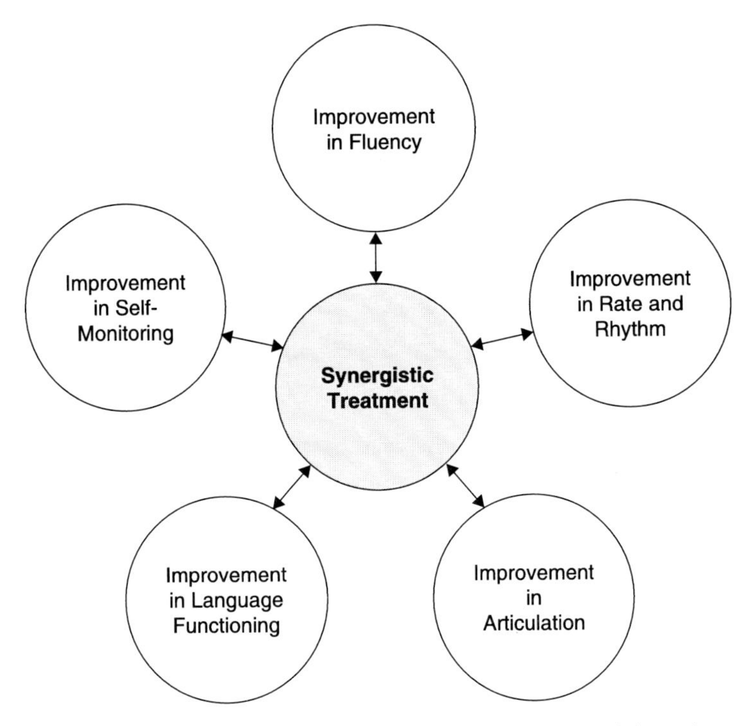

Figure 11.1 Myers' (1992) synergistic approach to the treatment of cluttering.

moves into monitoring/self-awareness, and advances into identification/modification of specific moments of cluttering. Figure 11.2 outlines Ward's protocol, including possible areas of treatment during speech modification.

Treatment effectiveness

Issues around the effectiveness of treatment must be considered by both the clinician and PWC. Two concerns related to this issue warrant the reader's attention: (1) lack of research on treatment efficacy and (2) poor client awareness. St. Louis and Myers commented on the lack of treatment research regarding cluttering. 'The state-of-the-art in the clinical treatment of cluttering is at roughly the same place the treatment for most other speech or language disorders was 20–25 years ago' (1995, p. 194). Fourteen years after St. Louis and Myers' comment, there is still very little in the way of treatment efficacy studies to guide the clinician in treatment decisions. Craig (2010) stressed the importance of conducting controlled clinical trials with an emphasis on cluttering, noting that what we have available to us is somewhat limited to the clinical nuggets from the experts in the field. For example, Daly (1993) noted that his treatment outcomes indicate that treatment takes longer

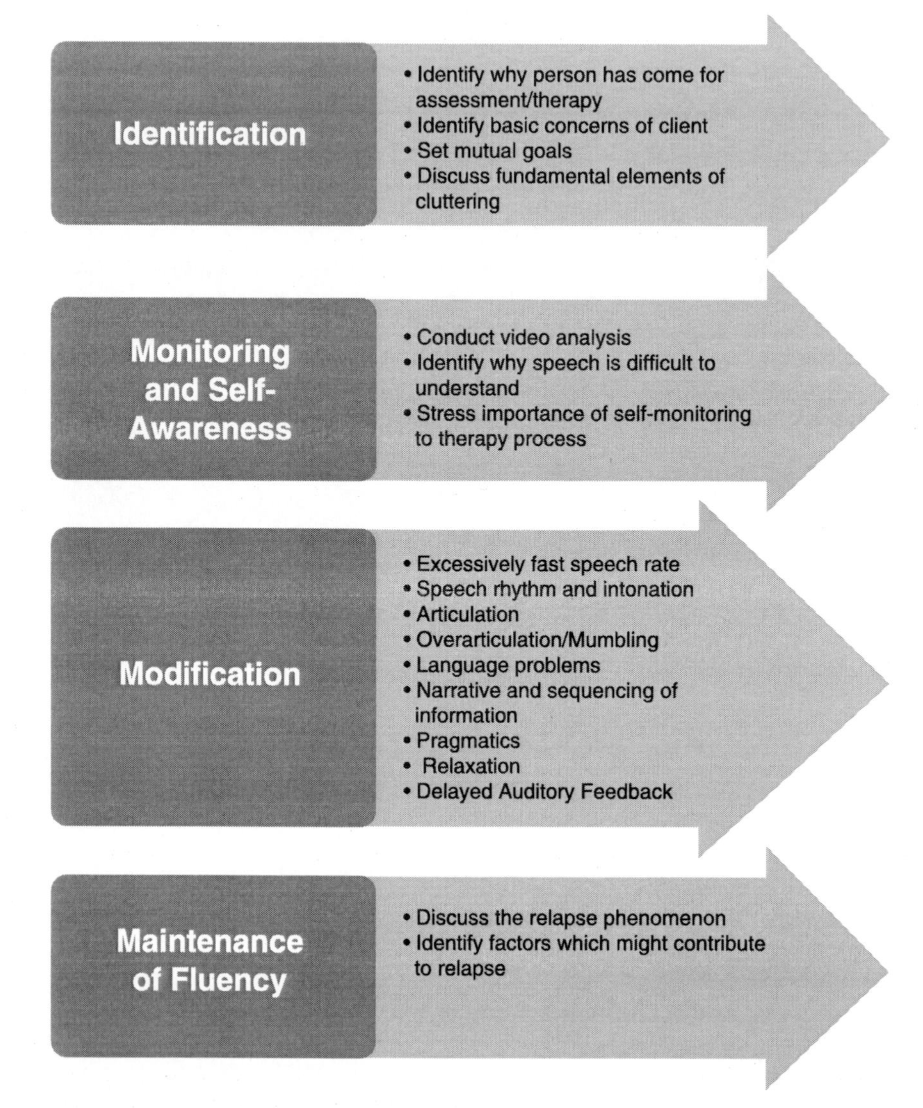

Figure 11.2 Ward's treatment protocol for the treatment of cluttering disorders.

for PWC than it does for clients who stutter, and that therapy should be highly structured.

Using a different perspective, through a review of clinical failures, Marshall and Karow (2002) provided insights into why some rate-control strategies are ineffective. The researchers suggested some clients might benefit from a 'top-down' treatment approach in which the client provides his listeners with more information during the communication exchange. Using a case study of an adult with the diagnosis of 'cortical cluttering', Marshall and Karow reflected on the changes in the treatment protocol that might have been useful in establishing more effective communication:

> Here he might have been taught (a) to inform listeners that he speaks fast and wants to know if he is not understood, (b) to provide topic alerts, (c) to attend to environmental cues (e.g., facial expression, body language) that signal he is not understood, (d) to verify when he feels he is not understood, and (e) to be sure communication partners pay attention.
>
> (2002, p. 13)

Such reports provide clinical insights; however, they are not systematically controlled research studies. Much of our knowledge regarding cluttering treatment comes from the 'clinical nuggets' of those who are practicing the art. To overcome the first hurdle, researchers and clinicians must agree on the key elements within the definition of cluttering. Ward (2006) noted that the field lacks a general consensus as to the core characteristics of cluttering. In years prior to Ward's comments, St. Louis et al. wrote:

> our long-term goal has been to 'put cluttering on the map' such that, first and foremost, a consensus on a standard definition of cluttering will emerge. After that occurs, we believe that improved understanding of the incidence, cause, diagnosis, and treatment of cluttering will no doubt follow.
>
> (2003, p. 22)

Bernstein Ratner expanded on this belief by writing that 'what we need to do is find some basic concepts to agree on. Among them might first be an agreement that we need to keep working on the problem' (2005, p. 181).

The second issue related to treatment efficacy is poor client awareness. Authorities in cluttering recognize the inherent difficulties in the treatment of PWC who do not exhibit self-awareness abilities or do not consider themselves as having a problem (Bennett, 2006a; Daly, 1992, 1996; Myers & Bradley, 1992; Myers & St. Louis, 1992; St. Louis & Myers, 1995; Ward, 2006). Myers and St. Louis (1992, p. 192) provided three explanations for this inherent weakness: (1) these clients are unaware of or unconcerned about their speech difficulties; (2) they may have disturbances in self-awareness, such as in time perception; and (3) many of their symptoms are due precisely to the fact that they do not or cannot exercise the normal degree of regulatory control of their speech and, often, nonspeech behavior. As clinicians attest, clients who are not aware of their communication deficits are more difficult to work with. Some clients may enter the therapy process with the underlying belief that they do not have a problem. Trying to convince an individual that help is needed challenges even the best therapist. Ward (2006) acknowledged that the prognosis for improvement is good only when the client is self-aware and has self-monitoring skills. For the more severe clutterer who does not have these skills, prognosis for improvement may be poor. In summary, without a clear definition and with clients who exhibit poor self-awareness, the measurement of treatment effects becomes confounded. But these issues should not stop researchers and clinicians from continuing work with PWC. Knowledge from clinical work helps develop a universally agreed-upon definition that enhances the ability to structure and conduct treatment studies.

Intervention paradigm

The treatment of cluttering presented in this chapter encompasses five major domains: rate, motor, language, pragmatics, and cognition. The following therapy activities draw on the writings discussed throughout this book. These ideas provide a foundation for the clinician and the client engaged in the treatment of cluttering. The criterion for selection of any one domain should be based on the differential diagnosis and establishment of an individualized treatment plan for each client. The concepts provided in Figure 11.3 may not be appropriate for all age groups and levels of severity of cluttering. These are presented as a place to start when treating this unique fluency disorder.

Rate

Rate of speech is believed to be the underlying, key component in the disorder of cluttering (St. Louis, 2010; St. Louis et al., 2003; St. Louis et al., 2007). Establishing rate control encompasses the areas of speed, tempo, and prosody. Manipulation of speed can occur through the structured practice and subsequent mastery of a variety of rate control strategies. Marshall and Karow (2002) outlined seven techniques clinicians may select to teach (see Table 11.3). These techniques have been shown to be effective with other fluency disorders, particularly stuttering (i.e., Gregory, 2003; Ingham, 1999; Onslow & Packman, 1997; Perkins, 1996).

Speed

Easy onsets, which manipulate the duration and transition between the first two sounds of an utterance, are one strategy that produces a decrease in speech rate. Gregory (2003) used easy onsets within the framework of his Easy Relaxed Approach-Smooth Movements. Clients are taught to start speech with an easy transition between the first two sounds of the word/phrase, with the rest of the utterance maintaining normal rate and prosody. Similar fluency techniques are soft contacts or light articulatory contacts. Here the client is asked to reduce the degree of pressure exerted during speech production (Perkins, 1996).

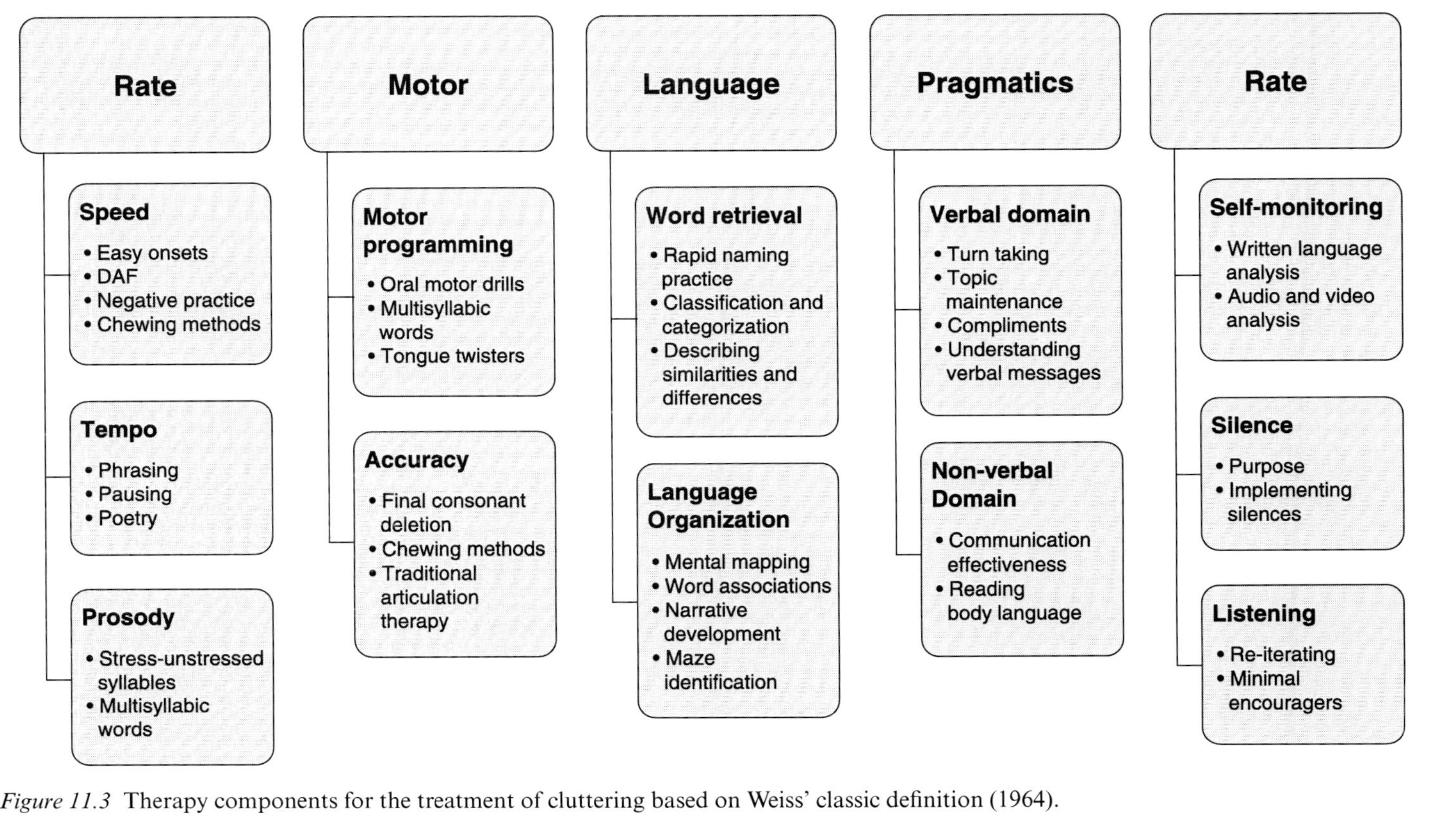

Figure 11.3 Therapy components for the treatment of cluttering based on Weiss' classic definition (1964).

Table 11.3 Marshall and Karow's (2002) strategies for rate control intervention

Technique	*Description of Technique*
Instructions to slow down	• Clinician modeling • Remind patient to slow down
Prolonged speech	• Prolonging vowels within syllables and words • Using continuous voicing • Clinician models
Rhythmic cueing	• Clinician points to words in passage • Rhythmically signaling desired speaking rate through finger tapping
Metronome	• Metronome set to 90 beats per minute
Finger/hand tapping	• Tap finger or hand in cadence with each word spoken • Clinician modeling
Pacing board	• Point to sections of board upon producing each word • Clinician modeling and demonstration
Delayed auditory feedback (DAF)	• DAF set at 250 ms • Clinician modeling and instruction

Several clinicians have used DAF to provide an opportunity for the client to experience a slowed speech rate with exaggerated enunciation (Bennett, 2006a; Daly, 1992, 1996; Myers & Bradley, 1992; St. Louis et al., 1996; St. Louis & Myers, 1997). DAF changes the speaker's auditory signal through a predetermined millisecond delay via an electronic device. The effects of DAF on the speech of the speaker are widely known. The reader is referred to the comprehensive review by Wingate (1988) for additional information. DAF can assist the client to 'feel' the difference between his habitual speaking rate and a more pronounced, slower rate. Daly (1992) noted that speaking under the DAF condition heightens the client's awareness of rate problems while facilitating the coordination of respiration, phonation, and articulation. Some clients may complain that their speech sounds 'strange' when using DAF. This reaction is not uncommon and may be attributed to the proprioceptive feedback routinely received when talking, i.e., fast, irregular rate feels 'normal' to the PWC. It takes time for the client to adjust to the delay and use DAF to create a slower speed. It is important to note that the usefulness of DAF for PWC must be evaluated on an individual basis, as few data exist and preliminary results are mixed for the long-term efficacy of use of DAF with PWC (see St. Louis et al., 1996).

Two additional strategies may be used to decrease speech rate: negative practice and chewing methods. Negative practice involves the production of speech at contrastive speeds, i.e., 50 miles per hour (mph) (regular), 75 mph (somewhat fast), and 100 mph (fast). The client chooses a written passage and reads out loud implementing each rate (rate is based on subjective estimates of speed). Myers (2010) added a unique twist to this exercise. She asks clients to produce speech at varying rates and then 'go even faster', having them exceed their maximum capacity. She stresses the importance of having the client 'feel the difference' and examine what happens when rate is manipulated (in both slow and fast directions). Clients can close their eyes when practicing rate control strategies to heighten awareness of other senses, such as tactile, kinesthetic, or proprioceptive feedback. Another rate control technique is the chewing method, a technique used for a variety of communication problems such as dysarthria, vocal dysfunction, and breathstream mismanagement. Bennett (2006a), Daly (1992), and Ward (2006) recommend this strategy to replace the mumbling characteristic of cluttered speech. Mumbling is defined as the consistent lack of articulatory movement with reduced volume (Ward, 2006). The chewing method involves having the client imagine chewing a piece of gum with exaggerated oral movements. The articulators begin moving in an open, relaxed manner, which facilitates clear articulation.

Tempo

Tempo, in musical terms, refers to the pace of a given piece measured in beats per minute. The greater the tempo, the larger the number of beats produced within a given time frame. Tempo, as related to speech production, refers to the number of phonemes produced during any given period of time. For PWC, tempo refers to the erratic spurts of fast speech accompanied by abrupt pauses and restarts. Therapy activities of phrasing, pausing, and using poetry will assist the client in regulating and varying tempo.

Phrasing involves teaching the client to speak in short, deliberate chunks of speech, i.e., three-to-four word utterances. Using a highlighter or red pen, the clinician and client read from a list of sentences and mark the most appropriate place to break the sentence into phrases. Providing visual cues helps the client prepare to stop. After marking the passage, the client reads each chunk aloud. Beginning with short sentences allows the client to self-evaluate his ability to implement this skill. Daly (1992) reported the tendency of PWC to ignore punctuation marks. Using visual cues delineating short, simple sentences helps the client create awareness of this habit. Gregory (2003) discussed the concept of daily practice of phrasing through the development of practice stimuli of words, phrases, and sentences. The client uses a speech modification strategy when producing the word, the phrase, and then the sentence, which is broken into two or three phrases. This exercise would benefit the PWC in efforts to modify speech tempo.

Pausing is an additional strategy designed to modify the client's tempo. Pausing involves instructing the client to pause when cued, typically at syntactically correct junctures, and silently count from one to two before continuing with the communication effort. Gradually the clinician reduces the frequency of cues and the client begins to self-cue. The client must learn to tolerate the silence during pauses (Van Riper, 1971). St. Louis and Myers (1997) recommend the use of pausing to decrease the demands placed on the speech production system, thus enhancing the client's ability to regulate speech rate and organize language output. Lastly, the majority of clinicians writing on the topic of cluttering recommend using poetry as a means of demonstrating tempo variability and regulation (Daly, 1992, 1996; Myers & St. Louis, 1992; St. Louis & Myers, 1995, 1997; Van Riper, 1971; Ward, 2006). Poetry allows the client to experience rhythmic speech characterized by appropriate use of pauses at linguistically correct units. The clinician can present a poem to analyze with the client. Together they can determine the number of syllables per phrase, as well as determine the most appropriate places to pause. Reading poems aloud while pausing and phrasing helps the client to modify speech tempo.

Prosody

Prosody is a suprasegmental feature of speech production related to the melody imposed on the communicative effort. Two prosodic features conveying meaning are word stress and rhythm, both influenced by speech rate. Speech rate has been found faster for questions than statements (van Heuven & van Zanten, 2005). For cluttering, the individual may not apply differential speaking rates for questions vs. statements, leaving the listener to infer the speaker's intent. Another prosodic variation to target in therapy is the prolongation of vowels as a feature of stress. An increase in speech rate produces the shortening of vowel segments resulting in the disruption of prosody. Therapy might include activities that help the individual differentiate between questions and statements, teach vowel prolongation as a stress marker, and educate the speaker on the role of pitch contours. Clients may benefit from educational activities that target stressed and unstressed syllables in multisyllabic words, the role of pitch changes in prosody, and vocal intensity as a prosodic marker. The most common strategy reported in the literature was contrastive stress drills in which the client engages in systematic practice of different stress patterns. Similar to negative practice exercises, the client produces one pattern and then another, attending to the differences in stress, rate, and/or intensity.

For CWC, direct therapy activities must be developed to teach these abstract concepts. Examples of two such activities will be described. First, the Stress Game is designed to demonstrate to CWC the role of stress in word meaning. Using contrast exercises, the clinician presents various sentences that have words underlined for emphasis. Next, a picture is drawn depicting the meaning behind the sentence. Clinician and client discuss the different connotations between the three sentences. After several examples, the client generates sentences and explains the meanings to the clinician. Table 11.4 provides an example of this activity.

Table 11.4 Activity to help children identify the role of stress in word meaning

Where's the emphasis?	
Sentence	*Picture depicting emphasis*
Do YOU want an apple?	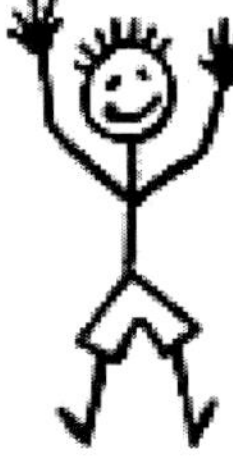
Do you WANT an apple?	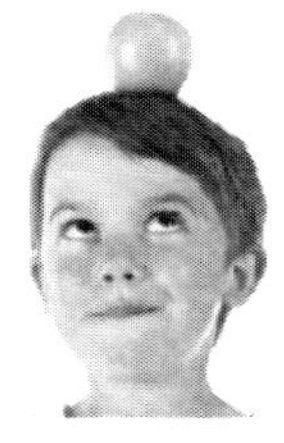
Do you want an APPLE?	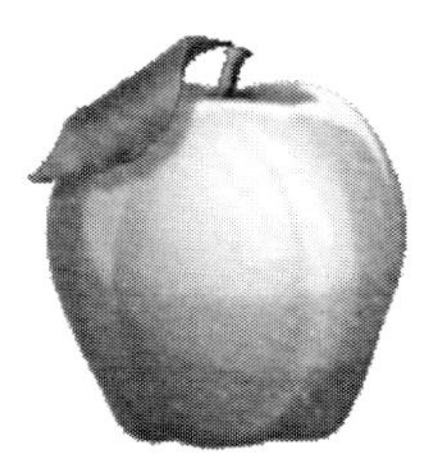

'Are you telling me or asking me?' is a therapy game where clients sort stimulus cards based on the clinician's production (i.e., question or statement). The client next generates a new sentence, and the clinician identifies the appropriate category. Gradually, the client says the sentence and identifies the appropriate category without clinician input. It is recommended that the clinician record the client's responses in case a discrepancy arises between the clinician and client's judgments. The recorded segment is available for replay and discussion. Therapy can also include contrastive drills to reinforce the prosodic differences between questions and statements (see Figure 11.4).

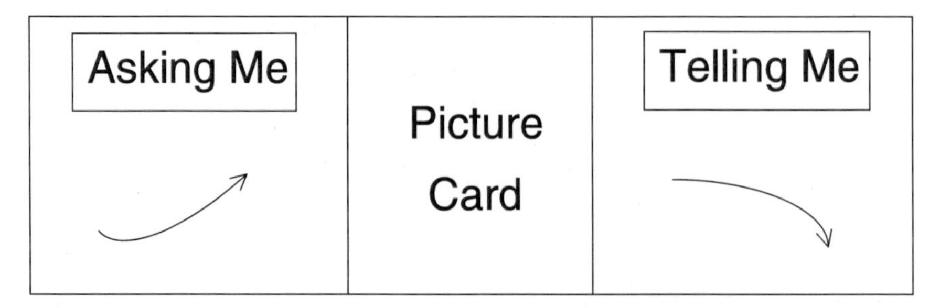

Step 1. Present the sentence strip and practice identifying questions and statements.

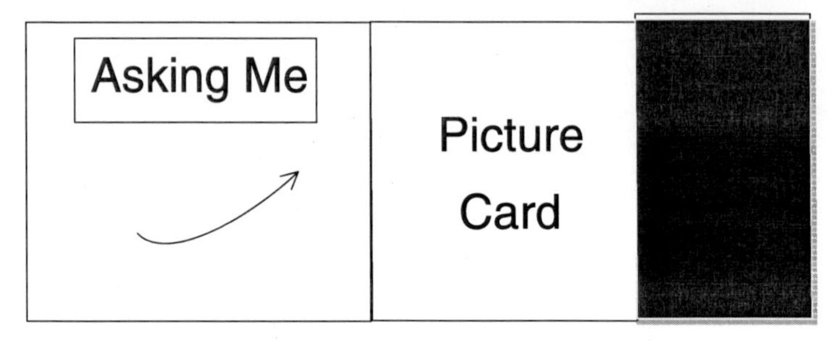

Step 2. Fold over one side (in this picture fold over the 'Telling Me' side). Have the client generate a question based on the picture card.

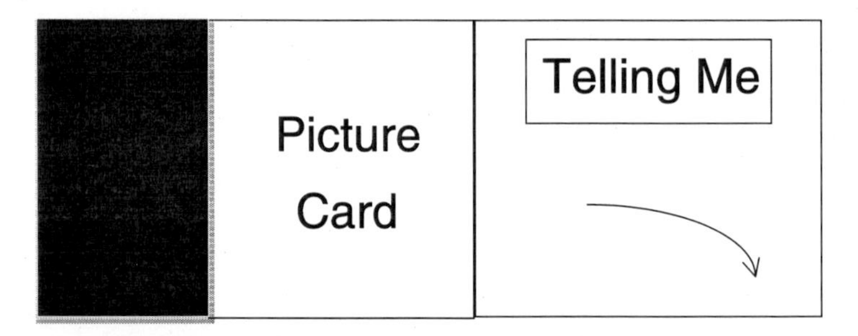

Step 3. Fold over the other side (in this picture, fold over the 'Asking Me' side). Have the client generate a statement based on the same picture card. Flip between the two types of sentenceforms by covering and uncovering the ends of the strip of paper.

Figure 11.4 Question versus statement therapy activity.

Motor

Cluttering has been characterized by inappropriate, usually excessive, degrees of coarticulation among sounds, as manifested in the deletion of stressed syllables and imprecise articulation (also see St. Louis & Schulte, chapter 14 and Ward, chapter 3 this volume). Both variables negatively impact speech intelligibility and need to be incorporated in therapy. Some principles of sound-specific articulation therapy may assist in improving sound accuracy.

However, treatment must go beyond sound accuracy drills. Although discussion of sound formation (i.e., place, manner, and voicing characteristics of each sound) enhances awareness, for clients who produce speech at excessive rates, therapy must teach strategies to change the overcoarticulation and deletions.

Overcoarticulation

St. Louis and Myers (1998) recommend having the client 'learn to exaggerate stressed syllables in longer words while being sure to include all the unstressed syllables (e.g., "par-tic-u-lar," "con-di-tion-al," or "gen-er-o-si-ty").' The authors indicate:

> Stressing a syllable in a multisyllabic word adds duration as well as increases both loudness and pitch of that syllable. The accentuation of a syllable often helps to organize the articulatory gesture, as if to provide the clutterer a 'center of gravity' or focal point in his speech.
>
> (n.p.)

Additionally, children can practice syllable awareness tasks, such as tapping out syllables. The clinician can make speech puzzles to demonstrate the number of syllables in a word. Here the clinician presents a picture of a four-syllable word (e.g., watermelon). Using craft scissors with different pattern edges, she cuts the picture into four pieces. Next, she demonstrates putting the puzzle back together, saying each syllable in a precise, clear manner.

Imprecise articulation

Daly (1996) utilizes oral motor drills to increase speech precision of PWC. Daly's three-step hierarchy to enhance motor programming skills includes accuracy, smoothness, and rate drills. These exercises help the client to produce multisyllabic words, a deficit common in cluttering. Strengthening the motor programming system also enhances the client's self-monitoring skills. The first component of Daly's program focuses on the production of accurate syllable strings controlled for the extent of movement within the oral tract. The client produces syllable shapes in a string of 10 repetitions. When the ability to produce a particular syllable sequence is established, the client then works on the smoothness or connectedness of these 10 sequences. The last aspect of this program involves the accurate and smooth production of syllabic strings within a given time frame, i.e., rate of production. Direct practice on multisyllabic units, starting from simple to complex, helps to develop clear, precise articulation (Riley & Riley, 2000). Tongue twisters are another therapy activity that will achieve the same goal. Stimuli, such as 'Susan sells shells at the seashore', force the client to reduce rate and overarticulate in order to maintain speech accuracy. Repetitive practice of tongue twisters will enhance the client's ability to monitor his speech through proprioceptive and auditory feedback.

Language

Difficulties in word retrieval and language organization may exist for a subgroup of PWC. Proposed theories and definitions, presented throughout this book, confirm the need to address language skills in some clients. The following is a brief discussion of word retrieval. The reader is referred to the literature on language disorders for more information.

Word retrieval

Daly (1996) observed that as PWC become more fluent, the emergence of word-finding difficulties becomes evident. Word-finding difficulties are observed when the individual cannot retrieve a specific noun, verb, adjective, etc. to match the communication intent. For example, the client might say 'light bulb' instead of 'light switch' or 'you know, the thingie'. The reader is referred to the literature on word retrieval for further elaboration of treatment guidelines (e.g., Bowen, 1998; German, 2000). Bennett (2006a), Bennett Lanouette (2007), Daly and Burnett (1999), Myers and Bradley (1992), and St. Louis and Myers (1997) have provided specific treatment goals for this particular subgroup of PWC. Table 11.5 summarizes the suggestions from these authors.

Table 11.5 Word-finding treatment ideas as applied to people with cluttering

Author	*Word-finding treatment suggestions*
Bennett	• Name key elements of description using graphic organizers • Use color coding to facilitate word associations • Sort words according to their proper classification • Perform compare/contrast activities • Complete analogies
Daly and Burnett	• Name attributes within given category • Categorize items or objects • Provide detailed description of objects with increased use of descriptors • Describe similarities and differences
Myers and Bradley	• Increase semantic classification and categorization skills • Increase speech and accuracy of word retrieval
St. Louis and Myers	• Work on word finding through reduced speech rate • Work on semantics and syntax, especially relational vocabulary (because, unless) • Use mental mapping of narratives to facilitate organization • Help clients identify 'maze' behaviors

Language organization

Another feature of cluttering is the lack of organized language production. The presence of maze behaviors, such as repetitions, false starts, and revisions, make speech difficult to comprehend. Evidence is needed to determine whether these repetitions, false starts, and revisions are the result of disorganized language or whether these behaviors merely make language *sound* disorganized. Adults who clutter may not be aware of the negative impact of mazing on the listener. A useful activity to demonstrate maze behaviors is to record the client generating a story from a set of sequence pictures. The clinician then transcribes the sample, highlighting the intended message. That which is not highlighted is maze behavior. The visual representation of how often the discourse is disrupted by these behaviors becomes more evident. Together, the clinician and client can listen to the discourse while following along with the transcript to create a better understanding of how cluttering impacts the flow of information. Other therapy activities designed to strengthen language organization can be found in the literature on language disorders.

Pragmatics

Pragmatics is the use of language within a given social context. It involves knowing what to say, when to say it, and how to say it in socially appropriate ways. Pragmatics involves three major communication skills: (1) using language for different purposes; (2) changing language according to the needs of the listener or situation; and (3) following rules for conversations and storytelling (ASHA, n.d.). Bowen (2001) identified eight pragmatics skills that might be relevant to some clients with cluttering: (1) knowing that you have to answer when a question has been asked; (2) being able to participate in a conversation through turn taking; (3) the ability to notice and respond to the nonverbal aspects of language; (4) awareness that you have to introduce a topic of conversation in order for the listener to fully understand; (5) knowing which words or what sentence type to use when initiating a conversation or responding to something someone has said; (6) the ability to maintain or change a topic appropriately; (7) the ability to maintain appropriate eye contact during a conversation; and (8) the ability to distinguish how to talk and behave towards different communication partners (i.e., formal with some, informal with others). The reader is directed to the social skills literature for examples of therapy activities that are designed to address pragmatic communication deficits.

Cognition

The term *cognition* is used to refer to the client's apparent lack of awareness of his communication problems. Some PWC may think listeners have the problem and don't attribute communication difficulties to any specific behavior they exhibit. As Dalton and Hardcastle noted, 'many just do not realize the speed at which they are speaking and are genuinely puzzled by their listeners' failure to understand them' (1989, p. 124). The ultimate goal of therapy for cluttering is for the client to self-monitor his speech production and take appropriate actions when a breakdown occurs. To achieve this goal, therapy should focus on the cognitive components of self-monitoring, use of silence, and enhanced listening.

Self-monitoring

Self-monitoring skills develop slowly and after much practice. The client is asked to repeatedly self-evaluate his performance and identify features needing change. This, again, is a difficult task for the PWC. Clinicians may use a written language sample of the client's narrative to demonstrate possible breakdowns. A written sample provides a concrete example of the client's cluttering that is difficult to refute. Listening and watching a videotaped sample of the client's communication is another way to enhance self-monitoring. Because listening to your own voice and watching yourself on video can be an uncomfortable exercise, it is recommended that the client view short video segments, typically one to two sentences at a time. This is particularly true when the client does not acknowledge or show awareness of his cluttering. After each segment, the client and clinician can evaluate the performance based on a Likert scale developed by both parties. Each participant rates the speech sample and then compares their rating with each other and/or with other communication partners, such as family members.

SILENCE

Use of silence is another potential cognitive skill deficit in PWC. Excessive talking has been observed clinically as a common feature of PWC. This author speculates that it is possible the verbosity occurs because PWC feel uncomfortable with periods of silence. The clinician can help the client understand the purpose of silence during the communication exchange. Silence can be used as a reflective period to think about the communication exchange and determine how to continue or terminate the conversation. Silence can aid in the accuracy of word retrieval by inserting a brief pause before commenting. Daly (1996) incorporated several cognitive strategies (relaxation, visual imagery, and breathing exercises) to enhance concentration and reinforce tolerance with silence. Additionally, Bennett (2006a) noted that teaching clients to monitor silent and talking periods may aid in reducing tangential verbosity. Clients must be able to verbalize what they are doing and why. A better understanding of their nonstop speech can enhance communication effectiveness.

Listening

The third cognitive component to treatment involves listening skills. Some PWC fail to attend to the verbal and nonverbal messages of their discourse partner. Overt work on identifying the verbal and nonverbal signals of 'misunderstanding' or 'confusion' can help the PWC. Work on nonverbal expressions helps clients 'tune in' to the listener. Teaching clients to use minimal encouragers, reflective comments, and direct questions may be required in therapy. Minimal encouragers are verbal signs that the listener is following the conversation. These include brief comments or interjections such as 'really', 'hum', or 'I see'. Head nodding and forward leaning of the body are two other strategies that convey listening. Reflective comments are interspersed in a conversation to demonstrate that the listener is following the discourse. For example, after the client mentions that he likes poodles more than shepherds, the clinician might comment, 'So you like poodles.' Learning to use direct questions related to comprehension can also facilitate communication effectiveness. The clinician demonstrates the use of questions to clarify that a break in communication has occurred ('I don't understand. Could you repeat that?' or 'Did you mean . . .?'). Again, using written cues of sample dialogues can help create an awareness of the need to request clarification.

Conclusion

Cluttering is a specific fluency disorder that warrants systematic intervention. Intervention should be tailored toward the client's needs, incorporating activities across the domains of rate, motor, language, pragmatics, and cognition. This chapter has provided several ideas for intervention that are appropriate for both adults and children with cluttering. Cluttering has recently received renewed interest in the profession of speech-language pathology. There exists a need for research in cluttering to establish a more comprehensive understanding of this communication disorder. Additionally, there is a lack of information regarding evidence-based practice in cluttering. Perhaps the future will remedy this situation.

References

ASHA. (n.d.). *Social language use (Pragmatics)*. Retrieved May 29, 2009, from http://www.asha.org/public/speech/development/Pragmatics.htm

Bennett, E. M. (2006a). Cluttering: Another fluency disorder. In E. M. Bennett, *Working with people who stutter: A lifespan approach* (pp. 484–507). Columbus, OH: Pearson Merrill Prentice Hall.

Bennett, E. M. (2006b). *Working with people who stutter: A lifespan approach*. Columbus, OH: Pearson Merrill Prentice Hall.

Bennett Lanouette, E. (2007). *Treatment in children who clutter: The language and fluency interface.* Presentation at the First World Conference on Cluttering, Katarino, Bulgaria.

Bernstein Ratner, N. (2005). Evidence based practice in stuttering: Some questions to consider. *Journal of Fluency Disorders, 30*, 163–188.

Bowen, C. (1998). *Stuck for words? Word retrieval activities for children.* Retrieved May 29, 2009, from http://www.speech-language-therapy.com/wordretrieval.html

Bowen, C. (2001). *Semantic and pragmatic difficulties and semantic pragmatic language disorder.* Retrieved May 29, 2009, from http://www.speech-language-therapy.com/spld.htm

Craig, A. (2010). The importance of conducting controlled clinical trials in the fluency disorders with emphasis on cluttering. In K. Bakker, L. Raphael, & F. Myers (Eds.), *Proceedings of the First World Conference on Cluttering, Katarino, Bulgaria* (pp. 220–229). http://associations.missouristate.edu/ICA

Dalton, P., & Hardcastle, W. J. (1989). *Disorders of fluency and their effects on communication* (2nd ed.). London: Cole & Whurr.

Daly, D. A. (1992). Helping the clutterer: Therapy considerations. In F. L. Myers & K. O. St. Louis (Eds.), *Cluttering: A clinical perspective* (pp. 107–121). Leicester, UK: FAR Communications (Reissued in 1996 by Singular, San Diego, CA.)

Daly, D. A. (1993). Cluttering: The orphan of speech-language pathology. *American Journal of Speech-Language Pathology, 2*, 6–8.

Daly, D. A. (1996). *The source for stuttering and cluttering.* East Moline, IL: LinguiSystems.

Daly, D. A., & Burnett, M. L. (1999). Cluttering: Traditional view and new perspectives. In R. F. Curlee (Ed.), *Stuttering and related disorders of fluency* (2nd ed.). New York: Thieme.

German, D. J. (2000). Basic concepts in child word finding. In D. J. German, *Test of word finding* (2nd ed., pp. 1–15). Austin, TX: ProEd.

Gregory, H. H. (2003). *Stuttering therapy: Rationale and procedures.* Upper Saddle River, NJ: Allyn & Bacon.

Ingham, R. J. (1999). Performance contingent management of stuttering in adolescents and adults. In R. F. Curlee (Ed.), *Stuttering and related disorders of fluency* (2nd ed.). New York: Thieme.

Marshall, R. C., & Karow, C. M. (2002). Retrospective examination of failed rate-control intervention. *American Journal of Speech Language Pathology, 11*, 3–16.

Mosheim, J. (2004, November 22). Cluttering: Specialists work to put it on the map of fluency disorders. *Advance Magazine*, 6–9.

Myers, F. L. (1992). Cluttering: A synergistic framework. In F. L. Myers & K. O. St. Louis (Eds.), *Cluttering: A clinical perspective* (pp. 71–84). Leicester, UK: FAR Communications. (Reissued in 1996 by Singular, San Diego, CA.)

Myers, F. L. (2010). Primacy of self-awareness and the modulation of rate in the treatment of cluttering. In K. Bakker, L. Raphael, & F. Myers (Eds.), *Proceedings of the First World Conference on Cluttering, Katarino, Bulgaria* (pp. 108–114). http://associations.missouristate.edu/ICA

Myers, F. L., & Bradley, C. L. (1992). Clinical management of cluttering from a synergistic framework. In F. L. Myers & K. O. St. Louis (Eds.), *Cluttering: A clinical perspective.* Leicester, UK: FAR Communications. (Reissued in 1996 by Singular, San Diego, CA.)

Myers, F. L., & St. Louis, K. O. (1992). *Cluttering: A clinical perspective*. Leicester, UK: FAR Communications. (Reissued in 1996 by Singular, San Diego, CA.)

Onslow, M., & Packman, A. (1997). Designing and implementing a strategy to control stuttered speech in adults. In R. F. Curlee & G. M. Siegel (Eds.), *Nature and treatment of stuttering: New directions*. Boston, MA: Allyn & Bacon.

Perkins, W. H. (1996). Fluency controls and automatic fluency. *American Journal of Speech-Language Pathology, 1*, 9–10.

Prins, D. (1997). Modifying stuttering: The stutterer's reactive behavior. Perspectives on past, present, and future. In R. F. Curlee & G. M. Siegel (Eds.), *Nature and treatment of stuttering: New directions* (pp. 335–355). Boston, MA: Allyn & Bacon.

Riley, G., & Riley, J. (2000). A revised component model for diagnosing and treating children who stutter. *Contemporary Issues in Communication Science and Disorders, 27*, 188–199.

Scaler Scott, K., & Ward, D. (2008, November). *Treatment of cluttered speech in Asperger's disorder: Focus on self-regulation*. A seminar presented at the annual convention of the American Speech-Language-Hearing Association, Chicago, IL.

Starkweather, C. W. (1987). *Fluency and stuttering*. Englewood Cliffs, NJ: Prentice-Hall.

St. Louis, K. O. (2010). A ten-year agenda for cluttering: Excerpt featuring seven key guidelines. In K. Bakker, L. Raphael, & F. Myers (Eds.), *Proceedings of the First World Conference on Cluttering, Katarino, Bulgaria* (pp. 20–30). http://associations.missouristate.edu/ICA

St. Louis, K. O., & Myers, F. L. (1995). Clinical management of cluttering. *Language, Speech, and Hearing Services in the Schools, 26*, 187–194.

St. Louis, K. O., & Myers, F. L. (1997). Management of cluttering and related fluency disorders. In R. F. Curlee & G. M. Siegel (Eds.), *Nature and treatment of stuttering: New directions* (2nd ed., pp. 313–332). Boston, MA: Allyn & Bacon.

St. Louis, K. O., & Myers, F. L. (1998). *A synopsis of cluttering and its treatment*. ISAD online conference. Retrieved May 29, 2009, from http://www.mnsu.edu/comdis/isad/papers/stlouis.html

St. Louis, K. O., Myers, F. L., Bakker, K., & Raphael, L. J. (2007). Understanding and treating cluttering. In E. G. Conture & R. F. Curlee (Eds.), *Stuttering and related disorders of fluency* (3rd ed., pp. 297–325). New York: Thieme.

St. Louis, K. O., Myers, F. L., Cassidy, L. J., Michael, A. J., Penrod, S. M., Litton, B. A., Coutras, S. W., Olivera, J. L. R., & Brodsky, E. (1996). Efficacy of delayed auditory feedback for treating cluttering: Two case studies. *Journal of Fluency Disorders, 21*, 305–317.

St. Louis, K. O., Raphael, L. J., Myers, F. L., & Bakker, K. (2003, November 18). Cluttering updated. *The ASHA Leader*, 4–5, 20–22.

van Heuven, V. J., & van Zanten, E. (2005). Speech rate as a secondary prosodic characteristic of polarity questions in three languages. *Speech Communication, 47*, 87–99.

Van Riper, C. (1971). *The nature of stuttering*. Englewood Cliffs, NJ: Prentice-Hall.

Ward, D. (2006). *Stuttering and cluttering: Frameworks for understanding and treatment*. New York: Psychology Press.

Weiss, D. A. (1964). *Cluttering*. Englewood Cliffs, NJ: Prentice-Hall.

Wingate, M. E. (1988). *The structure of stuttering: A psycholinguistic approach*. New York: Springer-Verlag.

12 Assessment and intervention of Japanese children exhibiting possible cluttering

Shoko Miyamoto

Introduction

Japan has recently witnessed an increased interest in interventions for people who have speech disorders with coexisting developmental disorders such as learning disabilities and attention deficit hyperactivity disorder (ADHD). In addition, there are frequent reports that some children exhibit rapid speech and repetition. Based on previous literature (Daly, 1993; St. Louis & Myers, 1997), I suggest the necessity to consider such children from the viewpoint of cluttering. Since at present in Japan, as elsewhere, there is no generally agreed upon definition of cluttering (see also St. Louis & Schulte, chapter 13 this volume), we cannot formally assess and treat children who suffer from this disorder. In this research, I will investigate the similarity between such cases and the international literature on cluttering, and discuss the feasibility of accepting a diagnostic classification of cluttering in Japan. Furthermore, I present two cases of children with suspected cluttering, where intervention was targeted using clinical methods that are specifically aimed at the treatment of cluttering.

Participants

The investigator selected two elementary school students, based on two criteria: (1) they had undergone treatment for stuttering in a special class for speech-language disorders and (2) their teachers regarded their speech to be too rapid to understand. The first student (S1) was an 8-year-old boy with advanced academic skills; the second (S2), a 9-year-old boy. Since the results on S2's intelligence test demonstrated a considerable discrepancy between his verbal and performance intelligence, he was suspected to have a learning disability.

Participant S1

S1 was first assessed when he was 6 years, 7 months. He was a speaker of Japanese. In motor development such as stability of head, sitting, and walking, he presented normal process. He did not begin speaking until 2 years of age. When he started to talk, he began stuttering. His speech was unintelligible to the point that his family and friends sometimes could not understand the content of his speech. When he was 5 years old, his mother began to worry about his speech in general, and specifically about his sound substitutions and stuttering. The family consequently brought S1 to a speech therapist. His mother was advised that her son had no problem. At the end of first grade, S1's mother requested help with her son's speech disfluency, and he began to attend therapy for speech-language disordered children in elementary school. At the time, he exhibited no apparent awareness of his disfluencies. With regard to academic skill, his ability of mathematics was excellent, and the other subjects were sufficient as well. Though speech characteristics were viewed as unintelligible and unorganized, writing and written composition were within normal limits. Grammatical skill was also within normal limits. Learning disability was not suspected. S1's classroom teacher reported that it was difficult for him to play with the other students in his class. Though he wanted to play with the other children, he couldn't communicate with them skilfully. Moreover, consistent with his lack of awareness of his disfluencies, he also had no awareness of his lack of intelligibility. In addition, his teacher indicated that he had a very short attention span.

In the initial assessment at 6 years, 7 months, final part-word repetitions accounted for the primary disfluency (24 percent) in S1's speech. (Note that the linguistic Mora unit involves syllable structures that differ in timing and stress patterning to those seen in syllables and words in English). Figure 12.1 shows the breakdown of disfluencies by type.

S1's speech fluency was re-evaluated at 8 years of age prior to enrolment in experimental sessions. Results of the evaluation revealed blocking and prolongations. No secondary behaviours were observed at this time. Notably, there were no disfluencies when reading aloud. The final part-word repetitions observed at 6 years, 7 months were still present, and occurred mainly in spontaneous speech on both content words and function words.

The Japanese checklist for possible cluttering (Miyamoto, Hayasaka, & Shapiro, 2006) was applied to S1 (Appendix A). This checklist comprises 24 items (where each item scores between 0 and 2 points) and is adapted from Daly's (1993) checklist. A score of greater than 20–25 points suggest possible cluttering. As is indicated in Appendix A, S1 received a score of 23 on this checklist.

Participant S2

S2 reportedly began talking rather late, and his speech was accompanied by stuttering. With regard to motor skills, S2 began walking late and he would climb up stairs with a stagger even as late as when he entered elementary school. From the time he entered school, he was treated in the special class for

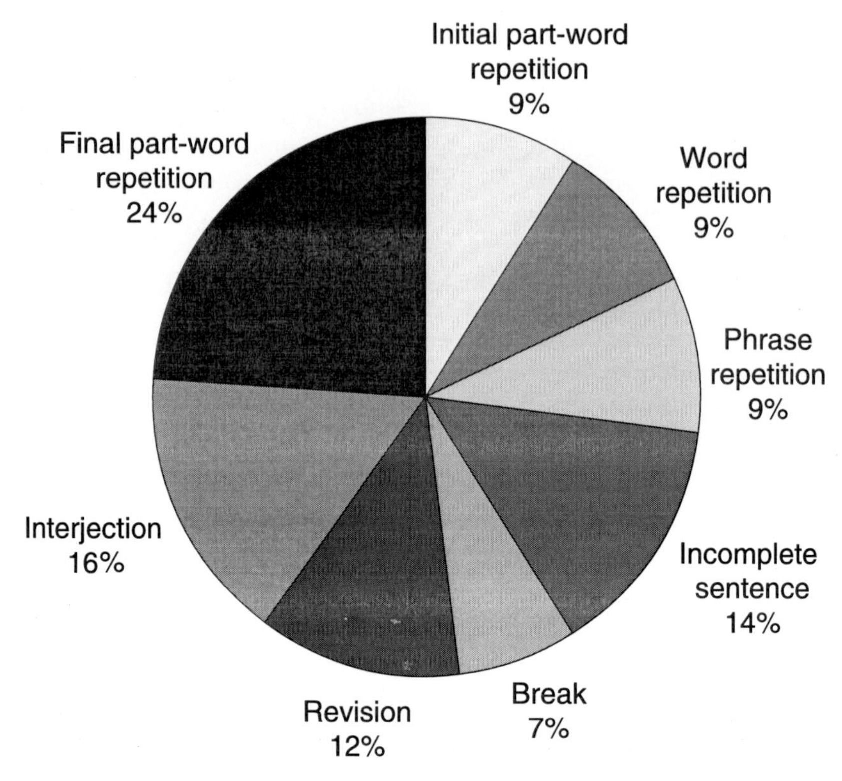

Figure 12.1 Percent of S1's disfluency in initial assessment.

children with speech-language disorders. At the beginning of the training, he was trained to focus on his articulation (over which there had been some concern, and there was subsequent improvement). Although S2 had been treated for stuttering, his stuttering was chronic and appeared untreatable because of the apparent lack of self-awareness about his speech. There was a discrepancy between S2's verbal IQ (VIQ) and performance IQ (PIQ). In addition, the results on the Japanese Picture Vocabulary Test (PVT) (Ueno, Utsno, & Inaga, 1991) and Illinois Test of Psycholinguistic Abilities (ITPA) (Ueno, Ochi, & Hattori, 1993) indicated that his verbal ability was lower than the average verbal ability of children his age. However, he was able to study with his classmates and adapted to school life. Difficulties with reading and writing were noted in class. With regard to academic skills, S2 made every effort to catch up with his classmates and his grades in mathematics were above average; his composition skills, however, were below average. S2's mother consulted some specialists on this matter, and his parents became aware that he exhibited tendencies of having a learning disability.

Classification procedure

The investigator recorded conversations with both participants on a mini-digital video tape and extracted 10-minute speech samples. Subsequently, five specialists—whose area of specialization was stuttering—freely described the children's verbal and nonverbal behaviour. The author made a note of all the verbal and nonverbal symptoms and compared them with Daly's Checklist for Possible Cluttering (1993). Appendix B lists the raters' qualifications.

Classification results

S1's speech received a total of 53 ratings classified as outside normal limits (RONL), out of which the five specialists assessed the largest number as pertaining to rapid speech rate (8 ratings). The remaining issues concerned repeated syllables, words, and phrases (6); poor articulation (6); and unintelligible speech content (6). S2's speech received a total of 59 RONL, wherein the specialists identified a self-righteous attitude in communication (6), improper wording (5), poor syntax skills (5), excessive repetitions (5), prosody and intonation problems (5), poor articulation (5), and tics (5). For both subjects, most of the descriptions corresponded to items in Daly's checklist (1993) (Table 12.1).

Table 12.1 S1 and S2's descriptions and the number of descriptions in each category

	Description and number of descriptions	
	S1	*S2*
1	Rapid speech rate (8)*	Self-righteous attitude in communication (6)*
2	Excessive repetitions (6)*	Improper wording (5)*
3	Poor articulation (6)*	Poor syntax skills (5)
4	Unintelligible speech content (6)*	Excessive repetitions (5)*
5	Self-righteous attitude in communication (5)*	Prosody and intonation problems (5)*
6	Poor syntax skills (5)*	Poor articulation (5)*
7	Lack of consideration toward others (4)*	Tics (5)
8	Slurred articulation (3)*	Prolongations, blocks, and associated symptoms (4)
9	High frequency of inappropriate reference using pronouns (2)*	Unintelligible speech content (3)*
10	High verbal output (2)*	High verbal output (3)*
11	Impatient, short-tempered (2)*	Clumsy, uncoordinated (3)*
12	Good communication skills (2)	Rapid speech rate (2)*
13	Good syntax skills (2)	Interjections, fillers, and stops (2)*
14		Left-handed (2)*
15		Limited interest (2)
16		Sunny disposition (2)

* Corresponds with Daly's Checklist for Possible Cluttering (1993).

Treatment

Each participant was treated based on individual needs and presenting symptoms. With S1, the investigator observed a prominent tic and high muscle tension in the participant's body in the initial sessions. These behaviours included mouth opening, licking lips, and moving his hands. Throughout, there was the impression of an inability to express his feelings. The participant also exhibited oversensitivity to touch, and moreover, displayed difficulties with intentional body movement; for example, he could not throw a ball. Given the presenting bodily symptoms, instead of treating his speech directly, for 1 year, the investigator engaged him in play therapy that encouraged body movement. The participant practised throwing in the play room. After his tic and muscle tension disappeared, treatment began to focus on his speech. While repeating the final parts of words, the participant would appear to prepare to initiate the following word. The author hypothesized that S1's frequent final part-word repetitions were caused by his poor ability to formulate sentences. Thus his clinical goal was to formulate sentences fluently. Subsequent therapy consisted of once weekly 40-minute sessions over an 11-month period. The first part of a session involved the classification of sentences into the subject and predicate parts (primary stage: from chronological age [CA] 8:6 to CA 9:0). Next, S1 had to continue to formulate the sentence when given the first part of the sentence (second stage: from CA 9:0 to CA 9:3) (e.g., Clinician: 'The ball is . . .'; S1: 'The ball is in my house.'). In the last period, the clinician suggested a longer subject part for a sentence, and S1 was asked to formulate the predicate part (final stage: from CA 9:3 to CA 9:4) (e.g., Clinician: 'The pool in winter is . . .'; S1: 'The pool in winter is cold; I don't want to be into the pool in winter, because my body may get cold.').

Treatment goals for S2 were: (1) fostering control in speech and (2) improving speech awareness. All 25 sessions were held within 15 months. Each session consisted of reading aloud a short paragraph for about 15 minutes and using cards to present the story of a rabbit and turtle in order to visually depict the speed of speech.

Data collection and analysis

Frequency of video tape recording was kept to minimum, in the consideration of the influence of each child's condition. Single recordings were made in each session except in the final stage, where two sessions were recorded in the beginning and last period randomly.

To measure treatment effect, the investigator analyzed percentage of disfluencies in both spontaneous and structured task situations. Following recording sessions, spontaneous speech was orthographically transcribed by the child until 200 clauses in Japanese sentences were obtained. In English-speaking countries, data collection usually involves a word count, but because it is difficult to count words in Japanese sentences, clauses were tallied.

Treatment results

Speech disfluencies

The results of the treatment tasks administered to S1 demonstrated a sharp decrease in all types of disfluencies collectively as well as in final part-word repetitions (a decrease from 20 percent to 11 percent for all types of disfluencies and from 13.5 percent to 5.5 percent for final part-word repetitions) (see Table 12.2). The results were observed under spontaneous speech situations. Figure 12.2 shows a great decrease of final part-word repetitions especially.

Relations between mean length of utterance (MLU) and speech disfluencies in task situations

Table 12.3 shows speech data under spontaneous speech and task situations in both the second and final stages. In structured task situations, MLUs were higher than in spontaneous situations (second stage: spontaneous speech situation indicated an MLU of 3.19, task situation indicated 4.09; final stage: spontaneous situation indicated an MLU of 3.21, task situation indicated 6.64). Frequency and percentage of disfluency in task situation were lower than in spontaneous speech situation in both stages (second stage: spontaneous speech situation indicated 18.4 percent disfluency, task situation 11.1 percent; final stage: spontaneous speech situation indicated 19.4 percent disfluency, task situation 12.3 percent). Correlation coefficients were determined to assess relationships between MLU and speech disfluencies in task

Table 12.2 Results of treatment tasks administered to S1: number (percentage) of disfluencies out of 200 clauses

	Primary stage	*Second stage*	*Final stage 1*	*Final stage 2*
Interjection	2 (1)	4 (2)	6 (3)	1 (0.5)
Initial part-word repetition	7 (3.5)	2 (1)	2 (1)	3 (1.5)
Word repetition	0 (0)	3 (1.5)	6 (3)	2 (1)
Revision	1 (0.5)	2 (1)	2 (1)	0 (0)
Incomplete phrase	3 (1.5)	2 (1)	5 (2.5)	1 (0.5)
Broken word	0 (0)	4 (2)	4 (2)	4 (2)
Total	13 (6.5)	17 (8.5)	25 (12.5)	11 (5.5)
Final part-word repetition	27 (13.5)	23 (11.5)	9 (4.5)	11 (5.5)
Total	40 (20)	40 (20)	34 (17)	22 (11)

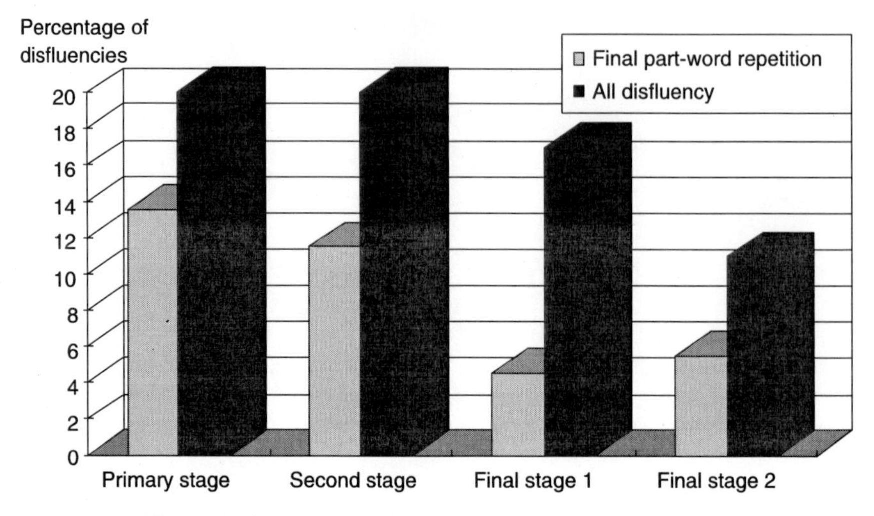

Figure 12.2 Change in frequency of disfluency.

Table 12.3 S1's linguistic vs. disfluency data in structured tasks and spontaneous speech

	Second stage		*Final stage 1*	
	Spontaneous speech situation	*Task situation*	*Spontaneous speech situation*	*Task situation*
Sentences (*N*)	62	11	56	11
Clauses (*N*)	201	45	180	73
MLU (*M*)	3.19	4.09	3.21	6.64
MLU (*SD*)	1.97	1.45	2.87	2.29
Frequency of disfluencies	37	5	35	9
% of disfluencies	18.4	11.1	19.4	12.3

N = number; *M* = mean; *SD* = standard deviation.

situations in the second and final stages. No significant correlations between MLU and speech disfluencies in task situation were observed for either stage.

Spontaneous speech situation

Correlation coefficients were determined to assess relationships between MLU and speech disfluencies in spontaneous speech situations in the second and final stages. A strong positive correlation was identified between MLU and speech disfluencies in the second stage, R=0.70, $F(1, 60) = 61, p < .001$). A strong positive correlation between MLU and speech disfluencies was also identified in final stage1, $R = 0.84$, $F(1,54) = 142, p < .01$) (see Figure 12.3).

Qualitative analysis

During S1's therapy sessions, awareness of his speech disfluency was increasing, and when he was in the latter part of the second grade (CA 9:3), he described why he went to the resource room for speech-language disordered students in his diary. He said, 'I go to resource room because I can't sometime communicate with other people well, because my words often stop. And I practice language and exercises moving my body to produce words easily.' Since increasing his awareness of his symptoms of speech, he devised methods for saying his words smoothly and efficiently. S1 was assisted by writing thoughts in his notebook before he said them. By the fourth grade, his disfluency had greatly reduced. Training was completed some 4 months later when he was 9 years, 8 months old.

Figure 12.4 presents the rate of reading aloud in all the sessions with S2. Initially, S2 was unable to discriminate among three presented reading rates. However, after the 7th session, he could read normally (3.732 syllables/second), slowly (2.093 syllables/second), and rapidly (7.226 syllables/second). Earlier, he showed difficulty in judging the author's speech rate. He did not express awareness of this difficulty until after the 14th session (Figure 12.4).

With intervention, S2 became aware of the speed of speech and after 10 sessions his disfluency in reading situations disappeared (see Figure 12.5).

Discussion

The characteristics of the two students who were hypothesized to exhibit possible cluttering were determined, through matching the specialists' descriptions of their speech, similar to many of the items on Daly's (1993) checklist. Such matches between descriptions and the checklist confirm that cluttering does occur in Japan, as it does in many other countries of the world. Henceforth, a definition for the diagnostic classification of cluttering is likely to help children who have not improved solely through stuttering therapy and are in need of specialized interventions to address their cluttering. The limitations to the specificity of such checklists in diagnosing cluttering should be kept in mind (see also Georgieva & Miliev, 1996; Scaler Scott, Grossman, & Tetnowski, 2010; Van Borsel & Vandermeulen, 2008; and Van Zaalen, Wijnen, & Dejonckere, chapter 9 this volume).

Treatment for cluttering was effective for both participants in decreasing patterns of disfluency. Part of the effectiveness seemed to lie in helping such children to become aware of their speech (also see Bennett Lanouette, chapter 11 this volume; Myers, chapter 10 this volume; Ward, 2006). While it was difficult for participants to control their speech quality in each and every situation, it is reasonable to assume that it is helpful for children who clutter to speak clearly, even if it is in just a few situations.

It is questioned whether S1 is considered to have other types of disorders as

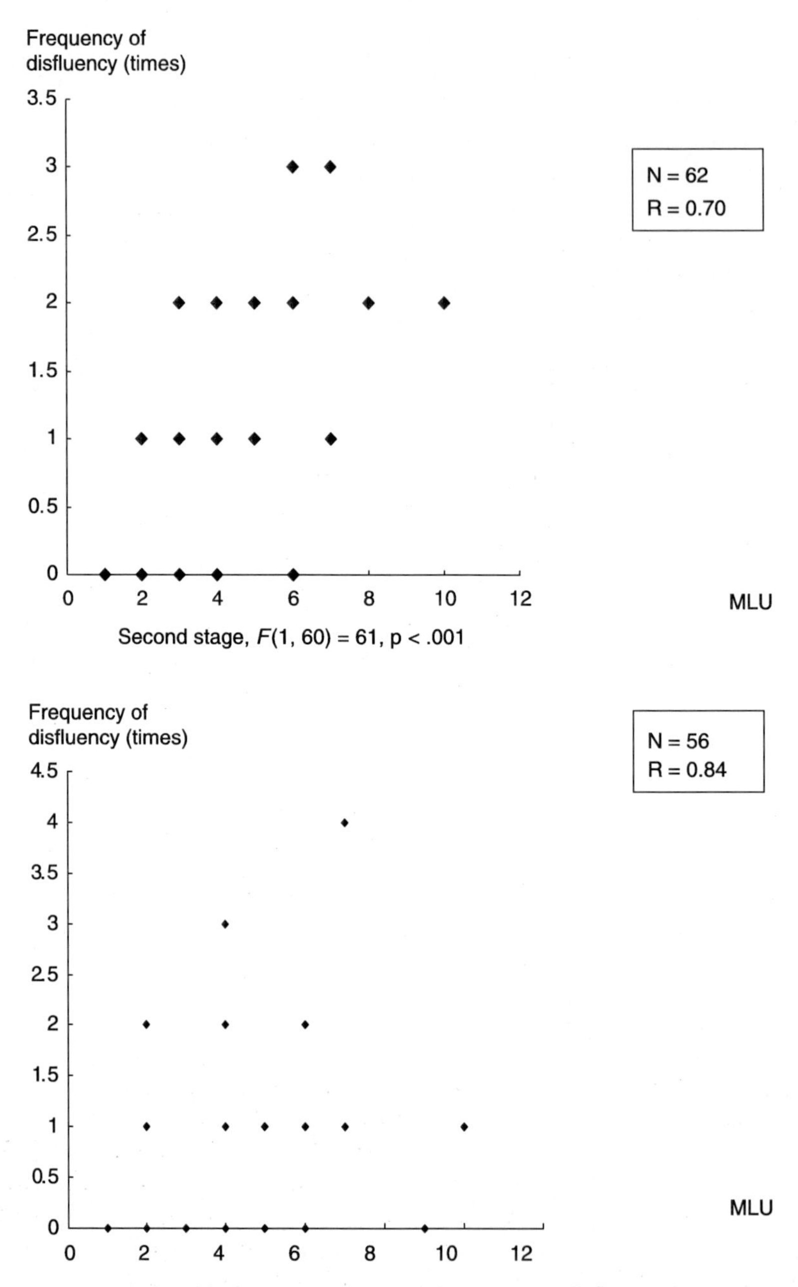

Figure 12.3 Relationship between MLU and frequency of disfluency in spontaneous speech situation for S1.

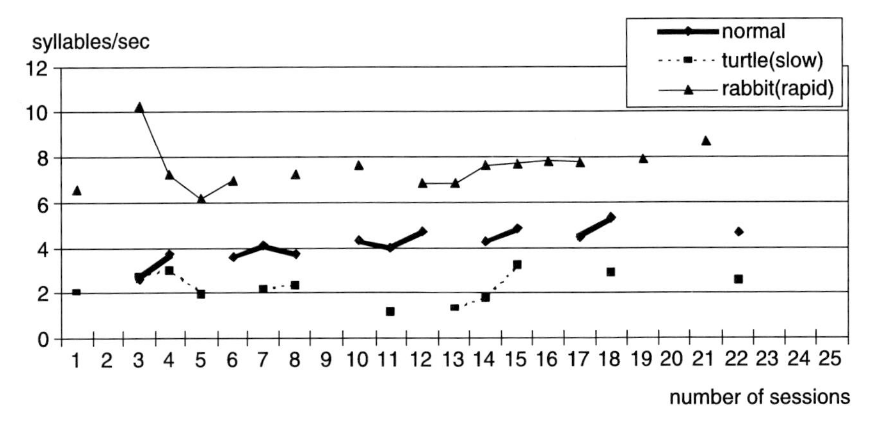

Figure 12.4 Discrimination between various speeds in reading aloud.

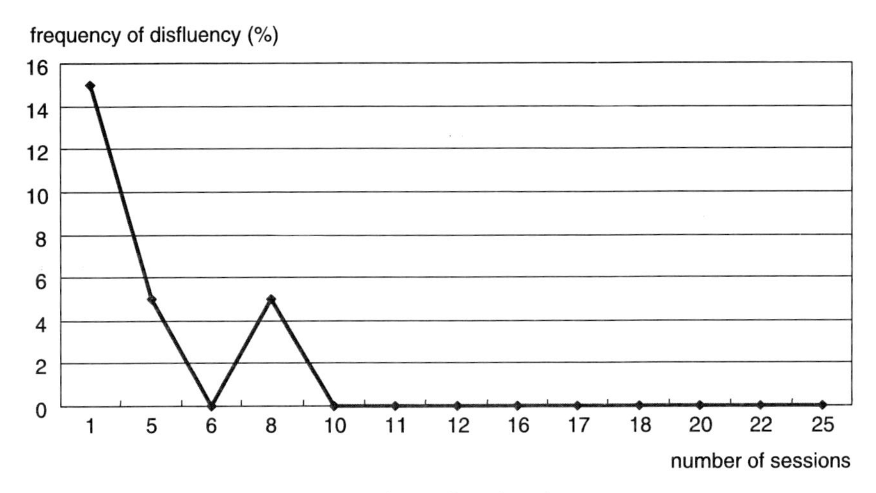

Figure 12.5 Frequency of disfluency in reading situations.

well as cluttering. He exhibited clumsiness in motor skills, poor interpersonal communication skills, and oversensitivity of touch. Though those kinds of features are discovered in children with learning disabilities, ADHD, or Pervasive Developmental Disorder Not Otherwise Specified (American Psychiatric Association, 2000), he had not been diagnosed with such developmental disorders. In treatment, it was also found that he could not perform sequentially. Speech disruptions were seen in writing; otherwise, the participant's ability of writing was kept at a normal level. It is important for improvement of speech disfluency to be assessed and diagnosed appropriately, considering all possible symptoms and diagnoses. In addition, these differences between the two participants call for differences in treatment techniques.

Summary

We have seldom seen reports on cluttering in Japanese articles, and rarely take notice of cluttering. But Japan has recently witnessed an increased interest in interventions for people who have speech disorders with coexisting developmental disorders such as learning disabilities and ADHD, and there are frequent reports that some children exhibit rapid speech and repetition. We hypothesized that using foreign definitions cluttering could be applied to such Japanese children. This hypothesis was supported by both Japanese specialist descriptions of the participants' speech matching definitions of cluttering, and by positive treatment outcomes when individual cluttering symptoms were targeted. Results call for re-examination of the current lack of emphasis on diagnosis and treatment of cluttered speech in Japan.

References

American Psychiatric Association. (2000). *Diagnostic and statistical manual of mental disorders* (4th ed., text revision). Washington, DC: American Psychiatric Association.

Daly, D. A. (1993). Cluttering: Another fluency syndrome. In R. F. Curlee (Ed.), *Stuttering and related disorders of fluency* (pp. 179–204). New York: Thieme.

Georgieva, D., & Miliev, D. (1996). Differential diagnosis of cluttering and stuttering in Bulgaria. *Journal of Fluency Disorders*, *21*, 249–260.

Miyamoto, S., Hayasaka, K., & Shapiro, D. A. (2006). An examination of the checklist for possible cluttering in Japan. In J. Au-Yeung & M. M. Leahy (Eds.), *Research, treatment, and self-help in fluency disorders: New horizons. Proceedings of the Fifth World Congress on Fluency Disorders*. Dublin, Ireland: International Fluency Association.

Scaler Scott, K., Grossman, H. L., & Tetnowski, J. A. (2010). Diagnosis of a single case of cluttering according to four different criteria. In K. Bakker, L. J. Raphael, & F. L. Myers (Eds.), *Proceedings of the First World Conference on Cluttering* (pp. 80–90). Katarino, Bulgaria. http://associations.missouristate.edu/ICA/

St. Louis, K. O., & Myers, F. L. (1997). Management of cluttering and related fluency disorders. In R. F. Curlee & G. M Siegel (Eds.), *Nature and treatment of stuttering: New directions* (pp. 313–332). Needham Heights, MA: Allyn & Bacon.

Ueno, K., Ochi, K., & Hattori, M. (1993). *Illinois test of psycholinguistic abilities, revised edition*. Tokyo: Nihon-bunka-kagakusha.

Ueno, K., Utsno, T., & Inaga, K. (1991). *Picture vocabulary test, revised edition*. Tokyo: Nihon-bunka-kagakusha.

Ward, D. (2006). *Stuttering and cluttering: Frameworks for understanding and treatment*. Hove, UK: Psychology Press.

Van Borsel, J., & Vandermeulen, A. (2008). Cluttering in Down syndrome. *Folia Phoniatrica et Logopaedica*, *60*, 312–317.

Appendix A

Japanese checklist for possible cluttering (Miyamoto et al., 2006; adapted from Daly, 1993) with scoring for participant S1

1	Started talking late	2
2	Fluency disruptions started early	2
3	Silent gaps or hesitations common; interjections; many 'filler' words	2
4	Stops before saying initial words to recall	2
5	Rapid rate (speaks too fast); speaks in spurts	0
6	Extrovert; high verbal output; compulsive talker	0
7	Jerky breathing pattern, respiratory dysrhythmia	2
8	Slurred articulation (omits or substitutes sounds)	0
9	Speech better under pressure	2
10	Difficulty following directions; impatient/uninterested listener	0
11	Distractible; attention span problems; poor concentration	0
12	Story-telling difficulty (trouble sequencing events)	2
13	Inappropriate reference by pronouns is common	2
14	Improper language structure; poor grammar and syntax	2
15	Clumsy and uncoordinated	2
16	Disintegrated and fractionated writing; poor motor control	2
17	Writing shows transposition of letters and words (omits letters)	0
18	Left–right confusion; delayed hand preference	0
19	Seems to think faster than he can talk or write	0
20	Improper stress patterns of speech; poor melodic accenting of sounds	0
21	Appear younger than age; small and/or immature	1
22	Other family member with same/similar problem; heredity	0
23	Impatient, impulsive, and/or short-tempered (ADHD) or untidy, careless (ADD)	0
24	Lack of self-awareness; unconcerned attitude over inappropriateness of many behaviors and responses	0
	Total score	23

Not at all: 0; Just a little: 1; Pretty much: 2.

Appendix B

Specialists who described the children's verbal and nonverbal behaviour

Subject	*Specialist*	*Occupation*	*Career*
	A	Speech-language-hearing therapist at a hospital	More than 15 years
S1	B	Speech-language-hearing therapist at a hospital	More than 10 years
	C	Speech-language-hearing therapist at a hospital	More than 5 years
	D	Researcher on speech-language-hearing pathology at a national research institute	More than 5 years
	E	Assistant manager at a Japanese self-help group for people who stutter and student at a vocational school for speech-language-hearing therapists	More than 5 years
	F	Teacher of special classes for children with speech-language disorders at public elementary schools	More than 30 years
S2	G	Teacher of special classes for children with speech-language disorders at public elementary schools	More than 20 years
	H	Instructor who trains speech-language-hearing therapists at colleges	More than 25 years
	I	Instructor who trains speech-language-hearing therapists at colleges	More than 10 years
	J	Assistant professor of special education at a university	More than 10 years

13 Self-help and support groups for people with cluttering

Kathleen Scaler Scott and Kenneth O. St. Louis

The movement toward self-help and support groups

Introduction

Self-help and support groups vary in how much they are oriented toward behavior change, support, education, and/or advocacy. In the purest use of these terms, self-help groups are focused on personal change effected through a specific program, but not facilitated by professionals, whereas support groups tend to focus only on emotional support, advocacy, and education, and may be facilitated by professionals. Despite these differences, the goals of self-help and support groups tend to vary along continua of degrees of personal change orientation and professional involvement (Farris Kurtz, 1997). Modern self-help groups had their origins with Alcoholics Anonymous (AA) in 1935. The original impetus for AA groups was to help with a problem that the medical profession alone could not solve. Since the first AA self-help groups, the number and type of self-help and support groups has grown dramatically both within the United States and internationally (Farris Kurtz, 1997). Currently such groups are available for a large number of communication disorders providing adjunct and/or alternative help beyond traditional speech-language therapy and offering perspectives that are often not experienced in individual therapy. For example, although a speech-language pathologist (SLP) who does not clutter very likely can have some understanding of the struggles associated with cluttering, the SLP may lack authentic appreciation or empathy toward the subjective feelings and experiences of someone who clutters in daily life. Of course, this is also true of any communication disorder.

Although their structures vary widely, self-help and support groups that offer opportunities for members to meet face-to-face are typically organized into local or regional groups. Local/regional groups are typically part of larger national or international organizations. Often local support group members meet together on biweekly or monthly basis. Also, clusters of local groups or chapters may intermittently collaborate to sponsor larger, regional workshops on specific topics of interest. National and international meetings or conventions allow for the largest scale face-to-face meetings, and may occur annually or after a specified number of years. All of these possibilities provide opportunities for meeting and talking with others who share the same disorder or problem and, thereby, many common concerns.

With advances in technology and larger use of the World Wide Web, several support options have become available that, while not always allowing for face-to-face interaction, afford users the ability to experience support (often) in the comfort of their home and on their own schedule. Through online support, adults and children can connect and communicate in a variety of formats with others who share the same struggles and triumphs. In communication disorders, listservs now exist wherein discussions can occur between all members of the list via email messaging. Other online communication formats include chat rooms for real-time discussions of topics, and email penpals. Additionally, the offerings of the internet such as blogs, podcasts, and social networking sites allow for formal and informal discussions of experiences. The increased accessibility to webcams with free instant messaging services allow for simulated face-to-face interactions. The internet has also brought a convenient format for people to interact worldwide via formal online forums in communication disorders, such as the annual International Stuttering Awareness Day (ISAD) online conference, which occurs each October (Kuster, 2002). Through this three-week event, which culminates with celebration of International Stuttering Awareness Day, researchers, clinicians, and consumers from around the world can interact to share research, information, and experiences via formal paper presentations, threaded discussions of papers, and informal questions and discussions. With advances in technology, it is highly likely that new formats for interaction via the internet will continue to emerge.

Goals and activities of support and self-help groups

The purposes and activities of support and self-help groups are varied. While the primary purposes are behavior change, education, advocacy, and/or mutual support, an integral prerequisite for the groups is sufficient membership. Although strong support is possible among a small number of individuals (e.g., less than 5 participants), larger (e.g., between 8 and 20) and more diverse memberships allow for more wide-ranging viewpoints that may resonate with a greater number of individuals. In addition, practical concerns such as sharing of leadership roles and responsibilities involved with group membership can be more efficiently addressed with larger numbers of participants. Therefore, a secondary mission of support and self-help groups is outreach to potential new members. Larger numbers also increase the opportunities for advocacy on behalf of individuals with a specific communication disorder. Advocacy initiatives may take the form of training professionals such as SLPs; providing information to physicians, classroom teachers, and administrators; and encouraging lobbyists or politicians to support changes that would benefit people with the disorder in question. The greater the number of members available for such advocacy movements, the greater the possibilities for increased networking within public and government sectors, increased awareness, and advances in legislative action.

Cluttering self-help and support

Introduction

Recent interest in self-help and support for the fluency disorder of cluttering has emerged in the form of web-based forums. On the previously mentioned ISAD conferences, in most of its first 12 years, the number of articles devoted to cluttering was typically one or two each year after which time the first online conference solely devoted to the topic of cluttering was launched. Additionally, the International Cluttering Association (ICA) launched a website in 2007 devoted completely to the topic of cluttering. The ICA website provides information and resources for academicians, students, clinicians, and consumers (i.e., those who clutter). Although the website includes a multitude of information, it does not have the capability for communication through group messages. However, it does link consumers and families to an online support/self-help group for cluttering (see below).

Awareness of cluttering is limited among the general public (St. Louis, 1999; St. Louis et al., 2010). Also, in the vast majority of cases, persons with cluttering and/or parents of children with cluttering have received no formal training in speech-language pathology. Additionally, many trained speech-language pathologists regard their training in evaluating and treating cluttering to be weak and inadequate (St. Louis & Hinzman, 1986; St. Louis & Rustin, 1992). Therefore, because of general unawareness of cluttering and limited training available regarding its treatment, out of necessity, a few people who clutter have become experts in managing their own communication problems. One such person, Joseph Dewey, founded a Yahoo online support group in the late 1990s. Dewey (2007, Self-help section, para. 2) described the group as follows:

> Hi, I'm Joseph, and I started the cluttering group a few years ago as a friendly way for everyone to share information about cluttering. Three types of people are generally part of the group, 1) Parents of clutterers, 2) SLPs, and SLPs in training, and 3) clutterers. The discussions range from technical, to support, to therapies, to requests for information about cluttering. It's a very friendly, respectful group, and we entertain questions that range from: 'I'm writing a paper on cluttering. Is there someone with cluttering that would be okay with talking to me on the

> phone?' to 'Help! My son was just diagnosed with cluttering and I can't afford speech therapy. What can I do?' to 'I'm a clutterer, and I have a presentation next week at work. Any advice so I don't mess it up?' I invite everyone to be part of the group, and to contribute by asking questions or answering them.[1]

From Dewey's description, it is evident that the group is neither exclusively a self-help nor exclusively a support group, but some combination of the two. The group is free and open to anyone who is interested in cluttering. Consumers, clinicians, and researchers can benefit mutually from being involved with the same group. Consumers and the other members of the public can ask questions about the existing research regarding cluttering as well as hear professional opinions based on years of clinical experience and observation of people with cluttering. Likewise, clinicians and researchers gain valuable insight into consumer perspectives, insights that can spark ideas for new research projects and lead to more comprehensive treatment plans. Although understanding and appreciating consumer perspectives is virtually always beneficial to clinicians regardless of the communication disorder, in the case of cluttering specifically, its importance cannot be overstated. Many consumers report symptoms, such as 'racing thoughts', that either may not be readily apparent or are difficult to measure. Gaining insight into such symptoms and experiences of those with cluttering can assist researchers and clinicians with understanding and determining where these characteristics fit into the puzzle of cluttering (i.e., as part of the disorder itself or as commonly co-occurring symptoms).

For the consumer, the benefits derived from cluttering support groups are similar to those described by people who stutter involved with stuttering support. Among these benefits are meeting others who understand what they are going through and gaining new information about the disorder (Reeves, 2006; Yaruss et al., 2002). Consumers also report benefit from having a safe place to practice speech techniques, as illustrated in the following comments from adults with cluttering and parents of children with cluttering:

> In the beginning I was happy to finally have found someone like me. It was my first time having a place besides my speech therapist where people actually understood what it was like to 'be me'.
>
> (HBK, adult)

> With cluttering, it is overwhelming for us to really pin down how we as parents can help. As a result, I have reached out to others by joining the cluttering user group, contacting experts in the field and openly but selectively talking to others about Raymond and cluttering in hope that I will run across someone who has some information, experiences or contacts that can help.
>
> (DB, parent of school-age child)

> Being involved with other people certainly helps to build your confidence, you can talk to people who understand what you are going through, the group can devise therapy, we have regular visits from the local SLT [speech-language therapist].
>
> (PK, adult)

Just as contributors with the same communication disorders may have different experiences and perspectives, contributors vary in the reasons they participate in support groups. Some, like the author of the following example, benefit from helping others. The benefit described below is also reported for stuttering support groups (e.g., Yaruss et al., 2002):

> . . . now I try to function more as some kind of mentor, trying to tell parents of children with cluttering that having it does not have to be the end of the world. I also use it to publish new reflections, often after having tested them on people privately.
>
> (HBK, adult)

Partnering with other groups vs. independence

Although the cluttering self-help/support movement has been aided by partnerships with stuttering self-help and support initiatives, it continues to move toward independence from stuttering. Several reasons for this are based in cluttering's history of self-help/support, treatment, and research. Cluttering has been termed the 'orphan' of speech-language pathology (Daly, 1986, 1993; Weiss, 1964), often overshadowed by greater awareness and knowledge in the area of stuttering. This has resulted in misdiagnosis of cluttering, either as stuttering, or as no disorder at all. Such misdiagnoses are likely not intentional, but, instead, reflect a lack of sufficient knowledge of cluttering among clinicians. Once they have received training in cluttering, it is not uncommon for clinicians to reflect on their own prior misdiagnoses of cluttering. The experiences described by an adult and two parents of children with cluttering are examples of this unfortunate common experience for consumers:

> After some years, I again had problems in employment, no one would give me the chance of promotion, I was told that my speech was not conducive to liaising with customers but was a valued employee, if my speech improved maybe I could be considered for future positions. I again went to my GP and requested help for my speech and was referred to another SLT, this 'girl' still wet from university made the suggestion that there was nothing wrong with my speech at all, I walked out and felt alone again, but worse than before as I had been told I don't have a problem.
>
> (PK, adult)

> It was extremely difficult finding any SLP that was even aware of cluttering let alone knew how to treat it.
>
> (DB, mother of a school-age child)

> We have been trying to identify Jon's speech issues since the age of 3. Self help for a parent trying to find answers, services and resolutions have been a long and frustrating process. We have gone thru dozens of doctors and every possible type of testing from hearing, ADD, XY Chromosome, etc. He even had electrodes attached to his head for a day of monitoring brain waves. It wasn't until he was 12 yrs old and in 5th grade when his school speech therapist pondered the idea of cluttering. This was after 3 years of working with him. We spent 10 years of worries due to the lack of info on cluttering in the medical world. Knowing is half the battle. I believe if we had known sooner, my son would be much better off today.
>
> (JW, father of a teen)

A second possible reason that cluttering support seeks independence from stuttering relates to less than positive experiences of people with cluttering in self-help activities. Despite commonalities of experience between stuttering and cluttering, because the characteristics of cluttering differ from those of stuttering, it follows that some experiences may differ quite dramatically. If a support group is dominated by people with stuttering, there is the potential that such differences in perspective may not always be represented. One consumer reported such a difficulty:

> Yesterday there were eight people with stuttering and me with cluttering. Not one word about cluttering was said and when I tried to say something one of the persons in the group seemed to find it annoying saying 'this is not how we feel'.
>
> (HBK, adult)

To be sure, having support organizations solely devoted to the topic of cluttering might provide stronger support in many ways than would linking cluttering with stuttering. It is common, however, for stuttering and cluttering to co-occur, and in these cases, involvement in a group representing both disorders may be more beneficial to the consumer. Additionally, because many with cluttering are unaware of their communication difficulty and/or its specific name, small numbers of those with cluttering seeking support may necessitate linking with stuttering support groups to share resources and financial burdens:

> I met up with some other people in our area who stammered and we formed our own self help group . . . we practiced video speech recording, speaking circles, simple speeches, discussing our own speech problems

> and slowly we all seemed to gain confidence and the group grew from four people to over twenty, we were very pro active, I took on the secretaries position from inception, I used to bring the equipment each meeting, I initiated the newsletter and after a short while I took on the web site building and maintenance.
>
> (PK, adult)

If respect for differing perspectives among individuals is emphasized, regardless of participants' specific fluency disorder(s), people with cluttering and stuttering can work together in self-help and support activities. Whether or not groups maintain independence for cluttering or combine resources involves serious consideration of group members' goals, needs, and interests.

Personal stories of cluttering emerging through self-help

As noted earlier, the dearth of knowledge about cluttering as well as trained SLTs has motivated many with cluttering to devise their own therapy techniques, based on their readings about the disorder as well as trial and error strategies. We again emphasize the importance of understanding the experience of the *person* with the communication disorder. Moreover, we emphasize that dealing with cluttering and its various problems is an *individual* experience. The following quotes are from individuals with cluttering who have been kind enough to share their stories to illustrate these experiences. We first share these individuals' symptoms to set the background for our discussion of the impact of the disorder on their lives, and their insights about the most and least helpful strategies to overcome and/or manage symptoms.

Cluttering characteristics

While some people with cluttering report only speech-related symptoms, such as rapid speech or too many disfluencies, others report symptoms that are outside the current working definition of cluttering, such as difficulties with writing or auditory memory. Currently, insufficient evidence exists to be certain whether or not many of the non-speech-related symptoms would be considered cluttering according to the working definition advanced by St. Louis and his associates (St. Louis, Myers, Bakker, & Raphael, 2007)—and refined by St. Louis and Schulte (chapter 14 this volume)—or simply *associated* with cluttering.

Below we present symptoms consumers reported that fall both within and outside the realm of this definition. The symptoms are presented for informational rather than diagnostic purposes.

Characteristics included within the working definition

RATE AND SYLLABLE CHANGES

> My cluttering characteristics (I do not like referring to it as symptoms, as cluttering to me is not a disease) are mostly speech related. If I do not pay attention I tend to eat my letters and speak very fast . . .
>
> (HBK, adult)

> Jon's articulatory precision worsens with increases in length or coordinative complexity of a verbal task. Although many single and two syllable words are intelligibly produced, some are inconsistently modified by distortions, resequencing, or replacements of phonemes. As number of syllables increase in words or number of words increase in an utterance, syllable additions (telescoping) and deletions (condensing) also become apparent. Jon generally speaks with an overall low volume and limited oral motor movements. This gives an impression of his 'slurring' of his speech. His rate is generally within normal limits in short responses to questions, but becomes irregular in spontaneous lengthier utterances (as in monologue or explanation/description verbal activities).
>
> (SLP, evaluating Jon, a teenager)

> Raymond has an uneven rate of speech . . . He collapses multi-syllable words into slightly more than one syllable words. He drops off weak syllables such as 'nother' for 'another', 'usie' for 'usually', 'member' for 'remember' . . .
>
> (DB, mother of a school-age child)

> Excessively fast rate of speech, especially when excited, caught off-guard, or unsure of how to explain something . . . Condensing of syllables, e.g., 'therapy' might become 'terpy'.
>
> (AER, adult)

> . . . and could see that I was having trouble getting words out, my face would falter whilst trying to speak, I found that I could not say words with too many syllables in it very well, I learned that I could not speak long sentences very well, I could not read out from a book without extreme difficulties.
>
> (PK, adult)

DISFLUENCY

> I do not have any problems with the following, stuttering, reading, writing, so for me this is not something I worry about.
>
> (HBK, adult)

> Irregular repetitions of syllables, partial words, and phrases. Repetitions are not consistent with particular sounds/words or circumstances, as you

might expect from someone who stutters . . . If I'm caught in the moment of a major disfluency, I have a hard time getting it out right despite multiple attempts/strategies. It makes me wonder if that's what it feels like to someone who stutters. It's quite frustrating!

(AER, adult)

PROSODY

Additionally, he demonstrates minimal inflection and intonation patterns, further reducing his intelligibility.

(From SLP evaluation report on Jon, teen)

Other speech and language patterns not reflected in the working definition

WORD FINDING AND THOUGHT ORGANIZATION

In lay terms, Raymond has a tough time communicating his thoughts. He has a lot to say since he loves to talk. Unfortunately, he has trouble coming up with words, so it takes him a considerable amount of time to get out what he is trying to say . . . Can't always come up with the words that he needs, which makes speech more disfluent and he gets way off from the point that he is trying to make.

(DB, mother of a school-age child)

[I have] disorganized thoughts. [My cluttering] improves with familiarity (hence I can hide it well professionally!) [I am/tend to be??] rambling [and] talkative. [I have] difficulty maintaining a topic; . . . [I find myself] jumping back and forth between topics over the course of the conversation. Close friends can follow my thinking on this, but people who don't know me well are left confounded at the whole bit. [I have] difficulty 'getting to the point'.

(AER, adult)

My thought process is fast, I have trouble expressing myself, I say the wrong words at the wrong time, some people misconstrue what I say, but no one believes that it is my condition causing this problem . . . I act fast, I think fast, I (used to) work fast, my brain never stops, I always have thoughts in my mind.

(PK, adult)

ARTICULATION DEVELOPMENT

Developmentally later occurring phonemes are more distorted than earlier ones.

(From SLP evaluation report of a teenager)

SYNTAX

> In addition, sometimes what he would say would be garbled, i.e. Did I told you? Where buy that Mickey Mouse thing? Why her make, why her make um why her make her daughter let her go to her house? Do you know why?
>
> (DB, mother of school-age child)

PRAGMATIC LANGUAGE/AWARENESS

> Poor awareness of dysfluency and rate of speech (lifelong), but this is better now. It's still not great, though . . . Often impulsive with conversational turns . . . Difficulty interpreting cues that others are having a hard time following—what I often interpret as active listening is often the other person is overwhelmed at the rate or dysfluency.
>
> (AER, adult)

AUDITORY ATTENTION

> [I have an] inability to listen to one conversation in the background and holding another. I also can't have talk radio on in the car and talk to someone at the same time—my mind can't deal with the double language input.
>
> (AER, adult)

AUDITORY MEMORY

> Poor recall of verbal details despite excellent memory for things seen/done . . . Difficulty remembering names.
>
> (AER, adult)
>
> My memory is useless when it comes to what I have said to whom and who I have done what with. The first part does bother me a bit, as I tend to say exactly the same stories with exactly the same expressions and almost pauses. The only way I realize that I might have said this a lot of times before is when the people I am talking to get a extremely bored expression—they are usually too polite to tell me.
>
> (HBK, adult)

WRITING

> My writing is affected, I find it almost impossible to write neatly, and I find it almost impossible to read my own writing. I have difficulty typing, not for spelling as my spelling capabilities are not that bad, just pressing the correct keys in the right order as I get confused with which letter I

have pressed and which I need to press next, this is because I type fast, if I type slowly then I can get almost perfect composition.

(PK, adult)

Early impact of cluttering: response of others

While some Yahoo group contributors experienced deleterious effects on their achievements in life due to negative reactions from other people, others—while facing many challenges—reported more positive reactions of others to their disorder:

> Going back to the cluttering speech side, I know I have had problems since school days, peers used to make fun of me, teachers used to ridicule me, no one seemed to take me on face value, I was overlooked and not given the encouragement that other pupils had the advantage of. My own Father used to say I was good for nothing although I tried my hardest to please people and to get on with my life, it was not me holding myself back, it was others who would not allow me to get ahead or understand me or the problem that I had.
>
> (PK, adult)

> My family always joked about my 'motor mouth', being the family chatterbox, and I frequently heard things like 'my ears are tired from listening that fast'. It never occurred to any of us that things weren't right with my speech; my mom chalked it up to my being an outgoing, bubbly personality.
>
> (AER, adult)

> When I was little cluttering did cause a lot of discussions between my mother and me. I would get really angry when she did not understand what I was saying, as I thought I was talking well. I also suffered from extreme shyness and when I began understanding that I did in fact talk in a way that was difficult to understand, I would use this as an excuse in order to not deal with scary situations . . . One of my most painful childhood memories is also cluttering related. I was going to read a poem standing in front of the class and my teacher made me say 'one' between each word in order to slow down. I still remember how the pages looked . . . and what classroom I was standing in. Not exactly a proud moment . . . When I had my speech therapy evaluation my teacher had tried to send me to speech therapy for many years but I had denied, thinking I did not have a problem. When I finally gave in my father expressed concern talking to the speech therapist testing me. He wondered how his little daughter would be able to get an education and a job when no one understood what she was saying. Is it not funny how you remember those things so many years later?
>
> (HBK, adult)

> Jon's cluttering has affected him dramatically. It has hindered his social life considerably. As parents we are constantly worried about repercussions of this issue. He is kind of a loner at school and tends not to interact. Other children have made fun of his speech, but he takes it in stride the best he can. He does not participate in team sports, most likely due to the communication issues. He was seen by a neuropsychologist and she gave him a borderline Asperger's diagnosis. This was based mostly on the fact of his social skills, although the academic testing she performed was pretty much at average levels.
>
> (JW, father of teen)

> I feel with Raymond having cluttering and dyslexia, that his self-esteem becomes an issue. He is an amazing, brilliant boy and I don't want him to feel any different about himself. I have become angry and hurt when I see acquaintances avoid calling on Raymond when he has something to say. It may take him a long time to get his comments across but that doesn't mean that his opinions or thoughts are less valuable than those around him nor does his cluttering reflect on his level of intelligence or capabilities . . . When we moved the boys to a smaller school this year, and after I dropped the boys off at school, I would drive around the block that surrounds the playground so that I would grab a glimpse of Raymond in hopes that he was talking with someone. It would break my heart. Raymond would stand alone in the middle of the playground as children were running past him and as he watched other boys play basketball. I couldn't sleep at night.
>
> (DB, mother of school-age child)

Later impact of cluttering

Some with cluttering report that the misunderstanding of their communication disorder often had serious life consequences in terms of career advancement and feelings about communication in general:

> My problem has affected my life in many ways, socially, in education and employment, and even in old age I have many problems, mainly talking to people I do not know, talking to people for the first time, talking on the telephone, trying to order products on the telephone etc. . . . I was often in a position whilst speaking to someone that they would suddenly lose interest and leave, sometimes without a word, others used to question what I was talking about, some people used to say 'you are talking a load of rubbish', I am being evasive, and I used to get very upset and frustrated with these comments . . . I get so frustrated with my condition that sometimes I am afraid to approach people, I shy away from events where I do not know anyone, my social life has faltered, I am afraid to go anywhere now.
>
> (PK, adult)

Others reported that cluttering had little impact on their education, but had significant impacts on their careers, especially those involving communication:

> Before I was diagnosed by my fluency professor, I would say it didn't impact my life. I literally wasn't aware of how often people asked me to repeat myself, nor did I understand why I had to explain myself many times for someone to 'get it'. I always assumed it was because they just didn't understand the subject matter, were tired, or some other innocuous reason. I never thought that it had anything to do with how I was presenting the information, because *I* understood it and it was clear to me, so obviously it HAD to be clear to the other person, right? . . . This really hit home during my first off-campus clinical rotation. I was interning at an acute care hospital, where most of our clinical population was stroke patients. I adapted quickly to the pace of the environment with the short patient stays, jumping quickly from one patient to the next, adjusting my plans of care given the rapid progression of medical status with the patients, etc. My speech rate came up with my supervisor, Julie, early in the semester. She told me she knew that I understood the information well, as it came through in my written reports clear as a bell. However, she was able to see that the (cognitively/linguistically) impaired patients couldn't follow my rate OR my content because it was so verbally disorganized. Trying to slow down when speaking with patients felt excruciating to me, and Julie and I had to come up with a system for her to let me know if I was speaking slowly enough so I could adjust as needed. I had NO concept when I'd start speaking faster, or I would think that I was speaking slowly enough and it still wasn't slow enough. There were days that I'd try so hard, and just couldn't quite get everything to come together. I'm not one to get discouraged easily, but there were days that I felt gloom and doom about ever being able to be successful as an SLP.
>
> (AER, adult)

> In most of my education my speech has really not been too much of an issue. When I was studying to become an occupational therapist it was a different story. I had a very hard time being understood in my first practice being in a new town. I still remember my mentor from back then talking to my teacher in Trondheim telling me that I was impossible to understand. The way she said it, she came from my hometown and not even she could understand me, neither did the patients or her coworkers. That practice put me into a very unpleasant place regarding cluttering. For a very long time I felt like I was nothing except a person with cluttering. I still remember feeling like Donald Duck, having a gigantic beak trying to make sense when talking, and then the rest of me being nothing more than a tiny green pea . . . For some reason [now] my speech has

> never seemed to be a problem at work. To be honest I am not sure why. I am controlling it well or people do not seem bothered by it, it seems like it is just a part of me. Maybe part of the reason is that I always work at institutions, so I am usually surrounded by the same people every day. I have noticed that my new coworker asks me to repeat quite often, but I seldom repeat things in phone calls. Maybe I simply do not notice. I do not know, but it works ok that I guess that is all that matters. I do however know that at work I usually try to slow down, while I do not at all care when I am with friends and family.
>
> (HBK, adult)

Therapy techniques and cluttering

What follows are comments regarding what people with cluttering have and have not found helpful in improving their communication skills. The reader should bear in mind that the varied nature of the responses below reflects the fact that different strategies work for different individuals. Additionally, it is important to note that research is still sorely needed to validate the effectiveness or ineffectiveness of various speaking techniques. As noted, the information is provided to foster insights into consumer perspectives rather than to generate treatment plans.

Strategies that 'worked'

> The use of phrasing and Delayed Auditory Feedback using the Speech-Easy device in the sessions has worked for Jon to attend to his speech and self correct. The use of a metronome along with reading aloud has been effective. Non verbal cues agreed upon by Jon and the therapists have improved his ability to self monitor his speech rate with greater accuracy; I will sometimes touch my chin when he is using a good rate and this positive cue helps him to stay at a good speech rate. The use of over articulation and producing effort for the ending sounds in words has also been effective in slowing his rate without telling him to slow down all the time. This technique has been more effective than a negative comment.
>
> (SLP treating teen)

> I practiced recording my voice, I also came upon the idea that if I recorded my voice on camera I could watch the articulation whilst I was speaking. I learned a lot by carrying out this experiment.
>
> (PK, adult)

> I find that modifying my dialect is an efficient way to controlling my speech. My hometown's dialect was once described as the dialect with half words, so adding cluttering to the mix does not make it any easier to understand. I am often asked where I am from even though I have been

living in the same town for close to thirty years. I have noticed that I tend to modify it mostly when I talk about cluttering or when I deliberately make an effort to slow down.

(HBK, adult)

Listening to my own voice also works. When I remember to do so, I will often do something that seems like stuttering when I am trying to slow down and remember to say all the words. Then it gets easier and I am able to speak better.

(HBK, adult)

As with many other clutterers, I am capable of 'slowing down' for periods of time when the need is present. When I consciously think about my speech, then several strategies work well and consistently—over-articulation with a particular focus on consonant production, thinking about MOVING slowly, organizing what I want to say in my head before starting to talk, and watching my listener for visual/audio feedback (e.g., quizzical look vs. requests to repeat). However, if I fail to consciously self-monitor, then my speech goes downhill. I don't automatically register the confusion on the part of my listener, and the dysfluencies have to be really, really bad for it to spark those, 'Oh, right, I need to think about my speech' thoughts. Times like those I feel like my mouth is running on a motor in the other direction and I have no control whatsoever—because I don't.

(AER, adult)

Writing everything down when I have to make phone calls works well. Then I can read the text and I have a draft to overarticulate after . . . Another thing that works is to spend a lot of time to relax and slow down before things like oral exams and job interviews. I also find that breathing exercises work as it reduces extra stress . . . When doing oral presentations I also find it efficient to make my notes filled with little notes to remind me to slow down. They are usually '5' (talk in segments for about five words) 'pt' (prat tydelig—meaning something like overarticulate), and little dots of fluorescent colors—preferably pink as I associate these dots with cluttering and slowing down. Reading texts backwards also works. It seems to make it easier to remember all the letters when I speak afterwards. The same goes with overarticulating.

(HBK, adult)

Strategies that 'did not work'

Pacing (e.g. with a metronome) didn't seem to have a direct effect on my speech.

(AER, adult)

> What did not at all work was singing on the words instead of speaking them. When I was learning to change my way of speaking my new method felt extremely unnatural. In that phase I tried the 'singing-on-the-words' method when I realized it was going too fast. Even if it made it easier to understand it sounded really stupid so I was asked to quit . . . I have also tried putting a see-through red mark on my glasses hoping that it would remind me to slow down. I did not try this for very long, (a) it looked stupid, (b) it was annoying to look at, (c) it did not really work . . . I have tried to associate eyes with 'slow down' but it did not work. I would always forget within seconds . . . I have tried to make my mobile phone vibrate every hour in order to take a few seconds at work to analyze how it was going, but it did not work either.
>
> (HBK, adult)

What clutterers want clinicians to know

> One very important thing is that there is no cure for cluttering, it will never go away and searching for the holy grail of talking fluent in every occasion is a waste of time and energy. For me, it took about twelve years to finally realize this. I used to have a dream that I could stop repeating things. Now I have come to terms with it. I can fool people to believe I do not have this for some time, but I will always have my slipups, sometimes for just a few seconds, often for a lot longer.
>
> (HBK, adult)

> Another thing is that with practice it is possible to reach several layers of speech control. Personally I have found five levels of speech control namely the following:
>
> 1 Extremely controlled—the way I speak to foreigners, people with hearing difficulties, and people with a very different dialect than mine. This is *very* easy to understand, but so controlled that I hardly use it.
> 2 Very controlled—they way I speak when I talk about c[luttering], during presentations, and things like that. When I listen to my own voice during this I can hear that it sounds very 'normal', it sounds just like everybody else.
> 3 Semi controlled—the way I speak when I try to pay attention to it, but also speak as 'freely' as possible—one moment controlling it, one moment not and when it is challenging for me to figure out who understands me or not. It is in these occasions I can get frustrated, I know that I try to control it, but as I am not listening to my own voice, I do not know how good or bad it is.
> 4 Not controlled—my natural way. Not good, but my friends and family usually understands.

5 Not at all controlled—when I am stressed, enthusiastic or something like that. Then no one understands, not even my best friends.

(HBK, adult)

There is nothing scary about cluttering. The way I often choose to describe it is that the thing that is supposed to control my level of speech in my brain does not work. I also add that the only way for me to talk in an understandable manner is to deliberately make an effort to do so. With practice it is perfectly possible to have a regular education and job; it just requires that you always will have to remind yourself that you still have cluttering . . . Cluttering alone is not caused by social factors, but for me it gets worse by stress, lack of sleep, being hungry, and enthusiasm.

(HBK, adult)

While any SLP can help a PWC [person with cluttering] with their underlying issues one at a time, they will not fully understand the 'whole picture'. I believe it's most beneficial when treating each underlying issue that the SLP keep in mind how it affects the other underlying issues as a whole.

(JW, parent of a teenager)

Currently, the 3 SLPs we have contacted are smart enough not to deal with the hassles of the insurance companies. While this is great for them, it does cause financial burdens for the consumer.

(JW, parent of a teenager)

I would like to see social interaction classes for PWC. This type of therapy is non existent for PWC. It should also be part of the whole picture.

(JW, parent of a teenager)

For the therapist, we as parents feel out of our realm and are looking to you for guidance on how to help our children. Raymond and Anthony now love going to speech therapy. Their SLPs make it fun for them. They play games while they are learning. I hear them laughing all the time. These kids are working so hard to get through the day that making speech fun doesn't make it seem like work for them. We truly value advice and recommendations from our speech therapists.

(DB, mother of a school-age child)

Conclusion: Overcoming adversity through innovation

The personal struggles those with cluttering have faced combined with the lack of knowledge regarding this communication disorder have led to the expanding role of cluttering in the self-help and support group world. For many with cluttering, frustration with seeking services for themselves or their children has led to resilience and resulted in creative ways to pool resources and information. The inclusion of clinicians and researchers in support groups has opened the door to mutually rewarding collaborations between professionals and consumers. With mutual respect for differing perspectives, such partnerships can lead to new developments in cluttering research, diagnosis, and treatment. It is of major importance that clinicians work to understand not just the outward speech characteristics associated with cluttering, but the perspectives of those living with this communication challenge. Only with an appreciation for this consumer perspective can advances in cluttering diagnosis and treatment be maximized to their fullest potential.

Acknowledgments

This chapter would not have been possible without the willingness of Dalal Beacom, Joseph Dewey, Peter Kissagizlis, Helene B. Kvenseth, Anjea Ehrle Ray, and Jonathan Wong to share their experiences with cluttering. We sincerely acknowledge their significant contribution toward helping professionals better understand the communication disorder cluttering.

Note

1 For this chapter, most spelling, punctuation, and typographical errors have been corrected from the original email versions. Messages from virtually anyone who frequently uses email occasionally or frequently contain inadvertent errors that do not reflect the author's best spelling, grammar, punctuation, and so on. Moreover, some individuals with cluttering have reported difficulties with spelling and other writing errors such that constructing and typing a simple email message can take much longer than expected. We corrected these errors because it was not possible to discern the extent to which they were features of cluttering, its associated symptoms, or simple typographical errors.

References

Daly, D. A. (1986). The clutterer. In K. O. St. Louis (Ed.), *The atypical stutterer* (pp. 155–192). New York: Academic Press.

Daly, D. A. (1993). Cluttering: The orphan of speech-language pathology. *American Journal of Speech-Language Pathology*, *2*, 6–8.

Dewey, J. (2007). *Self-help*. Retrieved April 26, 2009, from http://www.associations.missouristate.edu/ICA/

Farris Kurtz, L. (1997). *Self-help and support groups: A handbook for practitioners*. Thousand Oaks, CA: Sage.

Kuster, J. M. (2002). Online conferences: A new way to reach out and around the world. *Acquiring Knowledge in Speech, Language, and Hearing*, *4*, 86–89.

Reeves, L. (2006). The role of self-help/mutual aid in addressing the needs of individuals who stutter. In N. Bernstein Ratner & J. Tetnowski (Eds.), *Current issues in stuttering research and practice* (pp. 255–278). Mahwah, NJ: Lawrence Erlbaum Associates Inc.

St. Louis, K. O. (1999). Person-first labeling and stuttering. *Journal of Fluency Disorders*, *24*, 1–24.

St. Louis, K. O., Goranova, E., Georgieva, D., Coskun, M., Filatova, Y., & McCaffrey, E. (2010). Public awareness of cluttering: USA, Bulgaria, Turkey, and Russia. In K. Bakker, L. J. Raphael, & F. L. Myers (Eds.), *Proceedings of the First World Conference on Cluttering* (pp. 180–189). Katarino, Bulgaria. http://associations.missouristate.edu/ICA/

St. Louis, K. O., & Hinzman, A. R. (1986). Studies of cluttering: Perceptions of speech-language pathologists and educators of cluttering. *Journal of Fluency Disorders*, *11*, 131–149.

St. Louis, K. O., Myers, F. L., Bakker, K., & Raphael, L. J. (2007). Understanding and treating cluttering. In E. B. Conture & R. F. Curlee (Eds.), *Stuttering and related disorders of fluency* (3rd ed., pp. 297–325). New York: Thieme.

St. Louis, K. O., & Rustin, L. (1992). Professional awareness of cluttering. In F. L. Myers & K. O. St. Louis (Eds.), *Cluttering: A clinical perspective* (pp. 23–35). Leicester, UK: Far Communications. (Reissued in 1996 by Singular, San Diego, CA.)

Weiss, D. A. (1964). *Cluttering*. Englewood Cliffs, NJ: Prentice-Hall.

Yaruss, J. S., Quesal, R. W., Reeves, L., Molt, L. F., Kluetz, B., Caruso, A. J., et al. (2002). Speech treatment and support group experiences of people who participate in the National Stuttering Association. *Journal of Fluency Disorders*, *27*, 115–134.

Part IV

Current and future directions in cluttering

14 Defining cluttering: the lowest common denominator

Kenneth O. St. Louis and
Katrin Schulte

Introduction

The root of the word 'definition' is the Latin 'definire', which means 'set limits to'. This chapter seeks to do that with the communication disorder called cluttering from a 'lowest common denominator' perspective. In mathematics, the lowest common denominator (LCD) is the smallest number that can be divided into the denominators of two or more fractions that are to be added or subtracted. One of its figurative meanings is the broadest and most widely applicable requirements for a given problem or issue. Another way to consider an LCD definition is to determine the minimum number of necessary and sufficient conditions in order that the problem or issue is de-limited or defined.

Speculations on cluttering definition

A plausible origin

We alert the reader to that fact that this section is—as the heading asserts—speculative. The assumptions therefore must be considered tentative, pending verification by careful research. Assuming that stuttering is typically more salient than cluttering, it is likely that identification and labeling of stuttering as a distinct entity preceded that for cluttering (Van Riper, 1992). Whereas exceptions would definitely exist, the saliency of stuttering is greater for both the speaker, as evidenced by the experience of clear instances of struggle, and the listener, who immediately recognizes abnormal ways of initiating and completing words.

It follows that stuttering was undoubtedly defined first, and it is therefore plausible that the recognition of cluttering grew out of clinical work with stuttering individuals. Some stutterers were probably singled out as being different from the typical cases, even though they may have believed that they did stutter. These atypical stutterers presumably did not struggle as much as their peers. They likely seemed to be faster talkers who were notable for not being concerned or even aware of specific words wherein difficulty occurred. As a result, those clinicians who treated many stutterers probably began to consider this subgroup, later identified as clutterers, to be a somewhat to completely different disorder, as in Van Riper's (1971) 'Track II' stutterers. In any case, the point to be made is that the roots of cluttering very likely originated within the group of speech disorders now known as 'fluency disorders'.

How would cluttering be recognized?

We speculate further that a suspicion of cluttering occurs in a predictable way. As with any disorder, certain perceptual cues initially signal a speech or language abnormality and alert the clinician to various possible diagnoses. Immediately on detecting an abnormality, it might be instructive to consider what probably will *not* cause a clinician to suspect cluttering. Cluttering is probably not suspected when a speaker seems to be struggling to get a word out, as would be true of stuttering. Similarly, cluttering is presumably not suspected as soon as a speaker demonstrates a few articulation errors, syntactic errors, or semantic anomalies. It is also not likely that cluttering would come immediately to mind if a speaker seemed not to be self-aware of her speech, e.g., not noticing that her voice loudness does not conform to the demands of the situation or not seeming to care if she was hard to understand. Neither would cluttering ordinarily be suspected when a speaker strays from the topic at hand, is a poor conversationalist, a poor listener, or seems to revise sentences more than usual (with a normal rate). And cluttering would not seem immediately apparent when a potential conversation partner demonstrates poor social graces, excessive fidgeting, or distractibility.

By contrast, we hypothesize that cluttering would be suspected if a speaker spoke much faster than expected, or in a more jerky, irregular rate than normal. Also, cluttering would be suspected if a clinician experienced difficulty understanding (intelligibility problems) that did not seem to be the direct result of common articulation or language problems. Instead, the listener would be struck that intelligibility problems were related to fast or jerky speech. Similarly, an experienced clinician might suspect cluttering after noticing more words than usual that were repeated, changed, restarted, or revised—all excessive normal disfluencies. Finally, the clinician might well think of cluttering immediately after hearing words being run together, especially those with several syllables.

In our opinion, the foregoing occurs rapidly in the mind of any clinician and often without clear awareness of all the steps. We speculate further that if clinicians are quite familiar with cluttering, they would probably not even notice that they considered the first list, e.g., articulation or language errors, poor self-awareness, compromised pragmatic skills, excessive movement, or distractibility, only *after* they suspected cluttering. They would probably ask themselves, 'Why is this person talking so fast?' or 'Why can't I understand him?' Then, they would probably unconsciously rule out the possibilities that these problems were due to not knowing the language, not knowing the topic, or struggling to get specific words out. If the foregoing is correct, then the first signs of cluttering are related to fluency and prosody more than to syntax, semantics, pragmatics, or cognitive ability.

Existing definitions

Why is it so hard to define cluttering?

It is well known, as we have implied, that individuals with cluttering frequently have many other disorders (St. Louis, 1996). Figure 14.1 shows a list of symptoms (ovals) and diagnoses (rectangles) that are frequently reported to be associated with cluttering. The list is not meant to be exhaustive. Since these and other symptoms frequently occur in individuals presumed to clutter, when the issue of definition is raised, the question of which symptoms should be considered obligatory or primary and which ones should be optional or ancillary quickly follows.

Common approaches to definition

There are at least six different approaches to integrate these and other symptoms and clinical conditions into a definition for cluttering. Before reviewing the approaches, we note that some definitions might aptly be regarded as clinical descriptions that seek more to account for the clinical symptoms commonly observed than to manage potential ambiguity in the resultant descriptive definitions. For example, one might include increased anxiety in one's 'definition' of stuttering, since anxiety is encountered frequently in the treatment of stuttering, yet not be concerned that such anxiety can and often does occur without stuttering.

Consensus definition

One approach to definition is through consensus, wherein the definition requires agreement or acquiescence from a number of stakeholders. Consensus-based definitions typically contain compromises that end up lacking in logical consistency. Three examples come from the World Health Organization (WHO), the American Speech-Language-Hearing Association (ASHA), and the American Psychiatric Association (APA). The WHO definition for cluttering is 'F98.6 Cluttering [has] a rapid rate of speech with breakdown in fluency, but no repetitions or hesitations, of a severity to give rise to reduced speech intelligibility. Speech is erratic and dysrhythmic, with rapid, jerky spurts that usually involve faulty phrasing patterns (e.g. alternating pauses and bursts of speech, producing groups of words

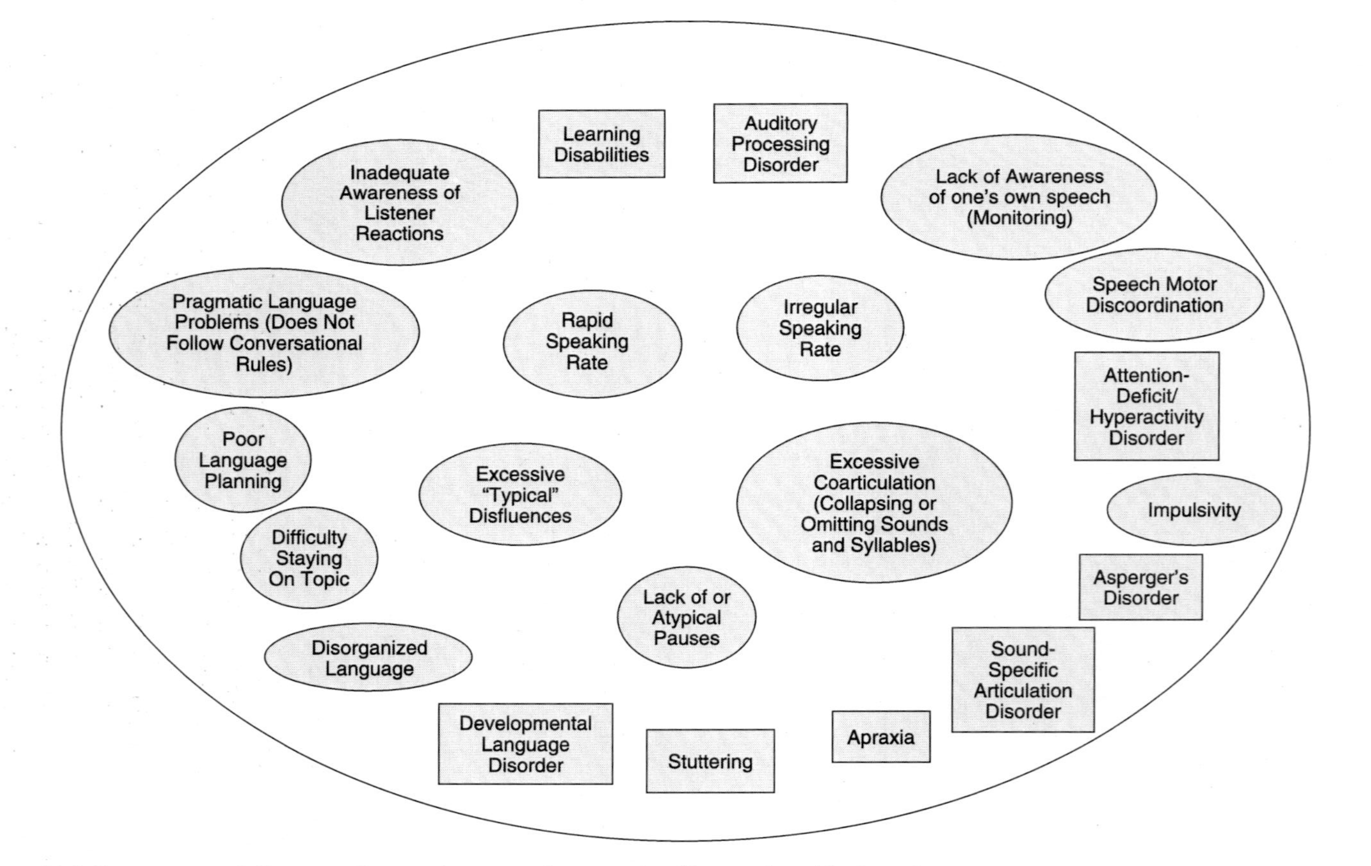

Figure 14.1 Symptoms and diagnoses frequently reported to occur and/or coexist with cluttering.

unrelated to the grammatical structure of the sentence)' (WHO, 1992, p. 290). The Special Interest Division of ASHA on Fluency and Fluency Disorders Guidelines on terminology stated: '3.11. Cluttering. Cluttering is a fluency disorder characterized by a rapid and/or irregular speech rate, excessive disfluencies, and often other symptoms such as language or phonological errors and attention deficits.' (ASHA, 1999). The *Diagnostic and Statistical Manual of Mental Disorders*, DSM-III-R reads, 'The essential feature of Cluttering is a disturbance of fluency involving an abnormally rapid rate and erratic rhythm of speech that impedes intelligibility. Faulty phrasing patterns are usually present so that there are bursts of speech consisting of groups of words that are not related to the grammatical structure of the sentence. The affected person is usually unaware of any communication impairment' (APA, 1987, pp. 85–86). The DSM-IV revision (APA, 1994) omitted cluttering, but presumably it would be subsumed under the entry for stuttering (Reid & Wise, 1995).

The newly formed International Cluttering Association has launched an initiative, driven jointly by professionals and people with cluttering (PWC), to develop terminology for cluttering (Scaler Scott et al., 2008). If this effort comes to fruition, it is possible that a consensus definition of cluttering, drawing heavily from clutterers themselves, will emerge.

Perhaps the primary advantage of the consensus definitions reviewed here is that they represent respected organizations that presumably reviewed the definitions carefully. This certainly was the case of the ASHA terminology guidelines definition. The first author led that effort, which invited comments from members of the Fluency and Fluency Disorders Special Interest Division on a draft written by the Steering Committee. At least four different sets of revisions of the terminology guidelines were circulated, but most of the disagreements focused on terminology for stuttering rather than for cluttering. There are disadvantages to consensus definitions as well. One is that they tend to be 'political' compromises rather than incisive, logical statements. Another is that they are influenced heavily by who writes the initial and final drafts, itself a 'political' issue.

Expert definition

A closely related approach to developing a definition or description by consensus is the strategy of developing one by experts. Stakeholders need not be experts, but they often are. As such, the definitions reviewed in the previous section could be regarded as expert definitions as well. Yet, two examples exist where experts were asked to identify symptoms or conditions often seen in clutterers and the results tabulated. St. Louis (1996) asked authors of data-based articles on 29 clutterers in a special edition of the *Journal of Fluency Disorders* on cluttering to evaluate their subjects according to 17 diagnoses and 29 abilities that might be impaired. The 10 items most frequently identified or rated most severe, in order, were: 'excessive disfluencies', 'rate of speech too fast'/'rate of speech too irregular' (tied rank), 'handwriting', 'pragmatic language abilities', 'interpersonal skills', 'speech motor abilities', 'sound/syllable (part word) repetitions', 'aware of fluency problem(s)', and 'irrelevant, confusing, or ungrammatical words or phrases'. Daly and Cantrell (2006) asked 45 fluency experts and 15 additional experts recommended because of their expertise in cluttering to rate 50 items taken primarily from the Checklist for Possible Cluttering (Daly, 1992–93; Daly & Burnett, 1999). The top 10 ranked items, in order, were: 'lack of effective self-monitoring skills', 'lack of awareness of communication errors or problems', 'telescopes or condenses words (omits, transposes sounds and syllables)', 'imprecise articulation (distorts speech sounds)', 'irregular speech rate: speaks in spurts', 'rapid rate (tachylalia) *with intact articulation*', 'interjections; revision; many filler words', 'compulsive talker; verbose or tangential; circumlocutions are common', 'poor language formulation; storytelling difficulty; trouble sequencing', and 'repetition of multi-syllabic words or phrases'. Based on the results of the expert ratings, Daly (2006) revised the instrument and renamed it the Predictive Cluttering Inventory.

The advantage of these two expert lists of symptoms is that they provide a relatively unbiased snapshot of what those who presumably are most familiar with cluttering consider to be essential features of cluttering. The two studies were quite different, however. St. Louis asked authors to describe their cluttering participants; Daly and Cantrell asked experts to rate various items or add new ones to those Daly identified as being commonly observed in cluttering. If several more such studies were reported, the most commonly reported items could be woven into a definition. As they stand now, however, the foregoing rankings provide some good ideas about what a definition should probably include, but not a definition per se. This is the major disadvantage.

Clinical symptoms definition

Another approach to definition is to base it on common clinical symptoms. Following are three examples. Weiss' (1964) definition of cluttering is among the most well known. He wrote:

> Cluttering is a speech disorder characterized by the clutterer's unawareness of the disorder, by a short attention span, by disturbances in perception, articulation and formulation of speech and often by excessive speed of delivery. It is a disorder of the thought processes preparatory to speech and based on a hereditary disposition. Cluttering is the verbal manifestation of Central Language Imbalance, which affects all channels of communication (e.g. reading, writing, rhythm and musicality) and behavior in general.
>
> (1964, p. 1)

Although Myers (1992) did not advance a specific definition, she described cluttering within a systems approach whereby rate, articulation, coarticulation, disfluency, language, and awareness are all interrelated. In her view, the symptoms of cluttering, e.g., disfluencies, are often surface manifestations of underlying processing difficulties, often related to breakdowns in normal synchrony of speech movements. Daly and Burnett wrote that 'Cluttering exists when an individual presents with one or more impairment(s) in each of five broad communicative dimensions reflecting cognitive, linguistic, pragmatic, speech, and motor abilities' (1999, p. 226). They then listed about 40 different symptoms, some repeated in more than one category, as sufficient examples of impairments.

A clinically oriented definition is attractive to clinicians, who face the problem of deciding how to categorize their clients and then decide what to attempt to remediate in therapy. This approach has the disadvantages that: (a) definitions may not be entirely logically consistent or (b) that symptom lists are long and unwieldy. An example of logical inconsistency might occur with Daly and Burnett's definition, wherein a person might manifest one of the pragmatic difficulties they list, e.g., 'verbose or tangential', but without specification of other obligatory symptoms, might be misdiagnosed a clutterer instead of a person with a pragmatic language disorder. In addition, if used to identify clients in the first place, these definitions may either include clients whom many would not regard as clutterers (e.g., individuals with apraxia or who are second-language speakers) or omit others whom many clinicians would regard as clutterers (e.g., individuals who manifest only fluency and prosody symptoms when being defined with a definition that lists lack of awareness as an obligatory symptom; Weiss, 1964).

Spectrum definition

Another approach to defining cluttering is in terms of a spectrum or continuum of related conditions, much as autism spectrum disorders are conceptualized. A number of European logopedists and phoniatrists wrote extensively about the continuum from stuttering to cluttering (e.g., Weiss, 1964). Ward, acknowledging that there is as yet no agreed-upon definition of cluttering, asserted that 'Cluttering is likely to contain one or more of the following key elements: abnormally fast speech rate, or uncontrolled bursts of fast speech; reduced intelligibility due to overcoarticulation and indistinct articulation; disturbances in language planning; greater and expected number of disfluencies' (2006, p. 152). Nevertheless, he also emphasized that often a person may manifest symptoms typical of cluttering; yet, clinicians would not be comfortable making a firm diagnosis of cluttering. For such individuals, he proposed the term 'cluttering spectrum behaviour . . . as a descriptor for those who display cluttering characteristics or tendencies but do not warrant a diagnosis of "cluttering" ' (2006, p. 152). Unlike the earlier writers, Ward's conceptualization of the spectrum is not between stuttering and cluttering but between highly fluent speakers and highly cluttered speakers.

The advantage of placing cluttering on a spectrum of clear disorder to no disorder recognizes the current ambiguity in defining the problem. One disadvantage is that, because few limits are inherent in these classifications, spectrums can spread, with new variants being added without serious rationale or debate.

Frequency of symptoms definition

Cluttering could be defined post hoc in terms of its most common symptom clusters. Bakker (personal communication) has advocated such an approach, whereby a large number of suspected clutterers would undergo standard testing and measurement, and the resultant data subjected to a factor analysis. Loadings on a few factors would then identify those symptoms that typically vary together and those that do not. A symptom-based approach to definition has not been systematically carried out to date, partly because finding large numbers of potential clutterers and testing them all the same way would be a very difficult and costly project to carry out, no doubt requiring collaboration from many testing centers.

The advantage of this approach to identifying symptoms is that we would begin to develop an empirical rather than a clinical approach to quantifying and classifying symptoms. The primary disadvantage is that it would still require some sort of a priori definition to determine what participant pool would constitute the clutterers to be studied. Another disadvantage, as noted, is the difficulty and expense of finding participants, testing them, and analyzing the results.

Lowest common denominator (LCD) definition

A final proposed approach to defining cluttering is in terms of its LCD, the approach advocated in this chapter. St. Louis and his associates have advanced a number of LCD working definitions for cluttering with the purpose of limiting the population of 'clutterers' in such a way as to develop a reliable, valid body of research on the disorder. St. Louis wrote that 'Cluttering is a speech-language disorder, and its chief characteristics are (1) abnormal fluency which is not stuttering and (2) a rapid and/or irregular speech rate' (1992, p. 49). In 2003, the working definition was updated:

> Cluttering is a syndrome characterized by a speech delivery rate which is either abnormally fast, irregular, or both. In cluttered speech, the person's speech is affected by one or more of the following: (1) failure to maintain normally expected sound, syllable, phrase, and pausing patterns; (2) evidence of greater than expected incidents of

> disfluency, the majority of which are unlike those typical of people who stutter.
>
> (St. Louis, Raphael, Myers, & Bakker, 2003, p. 4)

The working definition was again updated in 2007:

> Cluttering is a fluency disorder characterized by a rate that is perceived to be abnormally rapid, irregular, or both for the speaker (although measured syllable rates may not exceed normal limits). These rate abnormalities further are manifest in one or more of the following symptoms: (a) an excessive number of disfluencies, the majority of which are not typical of people who stutter; (b) the frequent placement of pauses and use of prosodic patterns that do not conform to syntactic and semantic constraints; and (c) inappropriate (usually excessive) degrees of coarticulation among sounds, especially in multisyllabic words.
>
> (St. Louis, Myers, Bakker, & Raphael, 2007, pp. 299–300)

The primary advantage of using an LCD definition is that it allows researchers and clinicians to conceptualize cluttering in the same way (Scaler Scott & St. Louis, 2009). As a result, research or clinical data on cluttering would be comparable from one report to the next. Earlier definitions, such as 'central language imbalance' (Weiss, 1964) permit so much ambiguity that research based on them is not clearly comparable. A promising approach to further systematize an LCD definition is provided by Van Zaalen, Wijnen, and DeJonckere (2009), who developed and tested operational definitions of the following symptoms derived from the St. Louis et al. (2007) definition: rapid speaking rate; irregular speaking rate; excessive normal disfluencies; and errors in syllable, word, or sentence structure. We posit that a good LCD definition is likely to be a prerequisite for major grant funding of cluttering research. Also, clinical strategies that are directed at the core features of cluttering could be differentiated from those directed at coexisting disorders. Researchers could develop the a priori definition that might then be used in the aforementioned symptom-based definition approach. The primary disadvantage of an LCD approach is that, to date, the experts do not agree on what the necessary and sufficient symptoms of cluttering should be. In other words, they would question the validity of the definition. And if there is disagreement on what will be included, the LCD definition may not be widely adopted.

A refined working LCD definition

Our refined working LCD definition is similar to that of St. Louis et al. (2007), but hopefully is more robust and easier to understand.

> Cluttering is a fluency disorder wherein segments of conversation[a] in the speaker's native language[b] typically are perceived as too fast overall[c], too

irregular[d], or both. The segments of rapid and/or irregular speech rate must further be accompanied by one or more of the following: (a) excessive 'normal' disfluencies[e]; (b) excessive collapsing[f] or deletion of syllables; and/or (c) abnormal pauses, syllable stress, or speech rhythm.

[a] Cluttering must occur in naturalistic conversation, but it need not occur even a majority of the time. Clear but isolated examples that exceed those observed in normal speakers are sufficient for a diagnosis.
[b] This may also apply to the speaker's mastered and habitual non-native language, especially in multilingual living environments.
[c] This may be true even though syllable rates may not exceed those of normal speakers.
[d] Synonyms for irregular rate include 'jerky', or 'spurty'.
[e] These disfluencies are often observed in smaller numbers in normal speakers and are typically not observed in stuttering.
[f] Collapsing includes, but is not limited to, excessive shortening, 'telescoping', or 'over-coarticulating' various syllables, especially in multisyllabic words.

The definition reaffirms the primacy of rate in defining cluttering. It also adds the important provision that cluttering occurs primarily in conversational speech. Oral reading is not included because cluttering-like symptoms (e.g., irregular speaking rate and excessive disfluencies) can be *caused by* reading difficulties. This, of course, is not to assert that cluttering cannot occur in oral reading or other speaking tasks; it simply must also occur in conversation. The refined definition further adds the important criterion that conversation must be considered in a language wherein limited second or foreign language knowledge or facility is not an issue. A third important addition is that cluttering can occur intermittently, even in brief segments or 'spurts' of rapid/irregular rates with necessary disfluency, coarticulation, or prosodic features. This is especially important given the strong tendency of those who clutter to 'normalize' during formal evaluations or research protocols (Bakker, Myers, Raphael, & St. Louis, 2010; Daly & Burnett, 1999; Daly & St. Louis, 1998; St. Louis et al., 2007).

Based on this working definition, we conceptualize the relationships among the various symptoms and diagnostic categories that are shown in Figure 14.2. Consistent with the St. Louis et al. (2007) working definition, the current definition states that cluttering is a fluency disorder. Fluency disorders typically manifest as stuttering; yet, fluency disorders can also manifest as rate disorders (for a slightly different position, see Starkweather, 1987). Clutterers *always* manifest abnormalities in rate; they are perceived to speak too fast, too irregularly, or both. A rate disorder is therefore obligatory in cluttering. Importantly, as shown in the third footnote above, measured syllable rates for clutterers may not exceed those for the normal speaker; yet their rates are *perceived* by normal listeners to be too fast, irregular, or both.

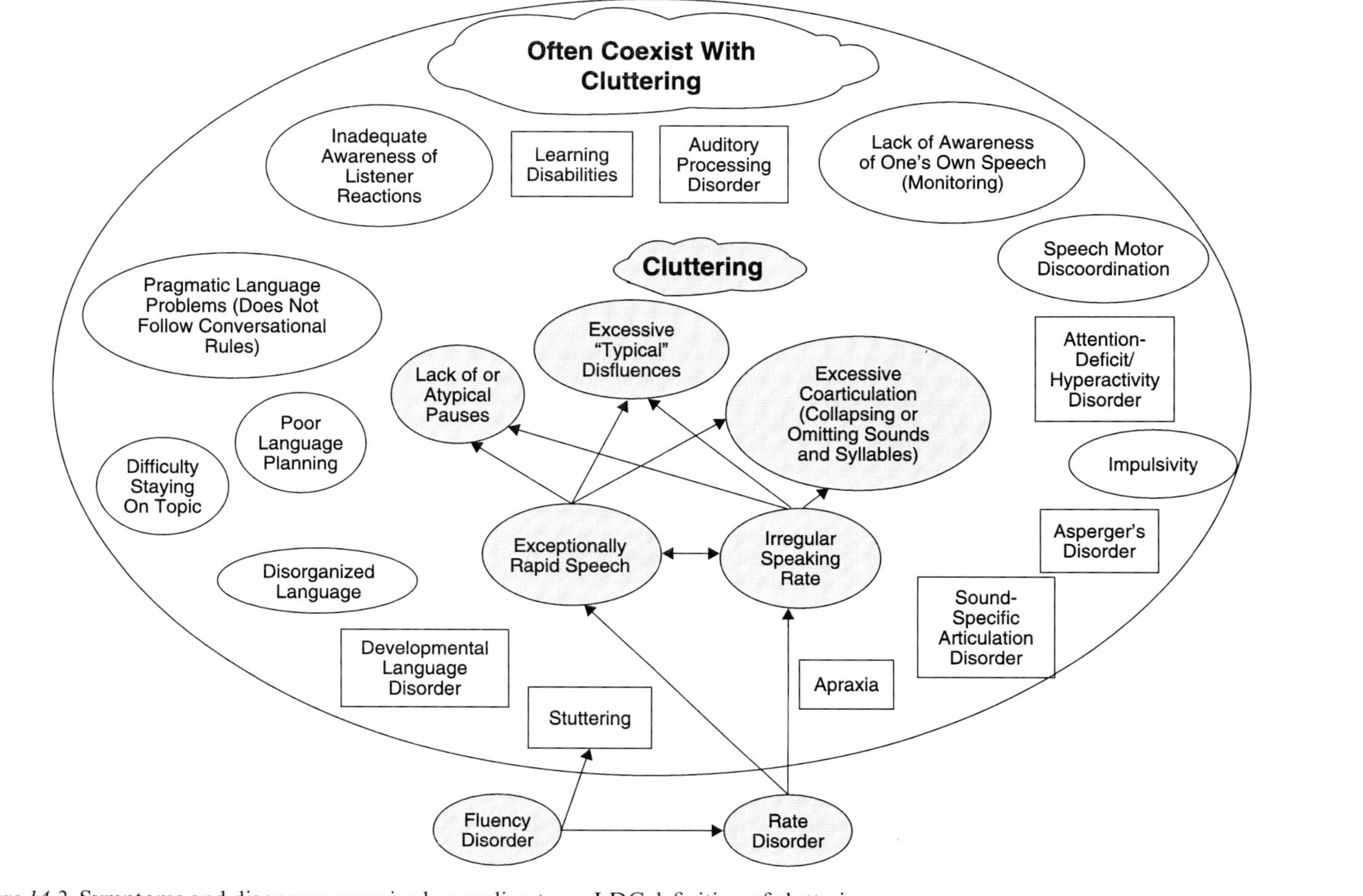

Figure 14.2 Symptoms and diagnoses organized according to an LDC definition of cluttering.

Also, consistent with the 2007 definition, an abnormally fast or irregular rate is presumed to *lead directly* to one, two, or three other obligatory symptoms. One rate-related consequence is too many disfluencies such as interjections, fillers, and revisions—not part-word repetitions, prolongations, and blocks seen in stuttering. Another is abnormalities in pauses that could be longer than usual breaks at non-syntactic boundaries, no pauses where they would ordinarily be expected (e.g., 'It's my turn (pause) not yours.'), or other abnormalities. A third consequence would either be collapsing or 'telescoping' syllables (e.g., 'smy birday' for 'it's my birthday') or deletion of all or parts of syllables (e.g., 'tmensly' for 'tremendously').

The above LCD definition does not address the reasons *why* one's rate is abnormal or *how* a rate anomaly causes problems in prosody, coarticulation, or continuity, it simply describes the necessary and sufficient symptoms. We believe that in order for an orderly progression of research to develop in cluttering to answer important questions such as these, investigators must study a population of individuals with a core of similar symptoms. The only way for that to happen is for researchers to start with the same or similar definitions of cluttering.

Profile of clutterers using an LCD definition

Study background, purpose, and procedures

The second author, KS, carried out an investigation in Germany (Schulte, 2009) designed to determine the likelihood of various coexisting conditions in a sample of individuals originally diagnosed or suspected to clutter, but also constrained as closely as possible by the St. Louis et al. (2007) LCD definition. Potential participants were referred to KS after she sent notifications by mail or email to approximately 1000 speech-language clinicians in Germany who specialized in treating fluency disorders, mainly stuttering. Instructions asked the SLPs *not* to refer stutterers since the intent of the study was to investigate those who cluttered but did not stutter. SLPs referred 18 persons from their caseloads whose speech, according to the referring clinicians, was characterized by rapid speaking rates and 'abnormal' speech. KS examined these participants in their homes.

The guiding rationale for the study was, using a battery of tests, questionnaires, and other procedures, to identify the presence or absence of other symptoms or disorders often frequently reported to be common among those with cluttering. The battery specifically targeted stuttering, articulation and language disorders, reading disorders, writing disorders, attention deficit hyperactivity disorders (ADHD), auditory processing disorders (APD), and oral motor abilities (for additional details, see Schulte, 2009). Constraints on the test battery included: (1) being sufficiently portable to carry and use at participants' homes; (2) being limited to 90 minutes to avoid overburdening the participants; and (3) containing elements that are practical and valid for participants from ages 9 to 65. Importantly, to rule out diagnostic ambiguities associated with stuttering, KS excluded from consideration individuals who stuttered, even if they also cluttered. In other words, KS's intent was to locate a nonstuttering sample of clutterers based on the 2007 definition and then test them to determine the prevalence of other associated conditions frequently reported to accompany cluttering.

Evaluations began with a videotaped interview with each adult participant or parent of a child participant designed to identify the likelihood of coexisting disorders. KS asked about medical history, previous treatment, and motor and language development from infancy to school age. She also asked about relatives who may have stuttered or had other speech and/or language disorders. To rule out stuttering, the Stuttering Severity Index (SSI-3; Riley, 1994) was scored from videotaped spontaneous and oral reading samples.

To screen for auditory processing disorders (APDs), KS asked a series of non-standardized questions. Thereafter, she administered the Mottier-Test, a standardized measure of auditory short-term memory and discrimination of sounds (Gomm, 2001; Welte, 1981). It requires the repetition of 30 nonsense words presented from a compact disk that vary in length from 2 to 6 syllables. Furthermore, a questionnaire for auditory processing disorders (Nickisch et al., 2006) was used to collect indicators for APD. Next, Döpfner, Lehmkuhl, and Steinhaus's (2006) Fragebogen zur Erfassung von ADHS [ADHD Questionnaire] for children and adults was administered as a self-assessment questionnaire to screen for symptoms of ADHD, developed from the ICD-10 (WHO, 1992) and DSM-IV (APA, 1994). To further measure abilities often compromised by ADHD, the Frankfurter Aufmerksamkeits-inventar (FAIR) [Frankfurter Attention Inventory] was also administered (Moosbrugger & Oelschlaegel, 1996). The FAIR measures one's directed attention and ability to concentrate, requiring precise and rapid discrimination of visually similar designs while simultaneous blocking out or ignoring irrelevant information. The person being tested must work with two goal items, e.g., marking all circles with three dots and all squares with two dots, as seen in Figure 14.3.

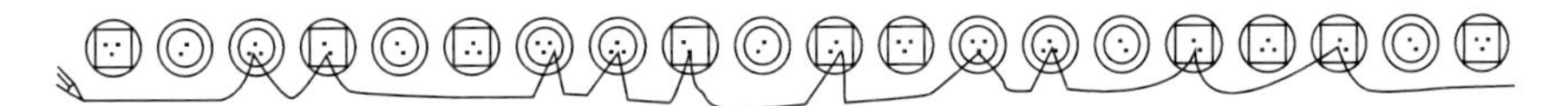

Figure 14.3 Sample sequence in the FAIR with complete marking of circles with three dots and squares with two dots.

Writing ability was examined using a standardized instrument known as the Rechtschreibungstest (RT) [Orthography Test] (Kersting & Althoff, 2004). Here, the examiner reads a short story while the participant follows with another copy of the text, and, during pauses in the examiner's reading, the participant is asked to write different frequently occurring words in spaces located on a worksheet. KS next carried out an assessment of participants' oral motor skills, that is, their abilities to move their mouths, tongues, and faces, e.g., touch their tongue tip to the corners of their mouths, click their tongues, and frown.

Thereafter, KS carried out a detailed examination of speech, language, and reading abilities consisting of: (1) reciting in rote fashion the days of the week and months of the year; (2) orally reading words; (3) orally reading sentences with increasing complexity; (4) orally reading faster and slower than normal; (5) orally reading nonsense words; (6) silently reading and then retelling a short story; and (7) conversing about hobbies, holidays, books, movies, and other topics to evoke spontaneous speech.

Participant results

As noted, KS visited homes of 18 potential participants, based on SLP referrals. Three were excluded because the case history and/or referral information indicated that they stuttered or manifested stuttering (on the SSI-3) and cluttering. These three did not receive the remainder of the test battery. As noted above, all of the referrals were for individuals with rapid speech rate and 'abnormal' speech symptoms. (This excluded the possibility of a speech rate that was not rapid but excessively irregular in the St. Louis et al. (2007) definition as one possible obligatory symptom.) Table 14.1 provides a brief summary of which cluttering symptoms, rapid rate, irregular rate, excessive non-stuttering disfluencies, unusual pauses or prosody, and collapsing syllables ('over-coarticulation') were observed for each participant. All 15 were reported to speak too fast, both from clinician referrals and from results of average speaking rates calculated during spontaneous speech. All rates exceeded the normal 250 syllables per minute rate reported by Sick (2004). Five of the fifteen (33 percent) also manifested irregular speaking rates. Even so, based on further analyses from the spontaneous speech samples, two participants (13 per cent; 10 and 13) did not manifest sufficient additional criteria to warrant objective definition of cluttering using the slightly modified St. Louis et al. (2007) definition. It is most likely that these individuals 'normalized' during the testing situation, a commonly reported characteristic of cluttering (Daly & St. Louis, 1998; St. Louis et al., 2007). The remaining 13/15 participants (87 percent) did manifest aspects of the rate-associated symptoms as follows: 6/15 with excessive normal disfluencies (40 percent), 9/15 with excessive coarticulation or collapsing of syllables (60 percent), and none (0/15) with unusual pauses or prosody (0 percent).

The total sample consisted of 12 males and 3 females (i.e., 4:1), consistent with previously reported sex ratios for stuttering and cluttering (Bloodstein & Ratner, 2009; St. Louis, 1996). Participants ranged from 11 to 44 years of age, with a mean of 22 years. Thirteen were monolingual native speakers of German, and two were bilingual (German and Thai or Polish). Nearly half (eight participants) were completing, or had completed, a high school diploma ('Abitur'). Based on self-reports from the interview, 13 (86 percent) were right-handed; one (7 percent) was left-handed (but later changed to

Table 14.1 Summary data for 15 persons who clutter

Participant	1	2	3	4	5	6	7	8	9	10	11	12	13	14	15
Age (yr)	37	15	29	16	37	18	15	14	22	14	25	44	21	14	11
Sex (m/f)	f	f	m	m	m	m	m	m	m	f	m	m	m	m	m
LCD definition															
Rate (+/–)[a] (faster than normal)	–	–	–	–	–	–	–	–	–	–	–	–	–	–	–
Regularity (+/–)	–	–	–	–	+	+	+	+	+	+	–	+	+	+	+
Nonstuttering disfluencies (+/–)	+	–	–	–	+	+	+	+	–	+	+	–	+	–	+
Coarticulation/collapsing in spontaneous speech (+/–)	+	–	–	–	+	–	–	–	+	+	+	+	+	+	+
Coarticulation/collapsing in oral reading (+/–)	–	+	+	+	–	+	+	+	+	+	+	+	+	+	–
Pauses & prosody (+/–)	+	+	+	+	+	+	+	+	+	+	+	+	+	+	+
St. Louis et al. (2007) Cluttering definition (modified)	y	y	y	y	y	y	y	y	y	n	y	y	n	y	y
Case history interview															
Family history speech-language problem (+/–)[a]	+	–	+	–	–	+	–	–	+	–	–	–	–	–	–
Handedness (R/L/A/ LR)[b]	LR	R	R	R	A?[c]	R	R	R	R	R	R	R	R	R	R
History of neurological problems (+/–)[d]	–	–	–	–	–	+	–	–	+	–	+	+	–	–	–
Problems in speech-language development (+/–)	U[c]	+	+	+	U[c]	–	–	U?[c]	–	–	U[c]	U[c]	U[c]	–	U[c]
Current cluttering therapy (y/n)	y	y	y	y	y	y	y	y	y	y	y	y	y	y	y
Childhood speech-language therapy (y/n)	n	y	y	y	n	y	y	n	y	y	n	n	n	y	n
Other therapy (y/n)[ef]	y	n	n	n	y	n	y[e]	n	y[e]	y[f]	n	n	n	n	n

continued overleaf

Table 14.1 continued

Participant	1	2	3	4	5	6	7	8	9	10	11	12	13	14	15
Speaking samples															
Rote speech (+/–)	+	+	+	+	+	+	–	–	+	+	+	+	+	+	–
Oral reading: nonsense words (+/–)	+	+	+	+	+	+	+	+	+	+	+	+	+	+	+
Oral reading: faster & slower (+/–)	+	+	+	+	+	–	+	+	–	–	+	–	–	+	+
Retelling story (+/–)	+	+	+	+	+	–	–	+	–	–	+	+	–	+	+
SSI-3 (+/Mi/Mo/Se)[g]	+	+	+	+	+	+	+	+	+	+	+	+	+	+	+
Questionnaires & tests															
Auditory processing questionnaire (+/–)	–	–	–	–	–	–	–	–	+	–	–	+	X[h]	–	–
Mottier Test (+/–)	+	+	+	+	+	–	–	+	+	+	+	+	+	–	+
ADHD questionnaire (+/Mi/Mo/Se)[f]	Se	Se	Se	Mo	Se	Se	Se	Mi	Se	Se	Se	Se	Se	Mo	Mo
FAIR (+/Mi/Mo/Se)[g]	+	+	Mi	+	Mi	Se	Se	Se	Mo	Se	Mo	+	Se	Se	+
RT (+/Mi/Mo/Se)[g]	+	Se	Se	Mo	Mo	Se	Se	Se	Se	Se	Mo	Se	Se	Se	X[h]
Oral motor screening (+/–)	+	+	–	+	+	–	–	+	–	–	–	+	+	–	+

a + indicates normal or no irregularities observed or reported; – indicates abnormalities or irregularities observed or reported.
b R indicates right-handed; L indicates left-handed; A indicates ambidextrous; L❐R indicates being changed from left- to right-handed as a child for writing.
c U indicates unknown; ?, indicates probable but not certain due to not being able to remember clearly.
d Indicates neurological problems not related to athletic injuries.
e Indicates psychotherapy.
f Indicates therapy for ADHD.
g + indicates none or normal; Mi indicates 'mild' deviation; Mo indicates 'moderate' deviation; Se indicates 'severe' deviation.
h X indicates missing data.

right-handedness for writing), and one (7 percent) was ambidextrous. Eleven participants (73 percent) reported relatives, both first degree and parents' relatives, with speech and language disorders, e.g., stuttering, cluttering, and problems in language acquisition. Of the 15 participants, 8 (53 percent) either were or had been in speech or language therapy, mainly from 4 to 6 years of age, as well as at the time of testing, for their cluttering disorders. No consistent connection between other treatments, e.g., psychotherapy, and their cluttering was reported or observed. Neither was there a consistent connection between a history of neurological disorders and cluttering.

No participants displayed cluttering symptoms or abnormalities while reading nonsense words. Nevertheless, in rote speech (e.g., reciting the months of a year in order without omissions, transpositions, or additions), 3 participants (20 percent) made errors. Of the 15 participants, 5 (33 percent) had difficulty varying their speech rates in oral reading. While retelling a short story after intervening testing, 5 participants (33 percent) manifested semantic errors (e.g., adding facts or propositions that were not part of the story), suggesting the possibility of higher demands on language processing.

In evaluating participants for auditory processing disorders, 12/14 (86 percent) showed suspected auditory processing difficulties on the case history questionnaire. (Case history data were missing for participant 13.) Of the 15 participants, 3 (20 percent) showed irregularities in auditory processing on the Mottier-Test. Similarly, in the area of attention, all 15 participants (100 percent) were scored as having irregularities on the ADHD questionnaire, 1 mild (7 percent), 3 moderate (20 percent), and 11 severe (73 percent). On the FAIR, 10 (67 percent) showed irregularities: 2 of the 15 were mild (13 percent), 2 were moderate (13 percent), and 6 were severe (40 percent).

On the RT, excluding participant 15 who had missing data, 13/14 participants (93 percent) demonstrated writing problems, 3 that were moderate (21 percent) and 11 that were severe (79 percent). Seven participants (47 percent) demonstrated problems in oral motor abilities, such as accurately moving the tongue tip outside the mouth to the left, right, up and down, or furrowing one's brow as in frowning after the examiner's model.

Concluding remarks

Most of what has been written about what does—and does not—constitute cluttering is speculative or theoretical; very little has been driven by evidence. This chapter provides a beginning effort to support views about definition with data from people who clutter.

All 15 participants examined by KS 'cluttered', according to their clinicians. The only diagnostic feature that was actually observed to characterize all 15 was a rapid rate of spontaneous speech, consistent with reports of the referring clinicians. That, alone, as we have pointed out, is not sufficient to diagnose cluttering, for there are numerous speakers who talk fast but would never be considered clutterers (see Bakker et al., 2010). On the other hand, according to the referring clinicians, all of these speakers did manifest other symptoms, at least intermittently, to warrant them being identified and treated for cluttering. In objective testing, the rate-related symptoms of excessive non-stuttering disfluencies, collapsing of syllables, and pause or prosody problems were present in 13/15 or 87 percent of the sample. Whether the remaining 13 percent normalized or perhaps should not be classified as cluttering cannot be determined with certainty. Nevertheless, we submit that the most likely explanation is that they did normalize based on experience with other clutterers who most certainly have done so (cf. Bakker et al., 2010).

We emphasize that KS made a serious attempt to isolate a sample of nonstuttering clutterers based on the St. Louis et al. (2007) LCD definition. If we assume that the 13 percent not clearly diagnosed by the modified definition were in fact clutterers but normalized during the testing, then KS's study provides estimates of the likelihood that some frequently reported disorders coexist with cluttering. She excluded the most commonly mentioned coexisting disorder, i.e., stuttering, because differentiating between stuttering and cluttering can be extremely difficult. The data presented here suggest the likelihood of coexisting abnormalities or irregularities relating to: (1) auditory processing (20–86 percent, as indicated by testing or case history, respectively); (2), ADHD (especially attention disorders) (67–100 percent, as indicated by testing or case history, respectively); (3) writing (93 percent); and (4) oral motor difficulties (47 percent). With this analysis, all of the participants manifested at least one coexisting disorder. Three participants presented with two coexisting disorders, and nine with three or more.

There are two important implications of this finding. First, confirming a plethora of reports (e.g., Daly & Burnett, 1999; St. Louis et al., 2007; St. Louis, Ruscello, & Lundeen, 1992), cluttering rarely occurs alone. Instead, it typically manifests with many other coexisting disorders. Second, the LCD definition does not deny any of these coexisting disorders; it permits a diagnosis of cluttering in the face of the entire wide range of clinical pictures. Importantly, if any of these 'other' disorders were used alone to define cluttering instead of the foregoing LCD definition, then not only would the pool of clutterers be reduced, several of the most clearly defined clutterers, and any 'pure clutterers' (based on the LCD definition), would be excluded.

As discussed above, consistent with Scaler Scott and St. Louis (2009), we submit that the LCD definition presented in this chapter or its precursor provides an optimal first step in maximizing research and clinical diagnoses for cluttering. Nevertheless, there are still problems. Clutterers who normalize during evaluations or research protocols will most certainly continue to occur in potential sample pools of people who clutter, just as covert stutterers occur in samples of persons who stutter. Testing procedures should be altered to include large samples of spontaneous and conversational speech, perhaps in unconventional settings (e.g., when the speaker does not know he or she is being monitored or recorded), and perhaps even with multiple examiners, to observe segments of cluttering. We submit that a great many more clutterers, sought and identified according to our LCD definition, should be evaluated to potentially confirm and expand the findings that cluttering usually coexists with other disorders. Eventually, evaluation protocols should determine relative percentages of common and uncommon coexisting conditions (see Figures 14.1 and 14.22). As a start, the data presented here suggest that auditory processing disorders, ADHD, oral motor difficulties, and writing problems clearly warrant additional study.

Acknowledgments

The authors, especially KS, gratefully acknowledge the guidance and assistance of Claudia Iven and Nitza Katz-Bernstein in the planning and analysis of the study herein reported.

References

American Psychiatric Association. (1987). *Diagnostic and statistical manual of mental disorders* (3rd ed., revised). Washington, DC: American Psychiatric Association.

American Psychiatric Association. (1994). *Diagnostic and statistical manual of mental disorders* (4th ed.). Washington, DC: American Psychiatric Association.

American Speech-Language-Hearing Association, Special Interest Division 4; Fluency and Fluency Disorders. (1999, March). Terminology pertaining to fluency and fluency disorders: Guidelines. *ASHA*, *41* (Supplement 19), 29–36.

Bloodstein, O., & Ratner, N. B. (2009). *A handbook on stuttering* (6th ed.). Clifton Park, NY: Delmar.

Daly, D. A. (1992–93). Cluttering: A language-based syndrome. *Clinical Connection*, *6*, 4–7.

Daly, D. A. (2006). *Predictive cluttering inventory*. David A. Daly. Available for download at http://associations.missouristate.edu/ICA/

Daly, D. A., & Burnett, M. (1999). Cluttering: Traditional views and new perspectives. In R. F. Curlee (Ed.), *Stuttering and related disorders of fluency* (2nd ed., pp. 222–254). New York: Thieme.

Daly, D. A., & Cantrell, R. P. (2006). *Cluttering: Characteristics identified as diagnostically significant by 60 fluency experts*. Paper presented at the 5th World Congress on Fluency Disorders, International Fluency Association, Dublin.

Daly, D. A., & St. Louis, K. O. (1998). Videotaping clutterers: How to do it and what to look for. In E. C. Healey & H. F. M. Peters (Eds.), *2nd World Congress on Fluency Disorders Proceedings* (pp. 233–235). International Fluency Association.

Döpfner, M., Lehmkuhl, G., & Steinhaus, H. (2006). *KIDS 1—Aufmerksamkeitsdefizit- und Hyperaktivitätsstörungen (ADHS)*. Göttingen: Hogrefe.

Gomm, B. (2001). *Mottier-Test. Audio-CD. Prüfmittel für Phonemdifferenzierung,*

Phonemidentifikation, artikulatorische Kinästhetik, auditive Sequenzierung bzw. auditives Kurzzeitgedächtnis. Retrieved June 8, 2009, from http://www.avws-bei-kindern.de/

Kersting, M., & Althoff, K. (2004). *Rechtschreibungstest (RT)*. Göttingen: Hogrefe.

Moosbrugger, H., &. Oehlschlaegel, J. (1996). *Frankfurter Aufmerksamkeits-Inventar (FAIR)*. Bern: Huber.

Myers, F. L. (1992). Cluttering: A synergistic framework. In F. L. Myers & K. O. St. Louis (Eds.), *Cluttering: A clinical perspective* (pp. 71–84). Kibworth, UK: Far Communications. (Reissued in 1996 by Singular, San Diego, CA.)

Nickisch, A., Gross, M., Schönweiler, R., Uttenweiler, V., Dinnesen, A., Berger, R., et al. (2006). *Auditive Verarbeitungs- und Wahrnehmungsstörung. Konsensus Statement. Überarbeitete und aktualisierte Version 2006*. Retrieved June 8, 2009, from http://www.dgpp.de/Profi/Sources/cons_avws.pdf

Reid, W. H., & Wise, M. G. (1995). *DSM-IV training guide*. New York: Brunner/Mazel.

Riley, G. D. (1994). *Stuttering severity instrument for children and adults* (3rd ed.). Austin, TX: Pro-Ed.

Scaler Scott, K., Bakker, K., St. Louis, K. O., Myers, F. L., Adams, C., Filatova, Y., et al. (2008). *Providing worldwide cluttering education: Accomplishments of the International Cluttering Association*. Poster presented at the Annual Convention of the Speech-Language-Hearing Association. Chicago, IL.

Scaler Scott, K., & St. Louis, K. O. (2009, July). A perspective on improving evidence and practice in cluttering. *Perspectives on Fluency and Fluency Disorders*, *19*, 46–51.

Schulte, K. (2009). *Communication and communication disorders: Empirical examination of characteristics and coexisting disorders on cluttering*. Doctoral dissertation, Dortmund: University of Technology, Dortmund.

Sick, U. (2004). *Poltern. Theoretische grundlagen, diagnostik, therapie*. Stuttgart: Thieme.

Starkweather, C. W. (1987). *Fluency and stuttering*. Englewood Cliffs, NJ: Prentice-Hall.

St. Louis, K. O. (1992). On defining cluttering. In F. L. Myers & K. O. St. Louis (Eds.), *Cluttering: A clinical perspective* (pp. 37–53). Kibworth, UK: Far Communications. (Reissued in 1996 by Singular, San Diego, CA.)

St. Louis, K. O. (1996). A tabular summary of cluttering subjects in the special edition. *Journal of Fluency Disorders*, *21*, 337–343.

St. Louis, K. O., Myers, F. L., Bakker, K., & Raphael, L. J. (2007). Understanding and treating cluttering. In E. Conture & R. Curlee (Ed.), *Stuttering and related disorders of fluency* (pp. 297–325). New York: Thieme.

St. Louis, K. O., Raphael, L. J., Myers, F. L., & Bakker, K. (2003, November). Cluttering updated. *The ASHA Leader*, *8* (21), 4–5 & 20–23.

St. Louis, K. O., Ruscello, D. M., & Lundeen, C. (1992). Coexistence of communication disorders in schoolchildren. *ASHA Monograph*, *27*.

Van Riper, C. (1971). *The nature of stuttering*. Englewood Cliffs, NJ: Prentice-Hall.

Van Riper, C. (1992). Foreword. In F. L. Myers & K. O. St. Louis (Eds.), *Cluttering: A clinical perspective* (pp. vii–ix). Kibworth, UK: Far Communications. (Reissued in 1996 by Singular, San Diego, CA.)

Van Zaalen, Y., Wijnen, F., & DeJonckere, P. (2009). Differential diagnostic characteristics between cluttering and stuttering—part one. *Journal of Fluency Disorders*, *34*, 137–154.

Ward, D. (2006). *Stuttering and cluttering: Frameworks for understanding and treatment*. Hove, UK: Psychology Press.

Weiss, D. (1964). *Cluttering*. Englewood Cliffs, NJ: Prentice-Hall.

Welte, V. (1981). Der Mottier-Test, ein Prüfmittel für die Lautdifferenzierungsfähigkeit und die auditive Merkfähigkeit. *Sprache–Stimme–Gehör*, *5*, 121–125.

World Health Organization. (1992). *The ICD-10 classification of mental and behavioural disorders: Clinical descriptions and diagnostic guidelines*. Geneva: World Health Organization.

15 Scope and constraint in the diagnosis of cluttering: combining two perspectives

David Ward

Introduction

The fundamental problem of how to define cluttering has concerned, and at the same time confused, researchers from around the world for a great number of years (for a review Reichel & Draguns, chapter 16 this volume). Readers new to the study of cluttering will, on skimming most chapters from this book, quickly become aware of the ubiquitous and sometimes contentious issue of definition. The issues raised by problems with definition appear in almost every chapter, perhaps most notably those by Bakker, Myers, Raphael, and St. Louis (chapter 4); Reichel and Draguns (chapter 16); Scaler Scott and St. Louis (chapter 13); Van Zaalen, Wijnen and Dejonckere (chapters 7 and 9), as well as those writing with a therapeutic focus in mind, such as Bennett Lanouette (chapter 11) and Myers (chapter 10). In addition to these chapters, diagnosis comprises the primary focus of St. Louis and Schulte (chapter 14). In this present short chapter, I will first offer my perspective on current thinking on the subject matter, and conclude by outlining a model that integrates two current conceptualisations of diagnosis. The intention is to present a framework for describing and defining cluttering that is both functional and constrained, but at the same time acknowledges the importance in considering the implications of a wider diagnostic criteria.

Some thoughts on the underpinnings of a theory of diagnosis in cluttering

As we can see from other chapters in this current volume, despite controversy and difference of opinion, much has been written on the subject of how to diagnose, or perhaps more pertinently when *not* to diagnose cluttering. Weiss's (1964) book is regarded by many as the first clear attempt to define the disorder, and nearly 50 years later, it is still referenced in almost all debates on diagnosis. Between then and now, many authors have speculated on the nature of cluttering: what might and might not be considered core to a diagnosis with regard to fluency-disrupted speech? What are the significant features of cluttering with regard to fluency, speech rate, and motor disruptions? What, if any part, does a language processing component play? Do people with cluttering (PWC) have different personality types? Do PWC show differences in executive functions such as attention and memory (Daly & Cantrell, 2006; Myers, 1992; St. Louis & Myers, 1997; St. Louis, Myers, Bakker, & Raphael, 2007; Van Zaalen, Ward et al., 2009; Ward, 2006; Weiss, 1964)? While some empirical data are available to help inform decisions on such matters, in many cases these possibilities have been built on speculations.

In the most recent attempt to answer such questions, St. Louis and Schulte (chapter 14 this volume) carefully review a range of approaches to the diagnosis of cluttering, ultimately, outlining their own 'lowest common denominator' (LCD) definition, which comprises a further distillation of earlier working definition hypotheses (St. Louis, Raphael, Myers, & Bakker, 2003; St. Louis et al., 2007). The premise is that until we have an objectively based diagnosis free from possible artefactual features that may simply 'co-occur' with cluttering, rather than being core to it, the subject area will continue to remain confused and lacking direction (for a thorough explanation of the LCD perspective, see St. Louis & Schulte, chapter 14 this volume).

Given the range of speculation and lack of data that have been pervasive in the study of cluttering, this call for constraint in definition and unity across researchers and laboratories is well motivated. There is little doubt that the value of much of the comparatively little research on the subject of cluttering has, since the days of Weiss, been compromised by researchers applying their own interpretations of different definitions of the disorder. The danger, also, in accepting a syndrome-type definition, such as proposed by Weiss, is that the range of symptoms and features is so broad as to make testing such a notion almost impossible in practical terms.

Constraints surrounding a definition of cluttering

With this in mind, it might be helpful, when evaluating the balance of theoretical constraint in diagnosis, to consider two possibilities observed in statistical theory that can be applied to hypothesis testing. Testing a theory involves, amongst other things, finding the best balance between avoiding two diametrically opposed error types. The so-called type-1 error occurs when the null hypothesis is rejected when in fact it should not be rejected. A type-2 error, on the other hand, is observed when the null hypothesis is not rejected when in fact it should have been. The idea is that a range of procedures can be applied to make sure a balance between these potential errors is maintained. One obvious procedure is the differential use of probability (or '*p*') values, where, for example, lower values must be achieved for drug efficacy studies than in some other areas, where the ramifications of accepting an experimental hypothesis that should not be accepted are likely to be less damaging. Although we are not directly testing a hypothesis when attempting a definition of cluttering, there is a potential analogue regarding the degree of constraint that one imposes on any given definition. As already stated, Weiss's (1964) perspective, where cluttering is perceived to be one aspect of a larger syndrome affecting multiple modalities, runs the risk of being too broad to realistically be subjected to proper scientific testing and verification. Instead, taking a contrary position, St. Louis and Schulte reduce the many features that have been considered as cluttering down to the absolute minimum required to diagnose the disorder. They do this from a perceptual basis; that is, beginning fundamentally with attributes they believe listeners would regard as cluttering as opposed to anything that might possibly be considered anything else, regardless of whether that might be normal or abnormal. Importantly, they arrive at their conclusions as to what constitutes 'LCD' behaviour in cluttering through findings from a data-driven study.

LCD and a language component

The problem for the LCD perspective, and any other approach to defining cluttering, is that there has never been a single universally agreed starting position with regard to what exactly core cluttering is. Of course this statement has more than an air of circularity about it, so let me explain by way of an example. Most would agree that 'jerky' speech and a perceived fast rate of speech would be core to a definition of cluttering, but some also consider that a deficiency in language organization is also implicated (Bennett Lanouette, chapter 11 this volume; Daly, 1986, 1996; Myers, 1992; Van Zaalen, Wijnen, & Dejonckere, 2009; Ward, 2006, 2010; Weiss, 1964). Now, there is little objective and data-driven evidence that a language component is central to diagnosis (though see Van Zaalen et al., 2009; Van Zaalen, Wijnen, & DeJonckere, chapter 9 this volume), but actually there is little other than empirical observation to link jerky speech rhythm to the disorder. Even features once almost universally thought to be core diagnostic indicators, such as increased speed of speech, have been shown to need careful qualification; for example, we now know that it is the *perception* of increased rate, rather than a rate that is consistently observed and measured as exceeding normal limits, that seems associated with the disorder (St. Louis et al., 2003). My point here is simply that, in the absence of any single agreed starting position as to what cluttering is, the notion of how or where to look for cluttering must to some degree itself be speculative. Because of this, there is a danger that the debate can become circular. Continuing with our example above, imagine we were to accept that core cluttering were to include language processing components as well as fluency and motor speech ones. In such a case, when looking for scientific participants, we would, by definition, only include speakers who displayed such features in their speech when it came to enrolling participants with cluttering. St. Louis and Schulte, for example, recruited their participants on the basis of the St. Louis et al. (2007)

working definition, which excludes a language component. It is important to note that under the LCD definition, even the core factors of irregular speech rate and increased rate need not co-occur within any one given individual to produce a positive diagnosis. These two features could, theoretically each arise in 50 percent of those cases diagnosed as cluttering. They could also present in other ratios by the LCD method, perhaps extending to a 30:70 percent split, or beyond. Extensive language testing was not formally undertaken in the St. Louis and Schulte study, yet even so, 33 percent of St. Louis and Schulte's cluttering group manifested language errors. This could be interpreted as indicative of an increased association between motor and language problems in cluttering. However, a language component does not feature as a component in the LCD definition. To place all this in the context of a type-1 versus type-2 error debate, syndrome diagnoses, where definitions might include a multiplicity of speech and non-speech features, may be seen to fall toward making a type-2 error. St. Louis and Schulte are, of course, absolutely right to highlight the very considerable potential gains in 'reining in' a diagnosis, both in terms of providing a consistent starting point for researchers to work from, and from a scientific perspective, where a controlled definition will be helpful in the disorder being taken more seriously by the scientific community, including those bodies responsible for issuing grant monies for research. It is indeed vital that there is unified agreement on core diagnostic criteria, in order to coordinate inter-laboratory efforts when it comes to progressing our understanding of the disorder. At the same time, however, we need to be careful that attempts to delimit the diagnostic criteria of cluttering to more manageable proportions do not result in too much of a fall toward a type-1 error.

So should language be considered as a core part of cluttering? Alongside the considerations mentioned above, there is emerging empirical evidence to suggest that language processing should be considered within the core of a definition both from a language study perspective (Van Zaalen, Wijnen et al., 2009) and from a neurological one (Van Zaalen, Ward et al., 2009). Alm, too, tacitly endorses the significance of a neurological position on language in cluttering when allowing for a faulty language processing component within his executive hub model of cluttering (Alm, chapter 1 this volume). As mentioned in the paragraph above, though, it is important that there is a unified perspective on core diagnostic features. Thus, while we must continue to fully explore the extent of disordered language processing in cluttering, for the moment, St. Louis and Schulte's working LCD definition should be allowed to stand.

That said, there may be strong advantages in eventually including language components under the umbrella of a revised LCD definition. In addition to the issues raised above, where a loss of linguistic fluency is seen alongside a loss of motoric fluency, we also need to know the mechanisms at work in order to make assertions about any potential causal relationship between the two elements (see also Ward, chapter 3 this volume). That is, whether a loss over motoric control could result in a disordered linguistic output, or conversely, if faulty language processing might actually underpin the motoric disruptions seen in core cluttering. It is possible that the latter situation might arise even in the absence of overt linguistic errors. Further well-controlled research is needed to better define the nature of any such linguistic disruptions.

The role of cluttering spectrum behaviour within a lowest common denominator definition of cluttering

St. Louis and Schulte provide an elegant overview of a range of approaches that have been applied to the study of definitions of cluttering. One perspective briefly covered in their review is Ward's (2006, 2010) concept of cluttering spectrum behaviour (CSB). Briefly, CSB refers to the idea that while obvious cluttering may be readily observed when in pure and severe form, there may be a great number of speakers whose speech may be cluttering-like, but for whom clinicians might be uncertain about a diagnosis of cluttering. Ward (2010, p. 264) defines it thus:

> The term cluttering spectrum . . . can be defined as a speech/language output that is disrupted in a manner consistent with cluttering, but where there is a) insufficient severity; b) insufficient breadth of difficulties; or c) both, to warrant a diagnosis of cluttering.

It is important to emphasize that there are two components to this framework: one that recognizes potential differences in levels of severity and another that considers breadth of symptoms. St. Louis and Schulte imply that a spectrum approach to cluttering is not consistent with an LCD concept, but I do not believe this to be the case. Let me offer two hypothetical examples, one relating to each of the two strands of CSB to illustrate how the two concepts can co-exist to mutual advantage.

CSB and consideration of insufficient severity of symptoms for diagnosis

It is highly unlikely that any clinician, on observing those behaviours identified as 'core' by St. Louis and Schulte, would have a problem in diagnosing cluttering when these features are expressed to any reasonable and obvious extent. That is, such behaviour would clearly constitute cluttering, under both LCD and CSB perspectives. Let us now consider a second speaker whose rate is perceived to be overly fast, and produces some telescoping of words. The fast rate occurs only in certain naturalistic settings and the telescoping occurs infrequently, but noticeably within these naturalistic settings, also. This speaker would also fit the LCD definition, even if the output may not be identifiable as cluttering for perhaps 90 percent of the time under the clarifying point (St. Louis & Schulte, chapter 14 this volume):

> Cluttering must occur in naturalistic conversation, but it need not occur even a majority of the time. Clear but isolated examples that exceed those observed in normal speakers are sufficient for a diagnosis.
>
> (p. 242)

Let us finally take a third speaker who, like our second example, speaks quickly but only telescopes three or four words over the course of a day's speaking. This person might or might not fit the LCD definition, ultimately depending on one's interpretation of the meaning of the phrase 'examples that exceed those observed in normal speakers' (p. 242). By extension, this problem implicates the difficult notion of defining the extent of what might be considered 'within normal limits'. Of course, the same issue of what constitutes normal speech and language arises when diagnosing a range of speech and language disorders, not least in stuttering, which is often considered a close relative to cluttering. Core stuttering, such as blocking, can be differentiated from non stuttering disfluency with relative ease. A different situation arises with cluttering, where the disfluencies (by definition) are not stuttering-like, but many of which, instead, may be more commonly observed among those regarded to have speech within normal limits.

CSB and consideration of insufficient breadth of symptoms for diagnosis

Consider now the case of a person who presents with a speech output that is consistently both abnormally fast and highly irregular. This does not fit the LCD definition of cluttering, because it does not contain any of the additional features that are prerequisite. This case offers the reverse of the situation presented in the preceding section: namely, a speaker who has strong cluttering core symptoms, and whose speech output we might speculate would sound cluttered to a clinician. However, there are simply not enough symptoms to 'activate' the LCD diagnosis. Here again, we can suggest that this speaker might demonstrate CSB, although acknowledging that speech falls short of being considered cluttering.

Overlap of cluttering symptoms in multiple diagnoses: LCD and CSB perspectives

It is commonly agreed that cluttering symptoms (as defined by the LCD) can often appear in or alongside other disorders, some of which are speech- and language-based, and others that are behaviourally based, but have implications for speech and language functioning. (For recent perspectives, see Scaler Scott, chapter 8; Van Borsel, chapter 6; Van Zaalen et al. chapter 7, all this volume.) The relationship between cluttering and many of these disorders is unclear, however. St. Louis and Schulte clearly state that the LCD perspective has nothing to say about causality of the symptoms that are outlined. It simply comprises a method for diagnosing a range of speech symptoms under a banner of cluttering.

That perspective is perfectly reasonable, but it does leave a potential gap when describing the speech of someone who has a multiple speech/language diagnosis (Ward, 2010). Again, let us take a hypothetical speaker, this time a 12-year-old child, diagnosed with attention deficit hyperactivity disorder and autism spectrum disorder, who presents with a variety of speech and language disturbances, including high-level language processing problems, but whose speech also qualifies for an LCD definition of cluttering. While we may be certain under the LCD definition that this child is cluttering, we cannot be sure whether this individual (when the speech is taken alongside other communication problems) might better be described as a 'person with cluttering' or a person with a range of symptoms that include cluttering amongst others (see also Scaler Scott, chapter 8 this volume). With our presently limited understanding of what cluttering in essence actually is, this rather obscure distinction may appear a minor point of 'semantics'. Nevertheless, as knowledge about the neurology of cluttering as a stand-alone disorder develops (Alm, chapter 1 this volume; Van Zaalen, Ward et al., 2009), such differences will be of considerable importance when it comes to both the diagnosis and treatment of cluttering.

St. Louis and Schulte express concern over the potential dangers in taking a spectrum based approach, pointing out that 'because few limits are inherent in these classifications, spectrums can spread, with new variants being added without serious rationale or debate' (chapter 14 this volume). This concern might seem particularly pertinent with cluttering, where a considerable range of behaviours and attributes, both speech and non speech, have already been associated with it by some researchers (e.g., Weiss, 1964). Nonetheless, a spectrum approach to definition can be applied successfully to certain phenotypes. Autism comprises one such example where a disorder can be defined and diagnosed, but where it also makes sense to associate those with related but variant symptoms (or strength of symptoms) to the core behaviour through use of an 'umbrella', or spectrum, approach (autism spectrum disorder or autistic spectrum disorder [ASD], as recognised in the USA and UK, respectively). Migraine headache offers a further non-speech example. Despite the difficulties with qualitative definitions, both autism and migraine are recognized as bona-fide disorders or conditions, and continue to be studied scientifically. The idea is that CSB would be of similar use with respect to cluttering. The LCD definition would be taken as a starting point from which to trigger research in related areas, but in a principled manner, as St. Louis and Schulte suggest. Recall also that the LCD definition represents the latest of the 'working definitions', and as such, is likely to be subject to revision and change as more evidence is gathered. Areas of investigation that would be regarded as potential CSB would overlap with many attributes and features occurring just outside the core of St. Louis and Schulte's revised LCD figure (St. Louis & Schulte, chapter 14 this volume). It is important that the scope of CSB would itself need to be rigorously monitored, and any additions to the spectrum validated through data-driven studies.

Conclusions

St. Louis and Schulte's data-driven LCD definition provides the best attempt yet to clearly capture the key features of cluttering. There will always be problems in trying to reduce a disorder like cluttering to a binary decision; that is, diagnosing either 'cluttering' or 'not cluttering'. Severe cluttering, like severe stuttering, can easily be diagnosed. However, although even mild stuttering, once established, may readily be identified, the same cannot be said for cluttering when the symptoms are either less obvious or less prevalent (or both). Many features, including those identified in the LCD definition, can be seen to exist as a part of a spectrum existing between extremes that identify cluttering when severe, but may be seen as representative of the natural variability characteristic of 'normal' speech when mild.

References

Daly, D. A. (1986). The clutterer. In K. O. St. Louis (Ed.), *The atypical stutterer* (pp. 155–192). New York: Academic Press.

Daly, D. A. (1996). *The source for stuttering and cluttering*. East Moline, IL: LinguiSystems, Inc.

Daly, D., & Cantrell, R. P. (2006, July). *Cluttering: Characteristics labeled as diagnostically significant by 60 fluency experts*. Paper presented at the 6th IFA World Congress on disorders of fluency, Dublin, Ireland.

Myers, F. L. (1992). Cluttering: A synergistic framework. In F. L. Myers & K. O. St. Louis (Eds.), *Cluttering: A clinical perspective* (pp. 71–84). Leicester, UK: Far Communications. (Reissued in 1996 by Singular, San Diego, CA.)

St. Louis, K. O., & Myers, F. L. (1997). Management of cluttering and related fluency disorders. In R. Curlee & G. Siegel (Eds.), *Nature and treatment of stuttering: New directions* (pp. 313–332). New York: Allyn & Bacon.

St. Louis, K. O., Myers, F. L., Bakker, K., & Raphael, L. J. (2007). Understanding and treating cluttering. In E. G. Conture & R. F. Curlee (Eds.), *Stuttering and related disorders of fluency* (3rd ed., pp. 297–325). New York: Thieme.

St. Louis, K. O., Raphael, L., Myers, F. L., & Bakker, K. (2003, November). Cluttering updated. *The ASHA Leader, 8* (21), 4–5 & 20–23.

Van Zaalen, Y., Ward, D., Nederveen, A. J., Lameris, J. L., Wijnen, F., & Dejonckere, P. (2009). *Cluttering and stuttering: Different disorders and differing functional neurologies*. Presentation at fifth International Fluency Association congress, Rio de Janeiro.

Van Zaalen, Y., Wijnen, F., & Dejonckere, P. (2009). Language planning disturbances in children who clutter or have learning disabilities. *International Journal of Speech and Language Pathology*, *11*, 496–508.

Ward, D. (2006). *Stuttering and cluttering: Frameworks for understanding and treatment*. Hove, UK: Psychology Press.

Ward, D. (2010). Stuttering and normal nonfluency: Cluttering spectrum behaviour as a functional descriptor of abnormal fluency. In K. Bakker, L. Raphael, & F. Myers (Eds.), *Proceedings of the First World Conference on Cluttering, Katarino, Bulgaria* (pp. 261–267). http://associations.missouristate.edu/ICA

Weiss, D. A. (1964). *Cluttering*. Englewood Cliffs, NJ: Prentice-Hall.

16 International perspectives on perceiving, identifying, and managing cluttering

Isabella K. Reichel and
Juris G. Draguns

Introductory remarks

Cluttering as a discrete fluency disorder attained recognition in Europe earlier than it did in North America. Until recently, there was only intermittent and haphazard interaction among speech therapists and researchers concerned with cluttering in various countries and continents. Thus, developments in various parts of the world proceeded apace in partial or complete isolation. In 2007, when the International Cluttering Association (ICA) was founded, the intent to increase global interaction was made explicit. ICA was envisaged as a forum for communication, interaction, and eventual collaboration between researchers, speech therapists, persons with cluttering (PWC), and their families around the world. Its founding marked the potential beginning of a global effort dealing with cluttering as a worldwide phenomenon that may exhibit cultural nuances and features.

In this chapter, we take initial steps towards describing the unified and varied trends in cluttering. Specifically, we address: (1) past and current developments in the prevailing attitudes toward cluttering worldwide; (2) the characteristic modes of diagnosis of and intervention in cluttering; and (3) present and future activities of the ICA.

Historical origins and developments

Throughout history, references to cluttering have appeared in the literature around the world. Weiss (1964) noted that cluttering was 'discovered' by various authors at different points in history, and was given different names. In *The Problems*, Aristotle (1927) introduced three categories of articulatory impairments: *traylos*, corresponding to the inability to produce a particular letter; *psellos*, pertaining to the deletion of a particular letter or syllable; and *ischnophonos*, referring to the failure to join one syllable to another at a normal speed. According to O'Neill (1980), the Oxford translation renders the above three terms as 'hesitancy in speech', 'lisping', and 'stammering'. O'Neill noted that Aristotle's descriptions of articulatory problems did 'not correspond to the modern syndromes designated by these terms' (1980, p. 39). The Harvard University Press translation renders stammering as the 'inability to add quickly one syllable to another' (Aristotle, 1937, p. 275). Defective speakers are described as those who omit some sounds or syllables, and lisping is explained as the inability to control a certain letter. It is entirely possible that Aristotle was referring to what we now define as cluttering when he combined stammering, lisping, and defective speech in one category by saying 'all these disabilities are due to a failure of power' (1937, p. 275), and comparing the speech of people from the above category to the speech of 'a drunken and old man' (p. 275). In contemporary usage, Ward (2006) would possibly place such a disorder on the 'cluttering spectrum'. Cluttering is one of the oldest communication disorders, which at various points in history kept appearing and disappearing in medical and other writings without, however, leaving a continuous or cumulative record until modern times.

Weiss (1964) also pointed out that writers from various parts of the world used terms for describing symptoms of cluttering with a scientific or Latin nuance, such as *tumultus sermonis* (i.e., chaotic speech), *agitophasia* (i.e., excited speech), *tachyphemia* (i.e., quick speech), and *paraphrasia praeceps* (i.e., distorted speech formulation due to hurrying). *Poltern* is the German term for cluttering, describing a disorderly noise. *Bruddeln* is the North German term, which suggests noises emanating spontaneously. The Hungarian *hadaras* implies hurried speech, with resulting lack of clarity. *Tartajeo*, the Spanish term for cluttering, means general 'precipitous disorderliness' (Weiss, 1964, p. 15). The Italian *tartagliare* indicates repetitiousness. The French have several terms for varieties of cluttering: *bredouillement* means embarrassing and hurried speech; *balbutiement* refers to hesitation and repetition; *bafouillement* stands for talking in circles, and lacking the ability to get to the point; and *anonnement* refers to interjections of vowels of speakers who are searching for the next word. In German, these interjections of vowels are identified by the rarely used word *gaxen*. British speech therapists began to use the word cluttering in the second half of the 19th century, referring to disorderliness (Weiss, 1964). Examples of other terms for cluttering include *broddelen* (Dutch), *yu shu zhang ai* (Chinese), *løpsk tale* (Norwegian), *getkot* and *mova bezladna* (Polish), and *dibur hatuf* (Hebrew). The process of finding a term for the communication disorder cluttering in various countries around the world is still evolving. Just recently, the Indonesian representative to the ICA created a new word for cluttering, *graya*, and a Jordanian representative described cluttering by creating an equivalent for the word 'scramble' in Arabic.

In literature, characteristics of cluttering were fictionally portrayed in the character of Miss Bates in *Emma* by Jane Austen (1988). Bottomer (2007) observed that Miss Bates spoke rapidly, and lost control of her speech rate the longer she spoke. Her speeches were long and extremely exhausting for any listener to follow. She moved fast from topic to topic, used incomplete sentences, and had difficulties with sentence formulation. 'Full of thanks, and full of news, Miss Bates knew not which to give quickest' (Austen, 1988, p. 172).

In the 20th century, interest in cluttering originated in several locations in Europe, more or less simultaneously and, at first, in isolation. Concern with cluttering proceeded to spread to other continents, gradually attracting the attention of physicians and scientists in various parts of the world (Reichel, 2010). Many experts have observed that American texts have been less concerned with cluttering than international writings (Weiss, 1964), and that most of the foreign literature has not been translated into English (Simkins, 1973). St. Louis, Myers, Bakker, and Raphael (2007) contend that European logopedists, orthophonistes, and specialists in phoniatrics have been more interested in cluttering than their counterparts in North America due to the fact that the field of speech-language pathology in North America was previously under the influence of behavioral psychology and empiricism, disciplines that generally have been reluctant to recognize any disorder unless it has a clearly identifiable pattern. According to Georgieva (2010), the countries in which cluttering is recognized in Eastern and Central Europe are Russia, Czechoslovakia, the former East Germany (GDR), and Bulgaria. The countries in Western Europe that have a strong tradition in investigating cluttering are Germany, Norway, France, French-speaking Belgium, England, and Denmark. In North America, cluttering came to be recognized more or less simultaneously in Canada and the United States after the 1930s.

Perceptions of cluttering

Negative stereotyping of PWC

Dalton and Hardcastle (1993) noted that negative personality traits were attributed to PWC by several early experts in the field, sometimes hastily and on an impressionistic basis. At the interface of speech and personality, Khvatsev (1937) in Russia described vividly how sounds and words rumbled from clutterers' lips, madly chasing one another, mixed and confused, swallowed and unfinished. Each cascade of sounds and words is pronounced without taking a breath, until a lack of air leaves the person breathless and the speech rate gets to be so fast that there is no time to swallow saliva.

Froeschels (1946) portrayed the personality of PWC as careless, impulsive, messy, and forgetful. Freund (1966) described people who clutter as aggressive, expansive, explosive, extroverted, impulsive, uncontrolled, and hasty. Freund also found that clutterers' speech had a variety of negative effects on listeners, who often experienced tension, frustration, and confusion, and required intense concentration in order to be able to follow what the clutterer said. Weiss (1964) characterized the personality of the clutterer as a poor listener, impatient to vocalize his or her own thoughts, superficial, lacking consideration for other people and for the consequences of his or her behavior. He noted that PWC take the lead in dialogue, and disregard thoughts and feelings of other people. They annoy people by their insensitivity and childlike egocentricity. Weiss also observed that adolescents who clutter tend to be angry, perhaps due to their persistent failures in school. They are described as worried, frustrated, short-tempered, explosive, and unmanageable at home.

Ward (2006) cautioned, however, that personalities of clutterers have not been rigorously, systematically, or objectively researched. Based on his experiences with many of his clients, Ward believes that inattentiveness and poor self-monitoring can lead to poor listening skills, thereby causing misunderstandings and inappropriate responses. According to Dalton and Hardcastle, '[L]isteners are usually spared the anxiety transmitted by many stutterers, but they often produce their own in their effort to grasp the clutterer's meaning' (1993, p. 127). Dalton and Hardcastle believe that the negative stereotypes of PWC have never been substantiated.

Early contributors to the study of cluttering based their impressions about the personalities of PWC solely on clinical observation. Their impressions represent an amalgam of observed behaviors confounded with the reactions to the stress of communicating, and negative expectations by their interlocutors. Mullet acknowledged forerunners in the field of speech pathology who, '[by seeking] to loosen the tongue . . . sought also to untie the mind' (1971, p. 149). He felt that they 'reflected the compelling and manifold urges of their time' (p. 149). Times, however, have changed. More people now realize that negative stereotyping, prejudice, and stigma result in pain, hurt, and hatred. This destructive potential may be virtually universal, even though it exhibits considerable variation across historical periods, countries, and cultures (Reichel & St. Louis, 2007).

Public awareness of cluttering

Pireira, Rossi, and Van Borsel (2008) posited that the awareness of a communication disorder may determine the attitude toward the person affected by it. In order to assess the awareness of cluttering and stuttering, an Experimental Edition of the Public Opinion Survey of Human Attributes (POSHA-E) was distributed to the general public in the United States, Russia, Bulgaria, and Turkey (St. Louis et al., 2010). The questionnaire included lay-oriented definitions of cluttering and stuttering. The participants were asked to name seven individuals who presented with either stuttering or cluttering. Next, the participants were requested to provide age, sex, relation to them, severity of the disorder, and coexisting disorders for every person named. The survey also requested respondents' opinions, beliefs, feelings, and reactions toward both fluency disorders.

Within the survey, 40 percent of the total fluency disorders identified by the respondents were combined cases of cluttering-stuttering, and 60 percent of the fluency disorders were cases of stuttering. Respondents from the four countries viewed cluttering and stuttering as different fluency disorders, and took the position that both of these disorders may coexist. However, when given a description of both disorders, people recognized cluttering as well as stuttering, which contradicted the prevailing impression that stuttering is better known than cluttering. The most common comorbid syndrome in children and adults with both cluttering and stuttering was believed to be attention deficit hyperactivity disorder. Other comorbid communication disorders reported were language disorders, articulation disorders, and unspecified conditions.

Public attitudes about cluttering

The negative image of PWC has not been entirely overcome to this day (Green, 1999). When having a conversation with a PWC, the listener may be annoyed and stop listening, due to the speaker's compulsive talkativeness, poor articulation, monotonous tone, and/or endless flow of 'verbal drive' (Simkins, 1973). Some of the negative beliefs and stereotypes can run across countries and cultures, while others, especially in non-Western countries, are culture-specific, notably those that attribute illnesses and disorders to an 'act of God' or 'ghosts, demons, or spirits' (Al-Khaledi, Lincoln, McCabe, Packman, & Alshatti, 2009; St. Louis et al., 2007).

A survey of attitudes of the general public toward cluttering and stuttering in the USA, Turkey, Russia, and Bulgaria (St. Louis et al., in press) was conducted simultaneously with the companion survey of public awareness described above. In the survey, the POSHA-E was also utilized in order to compare both disorders with eight other human conditions considered to be positive, neutral, and negative. The respondents from all four countries participating in this survey viewed cluttering and stuttering similarly. Both disorders were viewed as negatively as being overweight, using a wheelchair, or having a mental illness; more negatively than being older or left handed; and significantly more negatively than being intelligent, multilingual, or a good talker. The most likely suspected causes for cluttering were believed to be psychological and related factors, as, for example, emotional trauma and tension at home; however, all of these causes were believed to be less influential than for stuttering. In addition, there was a lack of a total rejection of the idea that cluttering is caused by a virus or a disease, or an 'act of God', ghosts, demons, or spirits. Results indicate the presence of negative stigma toward cluttering and stuttering in all four countries. Negative opinions were also expressed about the ability of PWC to work in jobs requiring a significant amount of talking and/or responsibility. Respondents also expressed the belief that PWC may be nervous, excitable, fearful, or shy. Such responses confirm a negative stereotype resembling the well-known negative stereotype toward people who stutter. Selected examples of attitudes of the respondents from the four countries toward cluttering are presented below.

Americans were least likely to attribute cluttering to a genetic cause, an 'act of God', demons, or spirits. The Russians indicated that they would feel surprise should they be confronted with speaking to a PWC. Feelings of pity, fear, and concern about cluttering by neighbors, doctors, or religious leaders were highest among the Turks. Turks were also the most comfortable around PWC, and the most optimistic about PWC holding jobs that require a lot of talking. Bulgarians were least likely to report feeling embarrassed, impatient, annoyed, angry, or pitiful when talking with a PWC. They had the highest concern if they or their son or daughter had cluttering. To an unknown degree, the responses obtained in the survey by St. Louis et al. (2007) may have been affected by social desirability, which may have been defined differently in the four countries. Overall, general differences in attitudes across countries and languages appeared to be more substantial than specific differences in attitudes toward stuttering and cluttering.

Awareness of cluttering by speech therapists in countries around the world

The term 'speech therapists' as used in this chapter identifies those who diagnose and treat communication disorders. Speech therapists may be referred to by various job titles, such as speech-language pathologists, logopedists, orthophonistes, etc., depending on the country and language of origin (Reichel & Bakker, 2009). Historically and currently, awareness of the existence of cluttering and/or of the methods for diagnosing and treating it is limited among speech therapists. Surveys of speech therapists' awareness suggest that cluttering is generally familiar, but not thoroughly well-known, in the United States (St. Louis & Hinzman, 1988) and in the United Kingdom (St. Louis & Rustin, 1986). Responses to these surveys indicate that speech therapists felt uncertainty and lacked confidence in planning and carrying out therapy for clients with cluttering. Another questionnaire was given to speech therapists in Bulgaria, Greece, Great Britain, and the United States, specifically inquiring about 'cluttering' as distinct from 'stuttering' (Georgieva, 2004). Results indicated that speech therapists were well acquainted with the symptoms and the etiology of cluttering, but lacked a clear understanding of the differences and similarities between cluttering and stuttering, and had little experience with applying therapeutic techniques in clinical situations. Bulgarian and Greek speech therapists were more uncertain, especially about the choice of therapeutic procedures for cluttering. Speech therapists in all four countries reported not feeling adequately prepared and fearful of working with PWC, due to weak academic preparation, lack of clinical experience, and insufficient published information. More recently, a nine-question International Cluttering Survey (ICS) of 25 international representatives of the ICA (many of whom were speech therapists with a special interest in cluttering) was conducted (Reichel & Bakker, 2009). Of the 25 representatives surveyed, 10 (Australia, Belgium,

Bulgaria, Canada, Denmark, England, Faroe Islands, Israel, Sweden, and the USA) reported that, in their countries, speech therapists are aware of cluttering, but do not consider themselves competent to recognize its symptoms, diagnose it, or provide treatment. Speech therapists were reported to lack awareness of cluttering in eight countries (Argentina, Indonesia, Japan, Lithuania, Netherlands, Russia, Sudan, and Thailand). Speech therapists were reported to be well aware of cluttering in seven countries (China, Germany, Iceland, India, Ireland, Nigeria, and Norway).

Identifying cluttering

Op't Hof and Uys (1974) and Langova and Moravek (1970) posit that identifying cluttering has always been a challenge, since most people who present this disorder do not consider its manifestations to be pathological, nor do they seek professional help. Wolk (1986) acknowledged frequent disagreement about the symptomatology for the diagnosis of cluttering, thus further complicating identification of PWC. St. Louis (1992) insisted on the importance of identifying specific symptoms of cluttering in order to diagnose and differentiate it from other disorders.

Definitions of cluttering across nations

According to Weiss, 'cluttering is one of the most important disorders, not only of speech, but of language and communication in general' (1964, p. xi). Definitions of cluttering are based on clinical observations, experiences, and impressions rather than on research or systematic theory (see also Preus, 1996; St. Louis & Myers, 1997; St. Louis & Schulte, chapter 14 this volume). There is a wide variety of definitions of cluttering, due to the heterogeneous nature of this disorder (Op't Hof & Uys, 1974). According to St. Louis (1992) and Bakker (1996), the lack of an adequate universally accepted definition of cluttering has impeded research, and has interfered with the development of successful clinical procedures.

In describing cluttering, most of the pioneers consider it to result from the disassociation between thinking and speaking (De Hirsch, 1970), with speakers racing 'ahead of themselves' (Weiss, 1968, p. 708), and experiencing a feeling of incongruity between the urge to express an idea and the need to convey it through speech. Cluttering occurs, Froeschels (1946) contended, when the speech rate is faster than the thought process. Weiss (1964) divided symptoms of cluttering into obligatory (present in every case), facultative (may or may not occur), and associated (comorbid, i.e., symptoms accompanying but not specific to cluttering diagnosis). According to Weiss, an excessive number of repetitions of syllables and words, a lack of awareness of the speech problem, inadequate attention and concentration, perceptual weakness, and disorganized thinking are obligatory symptoms. Facultative symptoms include tachylalia, interjections, stopping before producing an initial vowel, articulatory and motor impairment, grammatical deficit, monotonous quality, jerky respiration, and delays in the development of speech. Associated symptoms encompass a wide range of comorbid symptoms, such as reading and writing difficulties, deficit in rhythmic and musical skills, restlessness and hyperactivity. More recently, Ward (2006) suggested using the term 'cluttering spectrum behavior' (CSB) to describe those people who exhibit the symptoms of cluttering, but who do not present a strong case for cluttering.

To gather information on the more recent use of cluttering definitions, a question about them was included in the aforementioned ICS (Reichel & Bakker, 2009). Out of the 25 respondents, 13 (Argentina, Australia, Belgium, Bulgaria, Canada, China, Denmark, Faroe Islands, India, Ireland, Israel, Japan, and Nigeria) stated that in their countries there were no unique definitions of cluttering. The definition proposed by St. Louis et al. (2007; see also St. Louis & Schulte, chapter 14 this volume) was used in six countries: Germany, Great Britain, the Netherlands, Norway, Russia, and Thailand. Six representatives presented definitions of cluttering that originated in their respective countries, namely Germany, Indonesia, the Netherlands, Russia, Sudan, and the United States. In Norway, several definitions were used in the literature, including that of Weiss (1964) and Daly (1992). Icelandic and Swedish representatives reported that their countries use the following definition of cluttering:

> A rapid rate of speech with breakdown in fluency, but no repetitions or hesitations, of a severity to give rise to diminished speech intelligibility. Speech is erratic and disrhythmic, with rapid jerky spurts that usually involve faulty phrasing patterns.
>
> (World Health Organization, 2007, F98.6)

Differentiating cluttering from stuttering

Van Riper wrote that confusion between cluttering and stuttering has persisted in the field of speech pathology since the 'proverbial pre-dawn darkness' (1970, p. 347). Historically, cluttering was considered to be the same phenomenon as stuttering (Georgieva, 2010; Van Riper, 1970). However, several pioneering contributors from Germany (De Hirsch, 1970; Freund, 1966; Froeschels, 1946) and Austria (Weiss, 1964) who later worked in the United States believed that stuttering is caused by cluttering. De Hirsch (1970) maintained that children with cluttering-like behavior whose linguistic systems are disorganized and immature tend to become stutterers as a result of emotional conflict and stress. Eisenson (1986) identified cluttering as a 'cousin' of stuttering, with both disorders coming from the same family tree. In his view, differentiating between these two fluency disorders is hampered by the lack of an empiric, universally agreed on definition of cluttering.

According to Georgieva (2010), empirical studies in Eastern Europe have not unequivocally confirmed that cluttering exists separately from stuttering, although some attempts to differentiate the two disorders were undertaken in Russia and the Czech Republic. Missulovin (2002) traced the first reference to cluttering in Russia to 1889, when Sikorsky reported 32.5 percent of children in his clinic were combined cluttering-stuttering cases. Sikorsky described cluttering as stuttering of organic origin. In Western Europe, studies to differentiate cluttering and stuttering have been conducted in England, Germany, and Norway (Georgieva, 2010).

Assessment of cluttering

Preus (1996) noted that the lack of a clear definition of cluttering and its symptoms complicates the assessment of this disorder. A recent guide for assessment of cluttering was created by a collaborative effort of the ICA clinical committee. The primary contributors to this guide represented the Netherlands, the United States, and Great Britain (Van Zaalen-op't Hof, Myers, Ward, & Bennett, 2009). This committee acknowledges that PWC may exhibit a variety of speech and language symptoms, although the extent to which some of these may be central to the core diagnosis of cluttering remains under review (see St. Louis & Schulte, chapter 14 this volume; Ward, chapter 15 this volume). The assessment of cluttering includes the evaluation of the severity of the disorder along several parameters, encompassing the case history, assessment of fluency and speech rate, speech and language abilities, and cognitive/academic skills.

Additional instruments available to assess cluttering around the world include a Predictive Cluttering Inventory (PCI) (Daly, 2007), a Checklist of Cluttering Behavior developed by Ward (2006), and a Cluttering Assessment Program (CLASP) (Bakker, St. Louis, Myers, & Raphael, 2005). There is also a measure of Speech Motor Control at the word level (SPA Test; Van Zaalen-op't Hof, Wijnen, & Dejonckere, 2009) that originated in the Netherlands. In international surveys, clinicians have proposed the development of a screening instrument for cluttering, a checklist for cluttering for teachers in special education classes, and the creation of instruments differentiating stuttering from cluttering, as well as improvement of diagnostic tools in general (Georgieva, 2004; Reichel & Bakker, 2009).

Cultural and bilingual considerations in assessment of cluttering

Weiss (1964) emphasized the importance of the environment in the prevalence of cluttering. He ventured the hypothesis that cluttering is more prevalent than, stuttering in the warm southern countries with socially outgoing people, and stuttering occurs more frequently than cluttering in cold northern countries. He believed that blacks and 'temperamental Latins' in Europe, and South Americans also had a higher incidence of cluttering.

Dalton and Hardcastle (1993) pointed out that their bilingual clients with cluttering in India and Pakistan showed some rhythmic noncluttering patterns of their first language. Moreover, Dalton and Hardcastle's Asian clients were found to present cluttering patterns of speech more frequently than stuttering. It is well worth reiterating that these theories are based on clinical observation rather than empirical evidence. Dalton and Hardcastle suggest reexamining clutterers' first languages in order to adjust treatment strategies to their clients' particular problems. They also recommend assessing the relationship between the types of disfluencies presented by speakers of different languages and the characteristics of those languages, such as rhythm and articulatory patterns. According to Hernandez (2009), switching between languages results in a more effortful cognitive retrieval process. These increased demands may bring changes in symptoms of bilingual speakers with cluttering.

Managing cluttering

Treatment of cluttering around the world

Treatment of individuals with 'pure' cluttering is almost never discussed in the literature due to people with pure cluttering lacking awareness of the problem and not seeking help (Preus, 1996). Daly (1993) stated that the problems of PWC are as unique as the configuration of a snowflake. Therefore, management of cluttering is particularly challenging. Experts in the field have made treatment recommendations based on their clinical experiences. De Hirsch (1970) believed that clients with a predominance of cluttering over stuttering had a better prognosis. Froeschels (1946) claimed that every cluttering patient he treated was cured in a 3- to 6-month period. Froeschels suggested that the preferred treatment of PWC is to coordinate the thought and speech phases. Considering that the speech phase is more accessible than the thought phase, the author recommended that the patient be taught to control the rate of speech and articulation. Froeschels suggested the strengthening of kinesthetic speech, using a series of alphabetic drawings of the speech mechanism (teeth, lips, tongue, nose) and their position while pronouncing specific sounds. The patient is requested to transcribe written passages into this phonetic alphabet three times a day. In Belgium, Mussafia (1970) described the treatment of cluttering by correcting the pronunciation of each phoneme. His clients were taught to slow down their rate of speech and 'to read slowly and calmly, syllable by syllable and word by word' (1970, p. 339). Clients were also asked to tell a story back in a 'colorful' manner. The language and reading were practiced in a rhythmic way, with accentuation of syllables or words.

In the former Soviet Union, speech pathology was a part of what was called the field of defectology. Defectology overlaps with learning disabilities and the area of abnormal psychology that deals with visual, hearing, language, and communication deficits. Based on the responses to a questionnaire that was presented to 27 clinicians from Croatia, the Czech Republic, Estonia, Lithuania, Poland, Russia, Slovakia, and Slovenia, fluency disorders are treated by means of what in Eastern Europe is called the 'complex method'. It comprises physiotherapy, behavioral therapy, speech therapy, music therapy, remedial gymnastics, logorhythmics, breathing exercises, and medical treatment (Fibiger, Peters, Euler, & Neumann, 2008). Filatova (1997) described her goals in treating PWC as addressing rate-rhythm organization as well as impaired attention, motor-visual, and audio-verbal memory types. Her goals are as follows:

1 Development of psychological functioning: attention, motor, visual, and audio-verbal memory.
2 Development of rate-rhythmical characteristic of speech movements.
3 Development of planning of expressive language.
4 Specialized pedagogical work directed at sequencing of the actions, teaching self-control, and facilitating appropriate social behavior.

Affective and cognitive aspects of cluttering

Affective and cognitive aspects of cluttering have not yet been extensively considered in the international literature. Several authors (Bennett, 2006; Dalton & Hardcastle, 1993; Daly, 1986, 1993; Daly & Burnett, 1999) are in agreement in emphasizing that PWC may respond to their failure to speak clearly and to be understood by experiencing anxiety, frustration (Dalton & Hardcastle, 1993), negative thoughts (Daly, 1986, 1993), nervousness, sadness, and low self-esteem (Reichel, 2010). In Norway, Green (1999) proposed that clinicians consider providing positive psycho-social conditions in order to improve PWC's fluency and self-monitoring skills. Canadian clinicians Langevin and Boberg (1996) included cognitive-behavioral skills training in order to change attitudes, perceptions, and self confidence of cluttering-stuttering clients.

In the United States, Daly (1986, 1993) proposed a combination of cognitive training, counseling, attitude change, relaxation, affirmation training, and positive self-talk in working with PWC. Reichel (2010) adapted Bar-On's (2000) 10 emotional intelligence (EI) competencies for the use of clinicians who work with PWC. Individuals with a preponderance of cluttering-like symptoms are introduced to the following five skills: (1) emotional self-awareness; (2) impulse control; (3) reality testing; (4) empathy; and (5) interpersonal relationships. Such training is designed to improve the awareness of emotions and communication behaviors, to facilitate the ability to manage emotions for achieving self-control, to cognitively process emotions, to realistically assess situations, to consider the feelings of listeners, and to maximize clients' ability to give and receive emotional closeness in relationships, which in turn may result in increased responsibility for meeting expectations.

Challenges in managing cluttering in countries with a dearth of speech pathologists

In a recent survey of professionals from ten countries with a limited number of speech therapists (Reichel, Myers, & Bakker, 2010), the respondents identified the following challenges in managing cluttering in their countries: a shortage of effective evidence-based treatment and universal protocol of the diagnosis; lack of epidemiological data (Brazil); a limited number of professionals who are competent in cluttering (China, Indonesia, Japan, Jordan, and Nigeria); very little awareness about cluttering (China, India, Jordan); absence of theoretical and practical knowledge (India, Lithuania, Poland); difficulty in bringing awareness about cluttering to the client, and low motivation in the client (India); people do not look for help due to the high cost and long distances (Nigeria); the concept of cluttering is complex, and etiology includes many psychological and biological factors (Poland and Sudan); inability to acquire adequate support from specialized entities; lack of enough centers and the prohibitive cost of tuition for university students (Sudan).

Present and future of the ICA

The ICA emerged from a confluence of scholarly, clinical, and consumer communities, with the primary goals of increasing the awareness and understanding of cluttering as well as improving diagnosis and treatment in all parts of the world. The ICA now has representatives from 43 countries, circulates a newsletter, and maintains a website (www.associations.missouristate.edu/ICA), which is partially translated into several languages, including Arabic, Bulgarian, Chinese, German, Dutch, Indonesian, Russian, and Spanish. The ICA has also initiated active committees, and has generated a collaborative network of researchers, clinicians, and activists from among PWC and their families worldwide. Various research projects, seminars, and publications on cluttering are conducted under the aegis of the ICA. Continuation of such multinational initiatives is an ongoing mission of the ICA (Reichel & Ehrle Ray, 2008).

Conclusion

Cluttering has been observed in various regions of the world, and efforts to remediate it have originated in a variety of locations. In this review, we have taken stock of observations pertaining to cluttering from a wide variety of cultures and have shared the results of early, nonrepresentative and non-random surveys related to awareness and attitudes toward, incidence and manifestations of, and management of cluttering across nations. The surface has barely been scratched, but the door has been opened for a more systematic information exchange on a larger scale. The field may then proceed from informants to samples and from samples based on availability to those based on randomness and representativeness. A network of professionals has been established who are willing to pool and exchange information and eventually to collaborate in the implementation of systematic multinational research projects. Focused, hypothesis-testing investigations can be designed and executed across language barriers and national boundaries. Procedures developed in a particular locale can be tested in another part of the world, and treatment successes, as well as failures, can be rapidly disseminated for teaching and clinical purposes.

A major objective of international research on cluttering is to study it in its sociocultural contexts. To that end, the following lines of research are proposed:

1 Qualitatively, contextual descriptions of cluttering in the families, communities, and institutions of various countries should be provided, somewhat along the lines proposed by the social psychiatrist, Kleinman (1991). Specifically, information is to be sought about the social idioms of expressing distress associated with cluttering and about the cultural conceptions concerning the origin and consequences of this disorder.
2 Quantitatively, studies should be conducted about the incidence, prevalence, and manifestations of cluttering in as many countries around the world as feasible. On the basis of the findings on psychopathology across cultures (Draguns & Tanaka-Matsumi, 2001), the prediction is ventured that the incidence of cluttering would vary minimally across cultures. Facultative and associated symptoms of cluttering may, however, show a greater range of variation, and some stylistic aspects of remediation and therapy may also vary across cultures.
3 The suggestion by Weiss (1964) that cluttering is associated with extraversion should be empirically investigated. Extraversion-introversion has emerged as one of the fundamental ‘Big Five’ personality traits that, moreover, has been extensively researched and cross-culturally compared (McCrea & Allik, 2002).
4 Across cultures, the factorially based and intensively investigated dimension of individualism-collectivism (Hofstede & Hofstede, 2005) may be germane to cluttering. Are the manifestations of cluttering different in North America and Western Europe where individualism prevails, and in cultures that tend toward collectivism, such as those of Russia, Japan, Mexico, or India?
5 Caution is indicated in imputing uniform personality characteristics to people who clutter, within and across cultures. Cultural and personality

characteristics related to cluttering should be noted, but they should not be dichotomized nor reified. There is an urgent need for well-documented case studies of atypical PWC who differ from many of their counterparts within a given sociocultural milieu.

6 A combination of flexibility and rigor is called for, together with a readiness to pool and alternate between clinical and research data, to shift one's focus from a unique case to a panorama of quantitative findings, and vice versa, to accommodate unexpected observations, and to integrate disparate data.
7 Further research is needed highlighting the issues of bilingualism and differences across languages and cultures in relation to symptoms of cluttering.

References

Al-Khaledi, M., Lincoln, M., McCabe, P., Packman, A., & Alshatti, T. (2009). The attitudes, knowledge and beliefs of Arab parents in Kuwait about stuttering. *Journal of Fluency Disorders*, *34*, 44–59.

Aristotle. (1927). *Problemata* (Prob.), XI, 30, 02b (translated by E. S. Forster). Oxford, UK: Oxford University Press.

Aristotle. (1937). *Rhetorica ad Alexandrum* (translated by H. Rackham). Cambridge, MA: Harvard University Press.

Austen, J. (1988). *Emma*. In R.W. Chapman (Ed.) (3rd ed.). Oxford, UK: Oxford University Press.

Bakker, K. (1996). Cluttering: Current scientific status and emerging research and clinical needs. *Journal of Fluency Disorders*, *21*, 359–365.

Bakker, K., St. Louis, K. O., Myers, F., & Raphael, L. (2005). *A freeware software tool for determining aspects of cluttering severity*. Annual National Convention of the American Speech Language and Hearing Association, San Diego, CA.

Bar-On, R. (2000). Emotional and social intelligence: Insights from the emotional quotient inventory. In R. Bar-On & J. D. A. Parker (Eds.), *The handbook of emotional intelligence* (pp. 363–388). San Francisco, CA: Jossey-Bass.

Bennett, E. M. (2006). *Working with people who stutter: A lifespan approach*. Upper Saddle River, NJ: Pearson Merrill Prentice Hall.

Bottomer, P. F. (2007). A speech language pathologist journeys to Highbury. *Persuasions: The Jane Austen Journal*. http://www.articlearchives.com/science-technology/behavior-cognition-psychology/957029-1.html

Dalton, P., & Hardcastle, W. (1993). *Disorders of fluency* (2nd ed.). London: Whurr.

Daly, D. (1992). Helping the clutterer: Therapy considerations. In F. Myers & K. St. Louis (Eds.), *Cluttering: A clinical perspective* (pp. 107–124). Leicester, UK: Far Communications.

Daly, D. (1993). Treatment strategies for the cluttering syndrome: Planning your work and working your plan. *Clinical Connection*, *3*, 6–9.

Daly, D. (2007). *Cluttering: Characteristics identified as diagnostically significant by 60 fluency experts.* 10th International Stuttering Awareness Day Online Conference [J. Kuster, Conference Chair], Minnesota State University, Mankato. http://www.mnsu.edu/comdis/isad10/isadcon.html

Daly, D. A. (1986). The clutterer. In K. St. Louis (Ed.), *The atypical stutterer: Principles and practice of rehabilitation* (pp. 155–192). New York: Academic Press.

Daly, D. A., & Burnett, M. L. (1999). Cluttering: Traditional views and new perspectives. In R. F. Curlee (ed.), *Stuttering and disorders of fluency* (2nd ed., pp. 222–254). New York: Thieme.

De Hirsch, K. (1970). Stuttering and cluttering. Developmental aspects of dysrhythmic speech. *Folia Phoniatrica*, *22*, 311–324.

Draguns, J. G., & Tanaka-Matsumi, J. (2001). Assessment of psychopathology across and within cultures: Issues and findings. *Behaviour Research and Therapy*, *41*, 755–776.

Eisenson, J. (1986). Dysfluency disorders: Cluttering and stuttering. In A. Goldstein, L. Krasner, & S. Garfeld (Eds.), *Language and speech disorders in children* (pp. 57–75). New York: Pergamon Press.

Fibiger, S., Peters, H. F. M., Euler, H. A., & Neumann, K. (2008). Health and human services for persons who stutter and education of logopedists in East European countries. *Journal of Fluency Disorders*, *33*, 66–71.

Filatova, Y. O. (1997). *Cluttering*. Moscow: Prometey (in Russian).

Freund, H. (1966). *Psychopathology and the problems of stuttering*. Springfield, IL: Charles C. Thomas.

Froeschels, E. (1946). Cluttering. *Journal of Speech Disorders*, *11*, 31–33.

Georgieva, D. (2004). Professional awareness of cluttering: A comparative study (Part Two). In H.-G. Bosshardt, J. S. Yaruss, & H. F. Peters (Eds.), *Fluency disorders: Theory, research, treatment, and self-help: Proceedings of the Fourth World Congress on Fluency Disorders* (pp. 630–634). International Fluency Association, Katarino, Bulgaria.

Georgieva, D. (2010). Understanding cluttering: Eastern European traditions vs. Western European and North American traditions. In K. Bakker & L. Raphael (Eds.), *Proceedings of the First International Conference on Cluttering, Katarino, Bulgaria* (pp. 230–243). http://associations.missouristate.edu/ICA

Green, T. (1999). The cluttering problem: A short review and a critical comment. *Logopedics Phoniatrics Vocology*, *24*, 145–153.

Hernandez, A. E. (2009). Language switching in the bilingual brain: What's next? *Brain and Language*, *109*, 133–140.

Hofstede, G., & Hofstede, G. J. (2005). *Cultures and organizations. Software of the mind. International cooperation and its importance* (2nd ed.). New York: McGraw Hill.

Khvatsev, M. E. (1937). *Logopedia*. Moscow: State Educational Publisher (in Russian).

Kleinman, A. (1991). *Rethinking psychiatry: From cultural category to personal experience*. New York: Free Press.

Langevin, M., & Boberg, E. (1996). Results of intensive stuttering therapy with adults who clutter and stutter. *Journal of Fluency Disorders*, *21*, 315–327.

Langova, J., & Moravek, M. (1970). Some problems of cluttering. *Folia Phoniatrica*, *22*, 325–336.

McCrea, R. R., & Allik, J. (Eds.) (2002). *The five-factor model of personality across cultures*. New York: Kluwer Academic/Plenum.

Missulovin (2002). *Patomorphos on stuttering*. St. Petersburg: Soyuz (in Russian).

Mullet, C. F. (1971). 'An arte to make the dumbe speake, the deafe to heare': A seventeenth-century goal. *Journal of the History of Medicine and Allied Sciences*, *26*, 123–140.

Mussafia, M. (1970). Various aspects of cluttering. *Folia Phoniatrica*, *22*, 337–346.

O'Neill, Y. V. (1980). *Speech and speech disorders in Western Europe thought before 1600*. Westport, CT: Greenwood Press.

Op't Hof, J., & Uys, I. C. (1974). A clinical delineation of tachyphemia (cluttering): A case of dominant inheritance. *South African Medical Journal*, *48*, 1624–1628.

Pireira, M. M. de B., Rossi, J. P., & Van Borsel, J. (2008). Public awareness and knowledge of stuttering in Rio de Janeiro. *Journal of Fluency Disorders*, *33*, 24–31.

Preus, A. (1996). Cluttering upgraded. *Journal of Fluency Disorders*, *21*, 349–357.

Reichel, I., Myers, F. L., & Bakker, K. (2010). *Worldwide panorama on cluttering: non-western countries, the first online cluttering conference—it's about time: to recognize cluttering* [J. Kuster, Conference Chair. Minnesota State University, Mankato http://www.mnsu.edu/comdis/]

Reichel, I. K. (2010). Treating the person who clutters and stutters. In K. Bakker, L. Raphael, & F. Myers (Eds.), *Proceedings of the First World Conference on Cluttering* (pp. 99–107). Katarino, Bulgaria. International Cluttering Association.

Reichel, I. K., & Bakker, K. (2009). Global landscape on cluttering. *Perspectives on Fluency and Fluency Disorders*, *19* (2), 62–66. Special Interest Division 4, Fluency and Fluency Disorders, American Speech-Language-Hearing Association (ASHA).

Reichel, I. K., & Ehrle Ray, A. (2008). The ICA adopts the cluttering orphan. *Perspectives on Fluency and Fluency Disorders*, *18*(2), 84–86. Special Interest Division 4, Fluency and Fluency Disorders, American Speech-Language-Hearing Association (ASHA).

Reichel, I. K., & St. Louis, K. O. (2007). Mitigating negative stereotyping of stuttering in a fluency disorders class. In J. Au-Yeung, & M. Leahy (Eds.), *Research, treatment, and self-help in fluency disorders: New horizons: Proceedings of the Fifth World Congress on Fluency Disorders* (pp. 236–244), Dublin, Ireland. International Fluency Association.

Sikorsky, E. A. (1889). *About stuttering*. Moscow: CPb (in Russian).

Simkins, L. (1973). Cluttering. In B. B. Lahey (Ed.), *The modification of language behavior* (pp. 178–217). Springfield, IL: Charles C. Thomas.

St. Louis, K. O. (1992). On defining cluttering. In F. L. Myers & K. O. St. Louis (Eds.), *Cluttering: A clinical perspective* (pp. 37–53). San Diego, CA: Singular.

St. Louis, K. O., Filatova, Y., Coşkun, M., Topbaş, S., Özdemir, S., Georgieva, D. et al. (2010). Identification of cluttering and stuttering by the public in four countries. *International Journal of Speech-Language Pathology*, *12*, 508–519.

St. Louis, K. O., Filatova, Y., Coşkun, M., Topbaş, S., Özdemir, S., Georgieva, D. et al. (in press). Public attitudes toward cluttering and stuttering in four countries. In F. Columbus (Ed.), *Psychology of stereotypes*. Hauppauge, NY: Nova Science Publishers.

St. Louis, K. O., & Hinzman, A. R. (1988). A descriptive study of speech, language, and hearing characteristics in school-aged stutterers. *Journal of Fluency Disorders*, *13*, 331–355.

St. Louis, K. O., & Myers, F. L. (1997). Management of cluttering and related fluency disorders. In R. F. Curlee & G. M. Siegel (Eds.), *Nature and treatment of stuttering: New directions* (2nd ed., pp. 313–332). Boston, MA: Allyn & Bacon.

St. Louis, K. O., Myers, F. L., Bakker, K., & Raphael, L. J. (2007). Understanding and treating of cluttering. In E. G. Conture & R. F. Curlee (Eds.), *Stuttering and related disorders of fluency* (pp. 297–325). Stuttgart: Thieme.

St. Louis, K. O. & Rustin, L. (1986). Professional awareness of cluttering. In F. L. Myers & K. O. St. Louis (Eds.), *Cluttering: A clinical perspective* (pp. 23–35). San Diego, CA: Singular.

Van Riper, C. (1970). Stuttering and cluttering: The differential diagnosis. *Folia Phoniatrica, 22*, 347–353.

Van Zaalen-op't Hof, Y., Myers, F., Ward, D., & Bennett, E. (2009). *Cluttering assessment*. Retrieved from http://associations.missouristate.edu/ica/resources/cluttering_assessment.htm

Van Zaalen-op't Hof, Y., Wijnen, F., & Dejonckere, P. (2009). A test of speech motor control on word level productions: The SPA Test (Dutch: Screening Pittige Articulatie). *International Journal of Speech-Language Pathology, 11*, 26–33.

Ward, D. (2006). *Stuttering and cluttering*. Hove, UK: Psychology Press.

Weiss, D. A. (1964). *Cluttering*. Englewood Cliffs, NJ: Prentice-Hall.

Weiss, D. A. (1968). Cluttering: central language imbalance. *Pediatric Clinics of North America, 15*, 705–720.

Wolk, L. (1986). Cluttering: A diagnostic case report. *British Journal of Disorders of Communication, 21*, 199–207.

World Health Organization. 2007. *ICD-10*. Available at: www.who.int/classifications/apps/icd/icd10online

17 Cluttering in the academic curriculum

John A. Tetnowski and Jill Douglass

Introduction

A review of the largest on-line booksellers reveals at least 51 textbooks have been published on the topic of stuttering. Of the top 20 textbooks likely to be used as a textbook for a graduate course in fluency disorders (this was determined by eliminating biographies on stuttering, research on a single topic of fluency, books over 20 years old, and workbooks on a single philosophy), 6 of the texts have a single chapter related specifically to cluttering, and 3 more have a chapter on 'related fluency disorders', of which cluttering is a partial theme. In addition, a relatively new textbook on stuttering and cluttering devotes two chapters to cluttering (Ward, 2006). From this informal review, it is apparent that cluttering is a topic that most authors consider appropriate for inclusion in a course devoted to fluency disorders.

In a more formal study, Scaler Scott, Grossman, and Tetnowski (2010a) found that 96 percent of the speech-language pathology programs surveyed in North America and Europe include some component of cluttering in their fluency courses. The average amount of minutes spent on cluttering instruction in these courses was 100 minutes with a mode of only 60 minutes. In spite of this deficiency, almost no university training programs offer specific coursework in cluttering.

Since there is such limited instruction on cluttering in higher education, the purpose of this chapter is to describe one such course that was offered as a doctoral-level seminar exclusively devoted to cluttering. The chapter will describe how the course was developed, the available resources to teach a seminar in cluttering, the outcomes of an advanced seminar in cluttering, and future directions for the dissemination of information in the area of cluttering.

Development of a course on cluttering

A critical mass is certainly a requirement for coursework on cluttering. A reasonable starting point to find this critical mass would be to investigate the master's degree programs in speech-language pathology. A survey of master's degree programs indicated limited and insufficient training in all areas of fluency disorders (Yaruss & Quesal, 2002). To multiply this effect, Sommers and Caruso (1995) found insufficient in-service training opportunities for speech-language pathologists in the area of fluency disorders. These factors, along with the data compiled by Scaler Scott et al. (2010a), led to a discouraging picture for students in the area of fluency disorders, and specifically cluttering, which receives just a small amount of attention in the already limited fluency-disorder training of speech-language pathologists.

The next reasonable place to search for training in cluttering would be doctoral-level training. According to a notable expert, there were no doctoral-level seminars available to speech-language pathologists in North America that he knew of in 2006 (St. Louis, personal communication, July 26, 2006). The bottom line is simply this: there are extremely limited opportunities for advanced students to gain expertise in the area of cluttering.

The idea of leading a doctoral-level seminar in cluttering certainly seemed like an exciting opportunity when requested to do so by a group of doctoral students prior to the Fall 2006 semester at the University of Louisiana at Lafayette. The program had 22 doctoral students at the time, so it appeared that a critical mass could be achieved. When actually established, an enrollment of three doctoral students took part in what some believed to be the first doctoral seminar in cluttering in the United States (St. Louis, personal communication, July 26, 2006).

Resources available for a course on cluttering

From the instructor's point of view, the challenge of finding sufficient resources for a doctoral seminar appeared to be daunting. A quick search on Google, Yahoo, and more traditional academic sources, such as the Institute for Scientific Information's (ISI) Web of Science, and Med-Line search revealed over 1 million matches related to the search term 'cluttering'. While reviewing hits on cluttering, it was discovered, however, that a large number of matches were related to factors such as 'un-*clutttering* your household' and other issues not remotely related to the speech-language disorder in question. When the search was modified to 'cluttering and speech disorder', the search was limited to just over 20,000 hits. Within this search was an abundance of information on definitions of cluttering from sites like Wikipedia; however, numerous sites also listed 'cures' for cluttering. These sites were from a combination of individuals who had eliminated cluttering on their own, or with the help of speech-language pathologists and affiliated professionals. The obvious purpose of these sites was to promote their business for eliminating cluttering or its handicapping effects. Sorting through the search results produced a limited amount of scholarly information on cluttering. The ISI Web of Knowledge (now Thomson Reuters Web of Knowledge) at the time of this writing lists 39 matches for the terms 'cluttering and speech' and a Med-Line search lists 49 matches for the same terms. In both cases, this was slightly more than the search for 'cluttering and speech disorders' brought about. Searching for information through electronic resources does yield some helpful findings, but it requires a significant amount of filtering.

Another source of information on cluttering comes from the limited textbooks on cluttering, but also from the book chapters in edited texts related to fluency disorders. A search of the largest on-line booksellers found a total of five books on cluttering (and speech); however, three of these books were listed as being out-of-print. The network of sellers of used books makes these books available to the public (often at a cost prohibitive price), but it is apparent that there is not an over-abundance of textbooks related to cluttering. The first author has found that one of the best sources of academic information on cluttering comes in the form of edited chapters in textbooks on stuttering. Among those that I found to be the most helpful are St. Louis, Myers, Bakker, and Raphael's (2007) chapter in Conture and Curlee's text, Daly and Burnett's (1999) chapter in Curlee's text and St. Louis and Myers' (1997) chapter in Curlee and Siegel's text (1997). These chapters are informative and have diverse and complete background information related to cluttering within the theoretical, clinical, and research arenas. They can serve as the basic introductions to the study of cluttering. In summary, although not readily available, there are enough sources of information to complete a serious inquiry into the topic of cluttering.

Preparing the syllabus

In preparing the course, it was apparent that there were a number of topics which needed to be considered in a seminar on cluttering. The first and most obvious decision that had to be made related to the basic concept of cluttering. A quick review indicated that there were two very different and distinct views of cluttering. One view of cluttering is as primarily a disorder of speech, while the opposing view defines cluttering as having its basis in language formulation and processing. Definitions of cluttering, including those of Luchsinger and Arnold (1965), Perkins (1978), and Weiss (1968), define cluttering as a complex disorder marked by rapid speech or irregular speech. However, their definitions also include a 'central language' imbalance or disorder that has a significant impact on multiple modalities that include speech, learning, processing, reading, and writing disorders. In this philosophy and the resulting definitions, cluttering is viewed as a 'central language imbalance' that encompasses oral language, written language, and in some cases, even musical abilities. Within this philosophy, the central language disorder is the primary cause of cluttering, which can result in its primary symptom of rapid or hurried speech.

The opposing view sees cluttering as primarily a speech disorder. This view is taken by St. Louis et al. (2007, pp. 299–300) who define cluttering as:

> a fluency disorder characterized by a rate that is perceived to be abnormally rapid, irregular, or both for the speaker (although measured syllable rates may not exceed normal limits). These rate abnormalities further are manifest in one or more of the following symptoms: (a) an excessive number of disfluencies, the majority of which are not typical of people who stutter; (b) the frequent placement of pauses of prosodic patterns that do not conform to syntactic and semantic constraints; and (c) inappropriate (usually excessive) degrees of coarticulation among sounds, especially in multisyllabic words.

It should be noted that this definition was just a 'working definition' at the time. The definition most closely resembling this definition came in an earlier publication (St. Louis et al., 2004). Given the fact that there is currently no universally accepted definition of cluttering, in setting up the reading list for a course in cluttering, a reasonable goal seemed to be to establish a definition for cluttering. In preparing for such a doctoral seminar, the first topic of discussion was to review the major definitions of cluttering, with an end point being for the participants to form their own definition of cluttering and to justify why their philosophy was taken. This was implemented into the syllabus as both a starting and an ending point.

Having reviewed previous definitions of cluttering, the participants in this seminar were now able to establish a personal framework that would guide them through their future studies in cluttering. As the instructor of record, it became apparent that the definition of cluttering was the basis for determining the validity of the previous research in cluttering. That is, many studies have reviewed the symptoms of people who clutter and compared them to other disorders, such as stuttering. Other studies reported on the characteristics of individuals who reportedly were 'clutterers', henceforth 'persons with cluttering' (PWC). Without a unifying statement of definition, at least three major themes arose. These themes included: (1) cluttering is a complex disorder that affects many areas of cognition, thought, and communication; (2) cluttering exists with many concomitant disorders, and rarely exists in a pure form; and/or (3) cluttering is not yet sufficiently defined to warrant any consistent scientific findings. In order to address these issues a syllabus was constructed that covered as many aspects of cluttering that could be identified and reasonably investigated within one academic term of 15 weeks. An outline of the various topics is summarized in Table 17.1, along with suggested readings in each area.

Table 17.1 Outline of topics covered in a seminar on cluttering

Topic	*Reading*
Incidence and symptoms	Becker, K. P., & Grundmann, K. (1970). Investigation on incidence and symptomatology of cluttering. *Folia Phoniatrica et Logopaedica, 22*, 261–271.
	St. Louis, K. (1996a). A tabular summary of cluttering subjects in the special edition. *Journal of Fluency Disorders, 21*, 337–344.
Comparison to stuttering	DeHirsch, K. (1970). Stuttering and cluttering: Developmental aspects of dysrhythmic speech. *Folia Phoniatrica et Logopaedica, 22*, 311–324.
	Georgieva, D., & Miliev, D. (1996). Differential diagnosis of cluttering and stuttering in Bulgaria. *Journal of Fluency Disorders, 21*, 249–260.
Clinical diagnosis	Daly, D. A., & Burnett, M. L. (1999). Cluttering: Traditional views and new perspectives. In R. F. Curlee (Ed.), *Stuttering and Disorders of Fluency* (2nd ed., pp. 222–254). New York: Thieme.
	St. Louis, K. O., Myers, F. L., Faragasso, K., Townsend, P. S., & Gallaher, A. J. (2004). Perceptual aspects of cluttered speech. *Journal of Fluency Disorders, 29*, 213–235.
Language, learning, linguistic issues, and perception	St. Louis, K., & Hinzman, A. (1986). Studies of cluttering: Perceptions of cluttering by speech-language pathologists and educators. *Journal of Fluency Disorders, 11*, 131–149.
	St. Louis, K., Hinzman, A., & Hull, F. (1985). Studies of cluttering: Disfluency and language measures in young possible clutterers and stutterers. *Journal of Fluency Disorders, 10*, 151–172.
	Teigland, A. (1996). A study of pragmatic skills of clutterers and normal speakers. *Journal of Fluency Disorders, 21*, 201–214.
	Weiss, D. A. (1968). Cluttering: Central language imbalance. *Pediatric Clinics of North America, 15*, 705–720.
Motor issues	Freund, H. (1970). Observations on tachylalia. *Folia Phoniatrica et Logopaedica, 22*, 280–288.
	Hashimoto, R., Taguchi, T., Kano, M., Hanyu, S., Tanaka, Y., Nishizawa, M., & Nakano, I. (1999). A case report of dementia with cluttering-like speech disorder and apraxia. *Rinsho Shinkeigaku, 39*, 520–526.
	Lees, R., Boyle, B., & Woolfson, J. (1996). Is cluttering a motor disorder? *Journal of Fluency Disorders, 21*, 281–288.
	Seeman, M. (1970). Relation between motorics of speech and general motor ability in clutterers. *Folia Phoniatrica et Logopaedica, 22*, 376–380.
Rate and prosody issues	Hartinger, M., & Pape, D. (2003). An articulatory and acoustic study of cluttering. *Proceedings of the 15th ICPhS*, Barcelona (pp. 3245–3248).

Topic	*Reading*
	Hutchinson, J. M., & Burke, K. W. (1973). An investigation of the effects of temporal alterations in auditory feedback upon stutterers and clutterers. *Journal of Communication Disorders*, *6*, 193–205.
	Rieber, R. W., Breskin, S., & Jaffe, J. (1972). Pause time and phonation time in stuttering and cluttering. *Journal of Psycholinguistic Research*, *1*, 149–154.
Relationship to ADD/ADHD and central auditory processing disorders (CAPD)	Heitmann, R., Asbjørnsen, A., & Helland, T. (2004). Attentional functions in speech fluency disorders. *Logopedics, Phoniatrics, Vocology*, *29*, 119.
	Molt, L. (1996). An examination of various aspects of auditory processing in clutterers. *Journal of Fluency Disorders*, *21*, 215–226.
Cluttering and autism spectrum disorders (ASD)	Thacker, A., & Austen, S. (1996). Cluttered communication in a deafened adult with autistic features. *Journal of Fluency Disorders*, *21*, 215–226.
Neurological correlates	Blood, I., & Tellis, G. (2000). Auditory processing and cluttering in young children. *Perceptual and Motor Skills*, *90*, 631–639.
	Chalokwu, C. I., Ghazi, M. A., Foord, E. E., & Lebrun, Y. (1997). Subcortical structures and non-volitional verbal behaviour. *Journal of Neurolinguistics*, *10*, 313–323.
	DeFusco, E. M., & Menken, M. (1979). Symptomatic cluttering in adults. *Brain and Language*, *8*, 25–33.
	Lebrun, Y. (1996). Cluttering after brain damage. *Journal of Fluency Disorders*, *21*, 289–296.
	Thacker, R., & De Nil, L. (1996). Neurogenic cluttering. *Journal of Fluency Disorders*, *21*, 227–238.
	Van Borsel, J., Goethals, L., & Vanryckeghem, M. (2004). Disfluency in Tourette syndrome: Observational study in three cases. *Folia Phoniatrica et Logopaedica*, *56*, 358–366.
Treatment	Brady, J. P. (1993). Treatment of cluttering. *New England Journal of Medicine*, *329*, 813–814.
	Craig, A. (1996). Long-term effects of intensive treatment for a client with both a cluttering and stuttering disorder. *Journal of Fluency Disorders*, *21*, 329–336.
	Daly, D. (1992). Helping the clutterer: Therapy considerations. In F. Myers and K. St. Louis (Eds.), *Cluttering: A clinical perspective*. Leicester, UK: FAR Communications. (Reissued in 1996 by Singular, San Diego, CA.)
	Dewar, A., Dewar, A. D., & Barnes, H. E. (1976). Automatic triggering of auditory feedback masking in stammering and cluttering. *British Journal of Disorders of Communication*, *11*, 19–26.

continued overleaf

Table 17.1—continued

Topic	*Reading*
	Langevin, M., & Boberg, E. (1996). Results of intensive stuttering therapy with adults who clutter and stutter. *Journal of Fluency Disorders*, *21*, 315–328.
	Marriner, N. A., & Sanson-Fisher, R. W. (1977). A behavioral approach to cluttering: A case study. *Australian Journal of Human Communication Disorders*, *5*, 134–141.
	St. Louis, K. O., & Myers, F. L. (1995). Clinical management of cluttering. *Language, Speech, and Hearing Services in the Schools*, *26*, 187–194.
Case studies	Daly, D., & Burnett, M. (1996). Cluttering: assessment, treatment planning, and case study illustration. *Journal of Fluency Disorders*, *21*, 239–244.
	Williams, D., & Wener, D. L. (1996). Cluttering and stuttering exhibited in a young professional. *Journal of Fluency Disorders*, *21*, 261–270.
	Wolk, L. (1986). Cluttering: A diagnostic case report. *British Journal of Disorders of Communication*, *2*, 199–207.

* In addition, topics of discussion and reading included a definition of cluttering, research needs in cluttering, and special topics in cluttering.

Beginning the semester: Establishing a method of study

Although a significant amount of research is already published in cluttering, the lack of a unifying definition of cluttering impedes significant advancement in the field. As an example, let's look at the Hashimoto et al. (1999) article that defines cluttering as clearly a speech disorder. The authors' diagnosis of cluttering included a single case study that based cluttering on the following symptoms: (1) abnormally fast speech; (2) monotonous speech; (3) speech that became faster and faster at the end of utterances; (4) speech that contained several omitted sounds, syllables and words; and (5) speech that could not be corrected easily under conditions of direct instruction and pacing. In contrast, and as previously mentioned, numerous other investigators include language issues within their definition of cluttering. It is indeed difficult to study an area that has such diverse definitions of the same concepts (on this subject also see St. Louis & Schulte, chapter 14 and Ward, chapter 15 this volume). This led to an understanding by the instructor and all participants that when we report that 'research subjects were diagnosed clutterers', we must also add the diagnostic features by which the subjects were actually placed in the experimental group. Nonetheless, this issue was discovered early in the process and served as a unifying factor throughout the semester.

Another factor that was discovered and discussed throughout the semester was: 'What exactly does a PWC look like?' More appropriately, the question should have been: 'What does a PWC *sound* like?' or 'How does a PWC act?' Since a definition of cluttering does not allow for consistent answers to these questions, it was suggested that maybe a real clinical sample could reveal some findings. The instructor of this seminar had accumulated several tapes over the years of individuals who were either diagnosed as a PWC and sent to the first author for verification or a second opinion, or who came directly to the university clinic where the first author was employed and received a tentative diagnosis of cluttering. By the first author's estimate, he has seen over 1000 individuals with fluency disorders, and only 6 were potential PWC. Luckily, at least three of these clients' records were preserved on videotape and examined for a common theme. Table 17.2 includes a summary of symptoms associated with these cases.

Since the instructor was unable to make contact with these clients any longer, a consistent protocol could not be established. However, these three cases are prototypes of how PWC are often placed in studies. That is, PWC are often included in scientific studies based on their being 'classified as PWC'. Some studies do indeed delineate criteria for PWC diagnosis, as in Hashimoto et al. (1999); however, just as many studies do not include these valuable data. In summary, it was also apparent to this class that criteria for diagnostic decision making should be included in all studies of cluttering. Without this information, valid and consistent findings of cluttering are unlikely.

Table 17.2 Symptoms of presumed cases of cluttering

Client	*Age at evaluation*	*Speech symptoms*	*Other symptoms*
1	9	Rapid rate, irregular rate, inconsistent omissions of sounds/syllables, stuttering rate of 2.9% SS during monologue task, many non-stuttering disfluencies	Poor reading, poor writing, poor academic performance, sloppy, expressive language delay
2	21	Rapid rate, irregular rate, consistent articulation errors including a lateral lisp, stuttering rate of 1.1% during monologue task, many non-stuttering disfluencies	Poor academic performance
3	26	Rapid rate, irregular rate, stuttering rate of 4.3% during monologue task	Some pragmatic and conversational errors noted (poor turn-taking, unusual eye contact pattern), some inconsistent articulation errors

From the findings outlined in Table 17.2, it also became apparent to our small group that there were significant problems in the area of cluttering research, primarily based on consistent definitions and symptoms related to cluttering. Based on this discovery, we took a method of determining what St. Louis and Schulte have termed the 'lowest common denominator' associated with both clinical and research symptoms associated with cluttering (see St. Louis & Schulte, chapter 14 this volume). From our findings, the only common factors associated with almost all diagnoses of cluttering include: (1) rapid rate; (2) irregular rate; and (3) disfluency of some type. In our study, we found many associated and/or concomitant disorders associated with cluttering; however, it is impossible at this time to determine whether these are concomitant to cluttering or part of cluttering itself. A partial list of these include articulation/phonological disorders (St. Louis & Myers, 1995), language disorders (Daly & Burnett, 1999; Teigland, 1996), motor disorders (Freund, 1970; Seeman, 1970), central auditory processing disorder (CAPD) (Molt, 1986), autism spectrum disorder (ASD) (Scott, Grossman, Abendroth, Tetnowski, & Damico, 2007; Thacker & Austen, 1996), genetic disorders, such as Down syndrome, and fragile-X syndrome (Preus, 1973; Van Borsel & Tetnowski, 2007), and neurological disorders (Lebrun, 1996; Thacker & De Nil, 1996). Also included in this list was the potential overlap of stuttering and cluttering (Dalton & Hardcastle, 1989; St. Louis & Myers, 1995). It was apparent within our seminar that the best way to approach the validity issue related to cluttering was to factor it down into its 'least common denominator'. Our conclusion was that the only common factors for cluttering are breakdowns in fluency accompanied by a rapid and/or irregular rate.

As we stay consistent with this concept of 'common factors' related to cluttering, it is important to address the issue of disfluency type. Very often, cluttering is defined as a fluency disorder that is not 'stuttering'. One might ask, 'If it is not stuttering, then what is it?' With the onset of Yairi's (Yairi & Ambrose, 1999) term 'stuttering-like disfluency' (SLD), stuttering is characterized by speech behaviors most typically exhibited by people who stutter (PWS) and not by other types of disfluency. The defining speech behaviors in this classification system include part word repetitions, single syllable whole word repetitions (with tension), and dysrhythmic phonations that include prolongations and blocks. Thus stuttering, or SLD, is marked by the four primary speech behaviors of part word repetitions, single syllable word repetitions (with tension), prolongations and blocks. All other disfluencies, including interjections, restarts, revisions, multi-syllable word repetitions, single-syllable word repetitions without tension, and phrase repetitions, would not be considered stuttering or SLDs. Several authors have found that the speech patterns in those considered to be PWC may include SLDs, but are more often marked by disfluencies not typically considered as stuttering (St. Louis, 1992; St. Louis & Myers, 1995). These can include phrase repetitions, interjections, revisions, incomplete phrases and other non-stuttering disfluencies (NSLDs). In the case of cluttering, breakdowns in fluency are a key diagnostic component, but unless the client is stuttering and cluttering, these breakdowns in fluency are more often NSLDs. However, some of the research studies used as course material did not make the distinction between types of disfluency and diagnosis of cluttering, thereby complicating the matter of differential diagnosis of cluttering from stuttering.

By mid-semester, it became apparent that any type of meaningful academic exercise in cluttering research and understanding had to begin with exploring and quantifying: (1) a definition of cluttering to be used in research and (2) the validity of characteristics used to clinically diagnose cluttering. Although this was our self-generated reference point for this seminar in cluttering, it was apparent that we were not alone. There were clear needs to advance basic and clinical research in cluttering. Thus the additional topic, 'research needs in cluttering' was added to our syllabus and is summarized in Table 17.3.

Outcomes of an advanced seminar on cluttering

This seminar on cluttering demonstrated the need in general for more research and specifically for more focused research into cluttering. As a result, several studies were initiated to advance the knowledge-base in cluttering. Currently, there are no less than eight publications, and no fewer than nine conference presentations that have resulted as a direct consequence of either taking or leading this seminar. Among these publications are the current chapter, as well as two other publications on cluttering in higher education (Scaler Scott et al., 2010a; Tetnowski, 2009), an article on perceptual judgments of cluttering (Grossman, Scaler Scott, Trichon, & Tetnowski, 2010), an article on diagnostic characteristics of cluttering (Scaler Scott, Grossman, & Tetnowski, 2010b), an article on a treatment approach to cluttering (Scaler Scott, Tetnowski, Roussel, & Flaitz, 2010), an article on concomitant disorders associated with cluttering (Tetnowski, 2010), and direct contributions to at least one more article (Scott et al., 2007), plus no fewer than nine

Table 17.3 Research needs in cluttering

Topic	*Reading*
Research needs in cluttering	Bakker, K. (1996). Cluttering: Current scientific status and emerging research and clinical needs. *Journal of Fluency Disorders*, *21*, 359–366.
	Curlee, R. (1996). Cluttering: Data in search of understanding. *Journal of Fluency Disorders*, *21*, 367–372.
	Nelson, L. (1996). Critical review of the special edition on cluttering. *Journal of Fluency Disorders*, *21*, 345–348.
	St. Louis, K. O. (1996b). Research and opinion on cluttering: State of the art and science. *Journal of Fluency Disorders*, *21*, 171–371.

presentations at national and international conferences. It should be noted that one of the tasks listed as a final requirement for completion of this seminar was to complete an informational brochure on cluttering for consumers. One of these brochures is in the final preparation stage to be distributed by the National Stuttering Association (Scaler Scott, 2010). The research and clinical contributions of this seminar are already visible and should lead to improved instruction for the next generation of speech-language pathologists. Since this was a doctoral seminar, the insights gained from this seminar will impact the knowledge-base of at least four individuals who will teach coursework in fluency at different university training programs.

Finally, it must be noted that the timing of this course was nearly perfect. It was completed approximately one year before the First World Congress in Fluency Disorders in Katarino, Bulgaria. All four participants submitted papers to be presented at the conference and two participants attended the conference. This conference served as a groundbreaking event for leading authorities to come together for discussion, interaction, presentation of research, and planning that will shape the direction of issues related to cluttering for the future. One of the outcomes of this conference was the establishment of the International Cluttering Association (ICA), which has set as its goal as 'to increase public and professional awareness about this communication disorder, so that ultimately more effective treatments can be established' (ICA, 2009). The current coordinator of the ICA was a participant at this seminar and is author of several articles noted in this section. Clearly, a single doctoral seminar in cluttering has had a significant impact on the advancement of cluttering.

Future directions

As the first author of this chapter, and the instructor for this seminar on cluttering, it becomes my privilege to make suggestions for the future direction in academic issues related to cluttering. In this regard, I offer at least four pieces of advice for those who are charged with educating the next generation of speech-language pathologists. It is certainly my intention that future professionals have more than just a cursory knowledge about cluttering (and stuttering, for that matter) as they enter the world of either clinical treatment or the world of research in communicative disorders.

Therefore, I make these recommendations for the instructors that will hopefully lead future seminars in cluttering.

Recommendation 1: Provide a definition of cluttering

Students typically have a general idea about a definition of cluttering and it is rare they have an exact idea about a definition of cluttering. As noted earlier, there are at least two distinct definitions of cluttering. One is that cluttering is the 'microcosm' of speech-language pathology that includes all clinical facets of language and speech that might be reported as part of cluttering. This philosophy was espoused by Weiss (1964), Perkins (1978), and later by Myers (1992) and Daly and Burnett (1999). These definitions are mostly clinical observations of what we may see in a clinical case of cluttering. The emphasis is not on whether a combination of symptoms will meet an exact criterion for cluttering, but whether cluttering was observed within a group of individuals, or even in a single individual. This definition does not attempt to separate cluttering (in a pure form), from cluttering as a concomitant to other speech, language, learning, or cognitive disorders. Although this may help future clinicians understand what a PWC may look like in the real world, it can also potentially lead to errors in differential diagnosis, and thus errors in treating people diagnosed as PWC. The opposing view is that espoused by St. Louis et al. (2007) and St. Louis and Schulte (chapter 14 this volume), which attempts to identify cluttering by the common factors. This view is more conservative in diagnosing individuals with cluttering, but is less likely to misdiagnose PWC from among those who have a syndrome of symptoms that might result in speech similar to cluttering. This more conservative view should be the standard for research in cluttering, and thus could lead to more appropriate and descriptive terminology, such as 'a person who clutters' or a 'person who has cluttered speech'. In this way, we know exactly what is being defined. That is, a 'person who clutters' is simply a person who exhibits rapid and/or irregular speech with excessive disfluencies. The 'person who clutters' may have several concomitant disorders, but they are 'concomitant' to cluttering and not part of the definition of cluttering itself (Tetnowski, 2010).

Recommendation 2: Provide samples of cluttered speech

In a discussion with two experts in the field of cluttering (Daly, personal communication; St. Louis, personal communication), I asked each of them, 'How many pure PWC (i.e., with no concomitant stuttering or other disorders) have you actually seen in your life?' I was surprised to hear the responses. Between the two experts, they had reportedly seen fewer than 20 pure PWC. 'Pure cluttering' that reportedly exists in rare cases would be easy to define and describe. However, observing a 'person who clutters' can be confusing because it is so often associated with other symptoms or disorders. Many of the clients that have been sent to speech and language clinics over the years hardly meet anyone's definition of pure cluttering. Therefore, most speech and language professionals have never seen a 'pure PWC'. Thankfully, today's world of advanced technology and information sharing can provide powerful clinical observations that can allow professionals in training to easily view PWC. The ICA website, for example, has samples of several people who are using cluttered speech. Other examples can be accessed through the stuttering home page.

Recommendation 3: Know that the field of cluttering is new and ever changing

Although writings on cluttering date back to those of Deso Weiss in the 1960s, our knowledge of cluttering is limited due to its presumed relatively low prevalence. Texts such as this, or special issues of journals such as the 1996 special issue on cluttering of *Journal of Fluency Disorders*, or the upcoming proceedings of the First World Congress on Cluttering, will all add to the emerging research and understanding of cluttering. These resources should serve as important documents for cluttering sources or seminars in higher education.

Recommendation 4: Know that not all fluency disorders are stuttering, and that not all people with rapid rate are PWC

St. Louis and Hinzman (1986) have indicated that speech-language pathologists are limited in their current knowledge of cluttering. In addition, St. Louis and Hinzman (1988) found that it is very common for fluency disorders to co-exist with other speech, language, and learning disorders. Tetnowski (2010) has also shown that cluttering is concomitant to many other disorders. The basic understanding must be that *not all fluency disorders are stuttering, and that not all people with rapid rate are PWC*. This finding must be meshed with consistent definitions and measurement profiles for cluttering and other fluency disorders.

In summary, a seminar in cluttering has been a very successful experience for all four of its participants. It is our sincere wish that the needs of clients who clutter and the researchers and clinicians interested in cluttering will be met by leading authorities in higher education. It is apparent to us that there is definitely a need for cluttering to be included in the communicative disorders curriculum.

Acknowledgements

We thank Kathy Scaler Scott, Mitch Trichon, and Heather Grossman for participating in this seminar. Without your encouragement and dedication, none of this would have taken place.

References

Bakker, K. (1996). Cluttering: Current scientific status and emerging research and clinical needs. *Journal of Fluency Disorders*, *21*, 359–366.

Becker, K. P., & Grundmann, K. (1970). Investigation on incidence and symptomatology of cluttering. *Folia Phoniatrica et Logopaedica*, *22*, 261–271.

Blood, I., & Tellis, G. (2000). Auditory processing and cluttering in young children. *Perceptual and Motor Skills*, *90*, 631–639.

Brady, J. P. (1993). Treatment of cluttering. *New England Journal of Medicine*, *329*, 813–814.

Chalokwu, C. I., Ghazi, M. A., Foord E. E., & Lebrun, Y. (1997). Subcortical structures and non-volitional verbal behaviour. *Journal of Neurolinguistics*, *10*, 313–323.

Craig, A. (1996). Long-term effects of intensive treatment for a client with both a cluttering and stuttering disorder. *Journal of Fluency Disorders*, *21*, 329–336.

Curlee, R. (1996). Cluttering: Data in search of understanding. *Journal of Fluency Disorders*, *21*, 367–372.

Dalton, P., & Hardcastle, W. (1989). *Disorders of fluency* (2nd ed.). London: Cole Whurr.

Daly, D. (1992). Helping the clutterer: Therapy considerations. In F. Myers & K. St. Louis (Eds.), *Cluttering: A clinical perspective*. Leicester, UK: Far Communications. (Reissued in 1996 by Singular, San Diego, CA.).

Daly, D., & Burnett, M. (1996). Cluttering: Assessment, treatment planning, and case study illustration. *Journal of Fluency Disorders*, *21*, 239–244.

Daly, D. A., & Burnett, M. L. (1999). Cluttering: Traditional views and new perspectives. In R. F. Curlee (Ed.), *Stuttering and related disorders of fluency* (2nd ed., pp. 222–254). New York: Thieme.

DeFusco, E. M., & Menken, M. (1979). Symptomatic cluttering in adults. *Brain and Language*, *8*, 25–33.

DeHirsch, K. (1970). Stuttering and cluttering: Developmental aspects of dysrhythmic speech. *Folia Phoniatrica et Logopaedica*, *22*, 311–324.

Dewar, A., Dewar, A. D., & Barnes, H. E. (1976). Automatic triggering of auditory feedback masking in stammering and cluttering. *British Journal of Disorders of Communication*, *11*, 19–26.

Freund, H. (1970). Observations on tachylalia. *Folia Phoniatrica et Logopaedica*, *22*, 280–288.

Georgieva, D. & Miliev, D. (1996). Differential diagnosis of cluttering and stuttering in Bulgaria. *Journal of Fluency Disorders*, *21*, 249–260.

Grossman, H., Scaler Scott, K., Trichon, M., & Tetnowski, J. A. (2010). Perceptual judgments of cluttering. In K. Bakker, L. Raphael, & F. Myers (Eds.), *Proceedings of the First World Conference on Cluttering, Katarino, Bulgaria* (pp. 142–146). http://associations.missouristate.edu/ICA

Hartinger, M., & Pape, D. (2003). An articulatory and acoustic study of cluttering. *Proceedings of the 15th ICPhS, Barcelona* (pp. 3245–3248). Barcelona: UAB.

Hashimoto, R., Taguchi, T., Kano, M., Hanyu, S., Tanaka, Y., Nishizawa, M., et al. (1999). A case report of dementia with cluttering-like speech disorder and apraxia. *Clinical Neurology*, *39*, 520–526.

Heitmann, R., Asbjørnsen, A., & Helland, T. (2004). Attentional functions in speech fluency disorders. *Logopedics, Phoniatrics, Vocology*, *29*, 119.

Hutchinson, J. M., & Burke, K. W. (1973). An investigation of the effects of temporal alterations in auditory feedback upon stutterers and clutterers. *Journal of Communication Disorders*, *6*, 193–205.

International Cluttering Association. (2009). (*Home page*). Retrieved September 20, 2009, from http://associations.missouristate.edu/ICA/

Langevin, M., & Boberg, E. (1996). Results of intensive stuttering therapy with adults who clutter and stutter. *Journal of Fluency Disorders*, *21*, 315–328.

Lebrun, Y. (1996). Cluttering after brain damage. *Journal of Fluency Disorder*, *21*, 289–296.

Lees, R., Boyle, B., & Woolfson, J. (1996). Is cluttering a motor disorder? *Journal of Fluency Disorders*, *21*, 281–288.

Luchsinger, R., & Arnold, G. E. (1965). Cluttering: Tachyphemia. In *Voice–Speech–Language (Clinical communicology: Its physiology and pathology)* (pp. 145–153). Belmont, CA: Wadsworth.

Marriner, N. A., & Sanson-Fisher, R. W. (1977). A behavioral approach to cluttering: A case study. *Australian Journal of Human Communication Disorders*, *5*, 134–141.

Molt, L. (1996). An examination of various aspects of auditory processing in clutterers. *Journal of Fluency Disorders*, *21*, 215–226.

Myers, F. L. (1992). Cluttering: A synergistic framework. In F. L. Myers & K. O. St. Louis (Eds.), *Cluttering: A clinical perspective* (pp. 71–84). Kibworth, UK: Far Communications.

Nelson, L. (1996). Critical review of the special edition on cluttering. *Journal of Fluency Disorders*, *21*, 345–348.

Perkins, W. H. (1978). *Human perspectives in speech and language*. St. Louis, MO: Mosby.

Preus, A. (1973). Stuttering in Down's syndrome. In Y. Lebrun & R. Hoops (Eds.), *Neurolinguistic approaches to stuttering* (pp. 90–100). The Hague: Mouton.

Rieber, R. W., Breskin, S., & Jaffe, J. (1972). Pause time and phonation time in stuttering and cluttering. *Journal of Psycholinguistic Research*, *1*, 149–154.

Scaler Scott, K. (2010). *Stuttering vs. Cluttering* [brochure]. New York: National Stuttering Association.

Scaler Scott, K., Grossman, H. G., & Tetnowski, J. A. (2010a). A survey of cluttering instruction in fluency courses. In K. Bakker, L. Raphael, & F. Myers (Eds.), *Proceedings of the First World Conference on Cluttering, Katarino, Bulgaria* (pp. 171–179). http://associations.missouristate.edu/ICA

Scaler Scott, K., Grossman, H. G., & Tetnowski, J. A. (2010b). Diagnosis of a single case of cluttering according to four different criteria. In K. Bakker, L. Raphael, & F. Myers (Eds.), *Proceedings of the First World Conference on Cluttering, Katarino, Bulgaria* (pp. 80–90). http://associations.missouristate.edu/ICA

Scaler Scott, K., Tetnowski, J. A., Roussel, N. C., & Flaitz, J. F. (2010). Impact of a pausing treatment strategy upon the speech of a clutterer-stutterer. In K. Bakker, L. Raphael, & F. Myers (Eds.), *Proceedings of the First World Conference on Cluttering, Katarino, Bulgaria* (pp. 132–140). http://associations.missouristate.edu/ICA

Scott, K. S., Grossman, H. L., Abendroth, K. J., Tetnowski, J. A., & Damico, J. S. (2007). Asperger syndrome and attention deficit disorder: Clinical disfluency analysis. In J. Au-Yeung & M. M. Leahy (Eds.), *Research, treatment, and self-help in fluency disorders: New horizons. Proceedings of the Fifth World Congress on Fluency Disorders* (pp. 273–278). Dublin, Ireland: International Fluency Association.

Seeman, M. (1970). Relation between motorics of speech and general motor ability in clutterers. *Folia Phoniatrica et Logopaedica*, *22*, 376–380.

Sommers, R. K., & Caruso, A. J. (1995). In-service training in speech-language pathology: Are we meeting the needs for fluency training? *American Journal of Speech-Language Pathology*, *4*, 22–28.

St. Louis, K. (1996a). A tabular summary of cluttering subjects in the special edition. *Journal of Fluency Disorders*, *21*, 337–344.

St. Louis, K., & Hinzman, A. (1986). Studies of cluttering: Perceptions of cluttering by speech-language pathologists and educators. *Journal of Fluency Disorders*, *11*, 131–149.

St. Louis, K., Hinzman, A., & Hull, F. (1985). Studies of cluttering: Disfluency and language measures in young possible clutterers and stutterers. *Journal of Fluency Disorders*, *10*, 151–172.

St. Louis, K. O. (1992). In defining cluttering. In F. L. Myers & K. O. St. Louis (Eds.), *Cluttering: A clinical perspective*. Kibworth, UK: Far Communications.

St. Louis, K. O. (1996b). Research and opinion on cluttering: State of the art and science [Special issue]. *Journal of Fluency Disorders*, *21*, 171–371.

St. Louis, K. O., & Hinzman, A. R. (1988). A descriptive study of speech, language, and hearing characteristics in school-aged stutterers. *Journal of Fluency Disorders*, *13*, 331–355.

St. Louis, K. O., & Myers, F. L. (1995). Clinical management of cluttering. *Language, Speech, and Hearing Services in the Schools*, *26*, 187–194.

St. Louis, K. O., & Myers, F. L. (1997). Management of cluttering and related fluency disorders. In R. F. Curlee & G. M. Siegel (Eds.), *Nature and treatment of stuttering: New directions* (2nd ed.). Boston: Allyn & Bacon.

St. Louis, K. O., Myers, F. L., Bakker, K., & Raphael, L. J. (2007). Understanding and treating cluttering. In E. G. Conture & R. F. Curlee (Eds.), *Stuttering and related disorders of fluency* (3rd ed.). New York: Thieme.

St. Louis, K. O., Myers, F. L., Faragasso, K., Townsend, P. S., & Gallaher, A. J. (2004). Perceptual aspects of cluttered speech. *Journal of Fluency Disorders*, *29*, 213–235.

Teigland, A. (1996). A study of pragmatic skills of clutterers and normal speakers. *Journal of Fluency Disorders*, *21*, 201–214.

Tetnowski, J. A. (2009, July). Cluttering in the communicative disorders curriculum. *Perspectives on Fluency and Fluency Disorders*, *19*, 52–57.

Tetnowski, J. A. (2010). Cluttering and concomitant disorders. In K. Bakker, L. J. Raphael, & F. L. Myers (Eds.), *Proceedings of the First World Conference on Cluttering* (pp. 251–260). Springfield, MO: International Cluttering Association.

Thacker, A., & Austen, S. (1996). Cluttered communication in a deafened adult with autistic features. *Journal of Fluency Disorders*, *21*, 215–226.

Thacker, R., & De Nil, L. (1996). Neurogenic cluttering. *Journal of Fluency Disorders*, *21*, 227–238.

Van Borsel, J., Goethals, L., & Vanryckeghem, M. (2004). Disfluency in Tourette syndrome: Observational study in three cases. *Folia Phoniatrica et Logopaedica*, *56*, 358–366.

Van Borsel, J., & Tetnowski, J. A. (2007). Stuttering in genetic syndromes. *Journal of Fluency Disorders*, *32*, 279–296.

Ward, D. (2006). *Stuttering and cluttering: Frameworks for understanding and treatment*. Hove, UK: Psychology Press.

Weiss, D. (1964). *Cluttering*. Englewood Cliffs, NJ: Prentice Hall.

Weiss, D. A. (1968). Cluttering: Central language imbalance. *Pediatric Clinics of North America*, *15*, 705–720.

Williams, D., & Wener, D. L. (1996). Cluttering and stuttering exhibited in a young professional. *Journal of Fluency Disorders*, *21*, 261–270.

Wolk, L. (1986). Cluttering: A diagnostic case report. *British Journal of Disorders of Communication*, *2*, 199–207.

Yairi, E., & Ambrose, N. G. (1999). Early childhood stuttering I: Persistency and recovery rates. *Journal of Speech-Language-Hearing Research*, *42*, 1097–1112.

Yaruss, J. S., & Quesal, R. W. (2002). Academic and clinical education in fluency disorders: An update. *Journal of Fluency Disorders*, *27*, 43–63.

Author index

Subject index

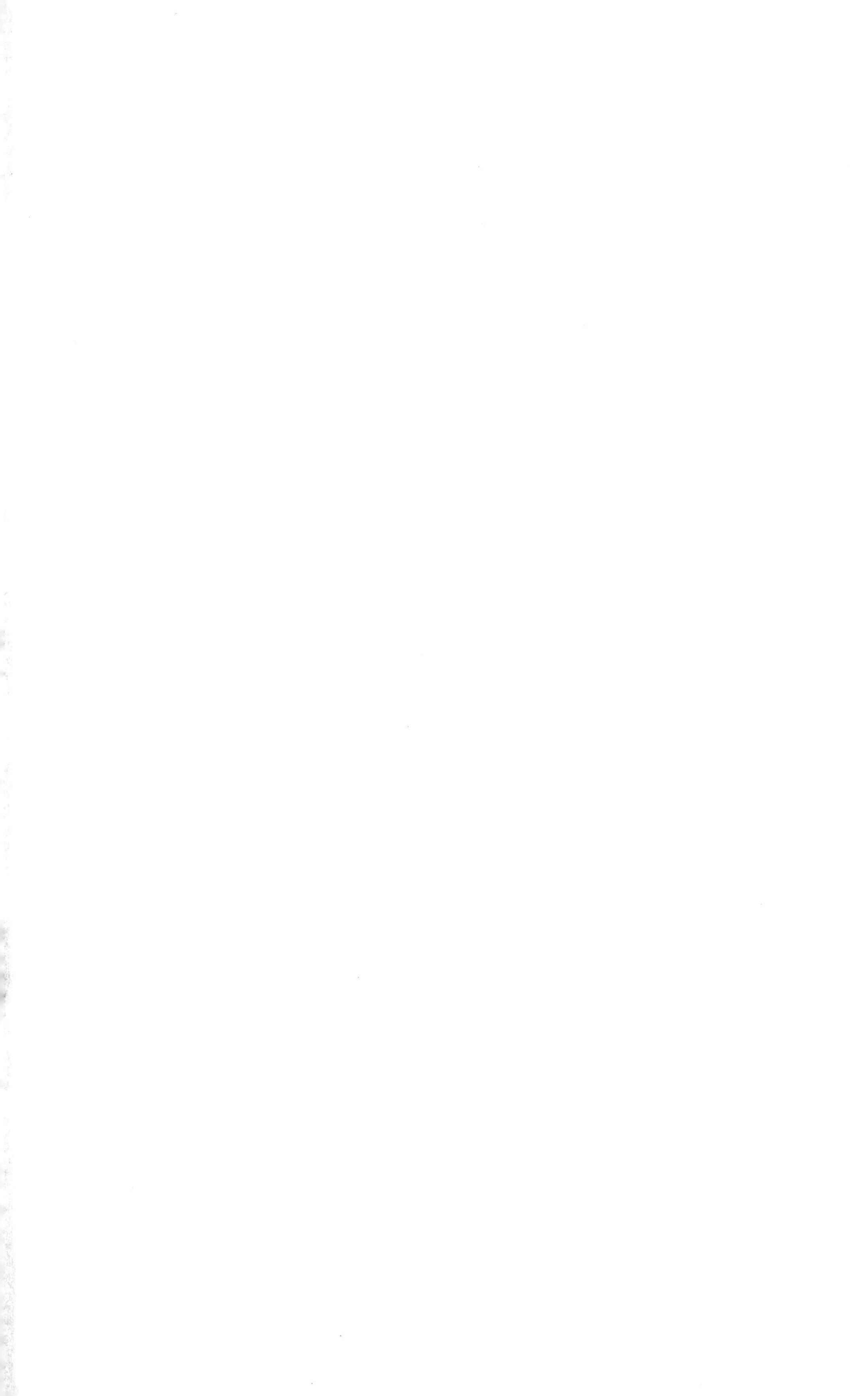